Clinical Manual of

MATERNITY AND GYNECOLOGIC NURSING

Clinical Manual of

MATERNITY AND GYNECOLOGIC NURSING

Susan M. Weiner, R.N.C., M.S.N.
Perinatal Clinical Nurse Specialist
The Family Center Program
Thomas Jefferson University Hospital
Philadelphia, Pennsylvania

The C.V. Mosby Company
St. Louis • Baltimore • Toronto   1989

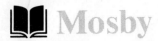

Editor: Nancy L. Coon
Senior developmental editor: Susan Epstein
Production editor: Stephen Dierkes
Designer: Rey Umali

The C.V. Mosby Company
11830 Westline Industrial Drive, St. Louis, Missouri 63146

Library of Congress Cataloging in Publication Data

Weiner, Susan M.
    Clinical manual of maternity and gynecologic nursing / Susan M. Weiner.
        p.   cm.
    Companion v. to: Maternity and gynecologic care / Irene M. Bobak, Margaret Duncan Jensen, Marianne K. Zalar, 4th ed. 1989.
    Includes bibliographies and index.
    ISBN 0-8016-5741-5
    1. Obstetrical nursing. 2. Gynecologic nursing. 3. Obstetrical nursing—Handbooks, manuals, etc. 4. Gynecologic nursing—Handbooks, manuals, etc. I. Bobak, Irene M. Maternity and gynecologic care. II. Title.
    [DNLM: 1. Gynecology—nurses' instruction. 2. Obstetrical Nursing. 3. Perinatology—nurses' instruction. WY 157.3 W423c]
RG951.B667 1989 Suppl. 2
610.73'678—dc19
DNLM/DLC   88-38432
for Library of Congress   CIP

C/VHP/VHP   9   8   7   6   5   4

Preface

The *Clinical Manual of Maternity and Gynecologic Nursing* was developed to meet the needs of both students and practitioners by presenting up-to-date, easily retrievable material on the clinical aspects of maternity and gynecologic nursing. For students, this manual serves as a resource to bridge the gap between theoretical classroom teaching and clinical practice. For maternity and gynecologic nurses functioning in traditional and expanded roles, it provides a convenient, practical reference.

Organized to parallel *Maternity and Gynecologic Care: The Nurse and The Family,* fourth edition, by Bobak, Jensen, and Zalar, this manual can in fact be used as a supplement to any comprehensive maternity text. The manual is comprised of eight units. Unit 1 reviews the anatomy and physiology of the human reproductive system and the basic gynecologic examination. Unit 2 deals with nursing care for the woman and family experiencing a normal pregnancy. Nutritional considerations and family dynamics are an important part of this unit. Normal labor and delivery are presented in Unit 3, including pharmacologic control of discomfort and techniques for fetal monitoring. Unit 4 provides guidelines for the assessment and care of the normal newborn, including nutrition and feeding. Nursing care during normal postpartum recovery is covered in Unit 5. Unit 6 focuses on high-risk pregnancy, labor, and delivery. Various conditions that complicate the childbearing process are discussed, including considerations for the pregnant adolescent. Care of the compromised neonate is presented in Unit 7, and includes assessment and interventions for the newborn with infections or drug dependence. The last unit focuses on women's health and gynecologic care. Fertility management, gynecologic and urinary concerns, violence, and neoplasia are presented in this unit.

The practical usefulness of this manual is enhanced by the liberal use of sample nursing care plans, summaries of nursing actions, guidelines for client teaching, step-by-step procedures, and information on laboratory tests and medications. This handy reference will prove invaluable to students and practitioners who care for women and their families in maternity and gynecologic settings.

Contents

Human Reproductive System

A woman is considered a gynecologic client for a far longer time than she is seen as an obstetric patient. For this reason it is most important for the nurse to understand gynecology-related anatomy and function and to know the reason the client is entering the health care system, the client's age, and social and religious factors that affect the client's care.

The gynecologic health assessment includes an interview, a physical assessment, and diagnostic testing.

This unit focuses on some of the essential pieces of the gynecologic examination process starting with an overview of anatomy and physiology, and finally the examination itself.

REVIEW OF ANATOMY AND PHYSIOLOGY

Basic knowledge about the female and male reproductive systems is a prerequisite to understanding the process of conception. A systematic investigation of the human reproductive system provides the maternity-gynecologic nurse with a firm foundation for gaining insight into the client's needs and health concerns. The nurse needs information on the similarities and differences of the female and male reproductive organs and their growth and development patterns. An understanding of immunology is also needed because of its important role in life's processes.

Female Reproductive System

The material in this section summarizes the anatomy and physiology of the female's internal and external genitals and breasts. Information is also provided regarding the menstrual cycle and the climacteric.

Table 1-1 *External Female Genitals (See Fig. 1-1)*

Structure	Function
Mons pubis (mons veneris)	Protects symphysis pubis during coitus
	Visually excites male
Labia majora	Protection for labia minora, urinary meatus, and vaginal introitus
	Sensitivity to touch and temperature important during sexual arousal
Labia minora	Swells with emotional or physical stimulation
	Glands within lubricate the vulva
Clitoris	"Key" to a woman's sexual feelings and female sexuality
	Sebaceous glands secrete smegma
Prepuse of clitoris	Protects glans clitoris
Vestibule	Encloses openings to urethra, paraurethral glands, vagina, and vulvovaginal glands
Urinary meatus	Carries urine from bladder to outside of body
Skene's glands (paraurethral glands)	Produces lubricating mucus
Hymen	Covers vaginal introitus
Bartholin's (vulvovaginal) glands	Secrete clear, viscid mucus during coitus
	Alkaline pH of mucus supports sperm
Fourchette	Connects posterior ends of labia minora
Perineum	Site of episiotomy
	Pubococcygeal muscle supports internal structures

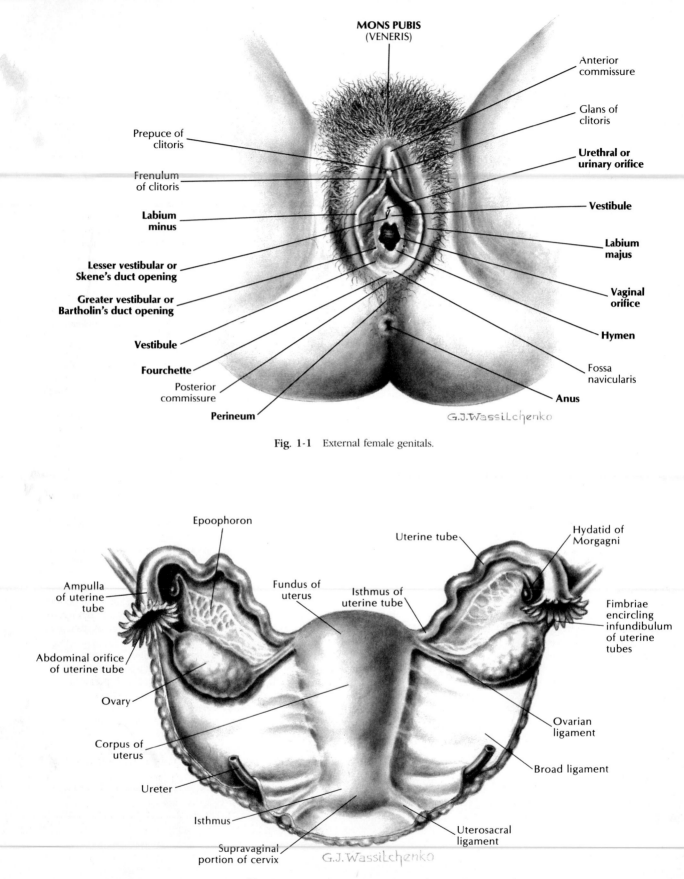

MONS PUBIS
(VENERIS)

Anterior
commissure

Glans of
clitoris

Prepuce of
clitoris

**Urethral or
urinary orifice**

Frenulum
of clitoris

Vestibule

**Labium
minus**

**Labium
majus**

**Lesser vestibular or
Skene's duct opening**

**Vaginal
orifice**

**Greater vestibular or
Bartholin's duct opening**

Hymen

Vestibule

Fossa
navicularis

Fourchette

Posterior
commissure

Anus

Perineum

G.J.Wassilchenko

Fig. 1-1   External female genitals.

Epoophoron

Uterine tube

Hydatid of
Morgagni

Ampulla
of uterine
tube

Fundus of
uterus

Isthmus of
uterine tube

Fimbriae
encircling
infundibulum
of uterine
tubes

Abdominal orifice
of uterine tube

Ovary

Ovarian
ligament

Corpus of
uterus

Broad ligament

Ureter

Isthmus

Uterosacral
ligament

Supravaginal
portion of cervix

G.J.Wassilchenko

Fig. 1-2   Uterus and adnexa, posterior view.

Table 1-2 *Internal Female Genitals (See Fig. 1-2)*

Structure	Function
Ovaries (female gonads)	Ovulates
	Produces hormones: estrogens, progesterones, androgens
Uterine tubes (oviducts-fallopian tubes)	Provides passageway for ovum; fimbriae pull ovum into tube; ovum propelled through tube by peristaltic motion and cilia
Ureters	Carry urine from kidneys to urinary bladder
Uterus	Menstruates cyclically and rejuvenates endometrium
	Supports fertilized ovum until development of full-term fetus
	During menstruation and after delivery, the functional layer sloughs off, and with aid of hormones cycle begins again
	Longitudinal muscle fibers in myometrium expel fetus during birth process
	Contraction of middle muscle layer produces hemostatic action after delivery (living ligature)
	Myometrium thins out, pulls up, and opens cervix to push fetus out

Uterine cervix
  Internal os: canal inside cervix that connects uterine cavity with vagina
  External os: narrowed opening between endocervix with vagina (rounded in nulliparous women, slit-like in gravid women)
	Sphincter action around internal cervical os helps retain uterine contents during pregnancy
	Elasticity allows for extensive stretchability during vaginal childbirth
	During labor, cervix effaces (thins out) and dilates to allow fetus to be pushed out of the uterus

Uterine canals Two types of epithelium meet at squamocolumnar junction, just inside external cervical os; squamocolumnar junction is the most common site of neoplastic cellular changes; cells from this junction are examined during Pap smear	Provide potential space Columnar epithelial cells produce odorless and nonirritating mucus in response to ovarian/endocrine hormones (estrogen, progesterone) Gives glistening pink color to cervix; deeper bluish red color is seen when woman is ovulating or is pregnant
Vagina	Organ of copulation in woman Birth canal Vaginal fluid maintains cleanliness of vagina

Pelvic floor and perineum
Upper pelvic diaphragm
  Resilient because of layers that are interwoven and interlaced
  (See Fig. 1-3 for structure of pelvis.)
	Support for pelvic structures
	Allows for dilation of vagina during birth and closure after delivery
	Assists with constriction of the urethra, vagina, and anal canal

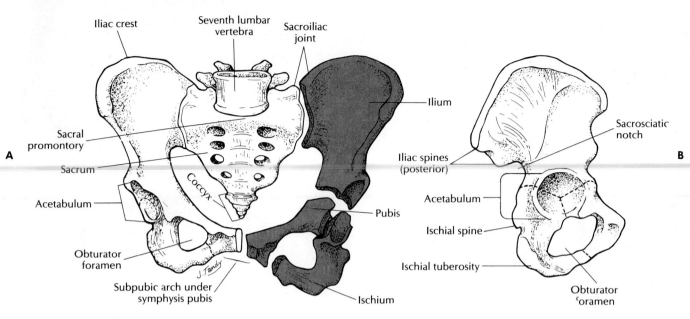

Fig. 1-3   Adult female pelvis. **A**, Anterior view. Three embryonic parts of left innominate bone are lightly shaded. **B**, External view of right innominate bone (fused).

Table 1-3   *Breasts (See Fig. 1-4)*

Structure	Function
Parenchyma	True glandular tissue
Stroma	Supports glandular tissue
	Estrogen stimulates growth and development of stromal tissue as well as of ductile system
Lobes	Each mammary gland is made up of 15 to 20 lobes
Acini (lobules, alveoli)	Secretes colostrum and milk; there should be *no* discharge from nipple except during pregnancy and lactation
	Myoepithelium below contracts to expel milk
Nipple (papilla)	Contains 15 to 20 openings from lactiferous ducts
	Surrounded by fibromuscular tissue (areola) and covered by wrinkled skin
	Directly below skin, Montgomery's glands secrete lubricant for nipple
Lactiferous sinuses	Serve as milk reservoirs
Cooper's ligaments	Provide support to mammary glands while permitting mobility of breast on chest wall

Menstrual Cycle. Menstruation is periodic uterine bleeding that begins with the shedding of secretory endometrium approximately 14 days after ovulation. **The first day of the menstrual discharge has been designated as day 1 of the cycle.** The average duration of menstrual flow is 5 days (range of 3 to 6 days), and the average blood loss is approximately 50 ml (range of 20 to 80 ml)—but there is great variation. During menstruation the average daily loss of iron is 0.5 to 1 mg.

I. Ovarian cycle: lasts approximately 29 days and is divided into two phases

  A. Follicular phase: day 4 to 14 (under the influence of follicle-stimulating hormone [FSH])

    1. Once ovum is ovulated, other follicles are less receptive to FSH and estrogen

    2. Estrogen levels increase, giving negative feedback to hypothalmus, which inhibits further secretion of FSH

    3. Progesterone surge after day 10 stimulates production of luteinizing hormone (LH), inhibits production of lesser follicles, and supports maturation of the graafian follicle

    4. On day 14, with the help of the progesterone surge, LH peaks and ovulation occurs.

    5. Follicular phase of the cycle causes the variation in each woman's cycle

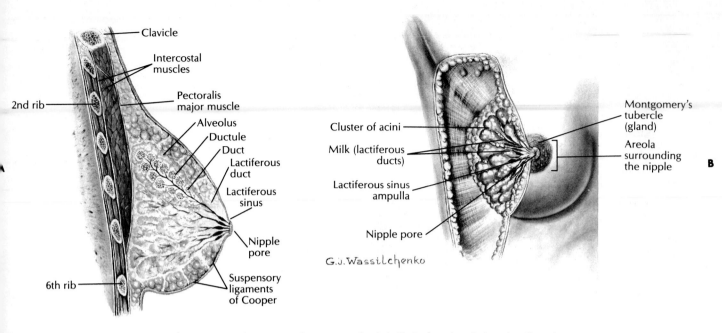

Fig. 1-4 Position and structure of mammary gland. **A**, Sagittal section. **B**, Anterior dissection.
(**A** from Seidel HM et al: Mosby's guide to physical examination, St. Louis, 1987, The CV Mosby Co.)

B. Luteal phase: approximately day 15 to day 28 (under the influence of LH, corpus luteum produces progesterone)
  1. Estrogen and LH levels decline
  2. Progesterone levels increase
  3. No fertilization of ovum causes the corpus luteum to degenerate and become corpus albicans (taking about 10 days); FSH levels increase again to prepare for a new cycle
  4. If fertilization occurs, corpus luteum is maintained beyond 14 days by the presence of human chorionic gonadotropin (HCG)
II. Endometrial cycle: divided into four phases
  A. Menstrual phase: lasts approximately 2 to 8 days
    1. Shedding of the functional two thirds of the endometrium; basal layer is always retained; regeneration begins near the end of the cycle from stromal and glandular cells in the basal layer
  B. Proliferative phase: day 5 to ovulation
    1. Period of rapid growth; endometrial surface is completely restored; stroma develops
    2. Occurs simultaneously with follicular phase of the ovary

  3. Is influenced by estrogen from ovarian follicles
  C. Secretary phase: from ovulation to about 3 days before next menstrual period
    1. Larger amounts of progesterone are produced
    2. Occurs simultaneously with luteal phase of the ovary
    3. Glands in endometrium become tortuous, serrated, and widened
    4. Cells lining the glands secrete a thin, glycogen-containing fluid
    5. Implantation (nidation) of the fertilized ovum generally occurs about 7 to 10 days after ovulation
    6. If there is no fertilization (implantation), progesterone and estrogen levels fall rapidly, and spiral arteries spasm
    7. Endometrium shrivels
  D. Ischemic phase
    1. Blood supply to functional endometrium is blocked, and necrosis develops
    2. Functional layer separates from basal layer
    3. Menstrual bleeding begins, marking day 1 of the next cycle

Table 1-4 *Climacterium*

Physiologic Change	Rationale	Signs/Symptoms
Decrease in primordial follicles in ovary	Women are born with a set number of primordial follicles in the ovary During reproductive years, 400 or more follicles mature; others atrophy	Anovulation
Decreased estrogen and progesterone production No endometrial growth to slough off	No ovulation of follicles or corpus lutea Decreased stimulation by gonadal hormones	Menstrual cycles become irregular or cease Menopause
Circulating pituitary gondotropin levels rise; FSH and LH remain high	No feedback mechanism from gonadotropins	Uterus becomes smaller and involutional
Reproductive organs and surrounding tissues shrink in size or slowly atrophy	Decreased ovarian estrogen affects target organs and supporting musculature	Loss of muscle tone in supportive structures (e.g., levator ani and pubococcygeus muscles)
Vaginal walls grow thinner, smoother, and shorter; vestibular glands produce less mucus; bladder walls become thin; calcitonin increases; calcium uptake decreases	Decreased estrogen	Lubrication during coitus may take longer; stress incontinence; increased bone density
Vasomotor instability; dilation of blood vessels	Surges of anterior pituitary hormones FSH and LH; hormonal disturbance in hypothalamus; release of prostaglandins	Hot flashes, hot flushes, night sweats, dizziness
Ovary's core produces androstenedione and weak male hormone converted into estrone, occurring in body fat; outer portion of ovary ceases production of estrogen; ovarian core also produces testosterone	Female hormones' influence declines, while male hormone influence remains static or increases in response to high levels of FSH and LH; obese women tend to have higher postmenopausal concentrations of estrone	Growth of dark, coarse facial hairs on chin; increased amounts of fuzzy facial hair

Male Reproductive System

To understand human sexuality and the process of fertilization and conception the nurse must also know about the male internal and external genitals.

Table 1-5 *Structures of External Male Genitals (See Figs. 1-5 and 1-6)*

Structure	Function
Mons pubis	Protects symphysis pubis during coitus
Penis	Organ of copulation and urination
Scrotum	Holds testicles and part of the spermatic cord; assists with optimum temperature control for sperm production

Table 1-6 *Structures of Internal Male Genitals (See Figs. 1-5 and 1-6)*

Structure	Function
Testes	Spermatogenesis; hormone production
Ducts (canals) of testes	Exit of sperm from body
Accessory glands: seminal vesicles (paired); prostate gland; bulbourethral (Cowper's) glands (paired)	Secrete fluids that support the life and function of the sperm
Semen	Vehicle for nutritional support and transfer of viable sperm

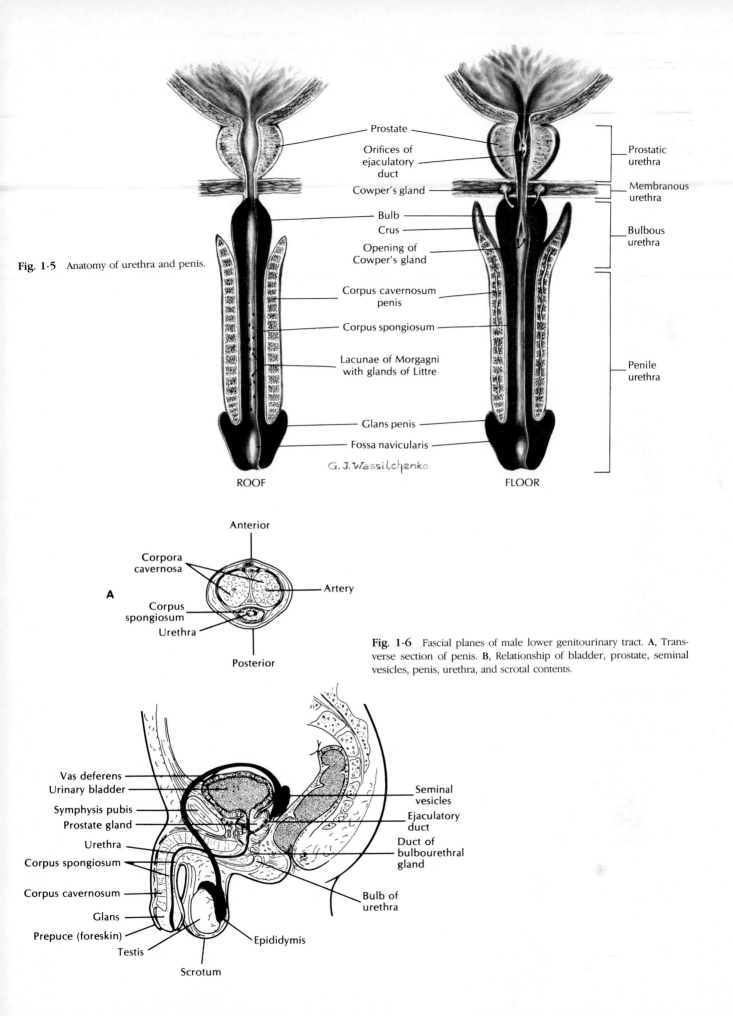

Fig. 1-5 Anatomy of urethra and penis.

Prostate

Orifices of ejaculatory duct

Cowper's gland

Bulb

Crus

Opening of Cowper's gland

Corpus cavernosum penis

Corpus spongiosum

Lacunae of Morgagni with glands of Littre

Glans penis

Fossa navicularis

G. J. Wassilchenko

ROOF

FLOOR

Prostatic urethra

Membranous urethra

Bulbous urethra

Penile urethra

Anterior

Corpora cavernosa

Artery

Corpus spongiosum

Urethra

A

Posterior

Fig. 1-6 Fascial planes of male lower genitourinary tract. **A,** Transverse section of penis. **B,** Relationship of bladder, prostate, seminal vesicles, penis, urethra, and scrotal contents.

Vas deferens

Urinary bladder

Symphysis pubis

Prostate gland

Urethra

Corpus spongiosum

Corpus cavernosum

Glans

Prepuce (foreskin)

Testis

Scrotum

Epididymis

Seminal vesicles

Ejaculatory duct

Duct of bulbourethral gland

Bulb of urethra

Table 1-7 *Comparison of Male and Female Sexual Response*

Male	Female
Vasocongestion:	
Sexual stimulation results in reflex dilation of penile blood vessels; erection and circumvaginal blood vessels; lubrication; engorgement and distension of genitals; venous congestion localized primarily in genitals and to a lesser degree in the breasts and other body parts	
Myotonia:	
Arousal is characterized by increased muscular tension and results in voluntary and involuntary rhythmic contractions	
Phases:	
Excitement	
1. Erection of penis (increase in length and diameter)	1. Vaginal lubrication (biologic function of preparing vagina for penile penetration)
2. Scrotal skin becomes thick and congested	2. Inner two thirds of vaginal barrel lengthens and distends
3. Testes elevate because of contraction of the cremasteric musculature	3. Cervix and fundus are pulled upward
	4. External genitals become congested and darker in color
	5. Clitoris increases in diameter and tumescence (vascular congestion and swelling)
Plateau	
1. Preorgasmic emission of 2 or 3 drops of mucoid substance released from Cowper's glands	1. Wall of lower third of vagina becomes greatly engorged, with labia minora forming the "orgasmic platform"
2. Testes continue to elevate until they are situated close to the body to facilitate ejaculatory pressure	2. Clitoris retracts under hood for protection from direct, intense stimulation
Orgasmic	
1. Testes held at maximum elevation	1. Strong rhythmic muscular contractions occur at 8-second intervals in orgasmic platform
2. Rhythmic contractions occur at 8-second intervals	2. Number of contractions ranges from 3 to 15
3. "Point of inevitability" (awareness of fluid's presence in urethra) occurs just before ejaculation and lasts 2 to 3 seconds	3. Uterus contracts
4. Ejaculation, with rhythmic contractions capable of expelling semen up to 60 cm (2 ft)	4. Phase may be described as: Sensation of suspension followed by intense sensual awareness, clitorally oriented and radiating upward towards pelvis Suffusion of warmth, especially in pelvic area Pelvic throbbing located in vagina and lower pelvis
Resolution	
1. First stage of resolution; 50% of erection is lost rapidly	1. Blood returns from engorged walls of vagina; labia majora and labia minora return to unexcited state
2. Second stage can last longer, depending on maintenance of physical condition	2. Clitoris rapidly returns from under hood; return to normal size may take longer
3. Refractory period (time necessary to complete cycle again) ranges from a few minutes to a few days	3. Uterus descends
	4. Cervix dips into seminal pool

Immunology

To administer comprehensive care, the nurse should know about the numerous and complex physiologic factors that serve to maintain the integrity of the body's organization when nonself cells or substances affect the body's patterns. When the human body's immune defense system is activated, the nurse must be aware of the implications for care.

Table 1-8   *Using Laboratory Test Data Regarding Activated Immune Defense System to Determine Approach to Health Care*

Test Performed	Purpose of Test	Nursing Care Implications
Agglutination and titer levels (blood test)	These two tests permit quantitative and qualitative determination of presence of antibodies to antigen. In quantitative phase, fact of clumping (agglutination) or no clumping is indicative of antibody-antigen reaction (depending on structure of test, absence or presence of clumping may be read as positive test for antigen-antibody reaction). *It is a test of this type that is performed as immunologic test for pregnancy (searching for antibody reaction to antigen known as human chorionic gonadotropin),* which is formed by fetal tissue. Qualitative or titration test indicates degree of response aroused in body by antigen. Commonly physician will order two tests of titration separated by a time interval *(as before delivery and after delivery, in case of indirect Coombs' test)* to determine if there has been a change—most notably a rise—in titer levels, which would indicate recent experience with antigen in question. *In case of testing for immunity (resistance) to rubella,* titration test is essential to determine if client has adequate number of antibodies to provide protection in event of repeated exposure to rubella virus. Most labs consider a titration at level of 1:10 as adequate to ensure a state of immunity against rubella. NOTE: The titration levels conferring immune status differ from disease to disease.	A positive test indicates that exposure has occurred to antigenic substance. *In case of direct Coombs' test* (for detection of specific maternal antibodies—IgG—on fetal erythrocytes, antigenic substances): positive test result should alert nurse to fact that neonate is at risk for hyperbilirubinemia, oxygen deficit (secondary to hemolysis of red blood cells), and all sequelae of erythroblastosis fetalis. *In case of indirect Coombs' test* (for detection of anti-Rh antibodies appearing in mother's serum): if test result is positive and if serial dilutions of serum indicate there is considerable anti-Rh antibody activity in mother's system, mother would not be a candidate for Rh_0 (Du immune) globulin, since she had already developed the IgM and IgG antibodies against Rh. *If pregnant woman has positive titration test for rubella at 1:4 dilution* (1 part serum to 4 parts diluent) but not positive test at 1:8 dilution, she does not have adequate antibody protection against rubella virus. Woman is then susceptible to acquiring disease if exposed to virus. Compounding risk is fact that rubella that can be demonstrated to have occurred during first trimester of pregnancy (on basis of interval-titration tests) poses a hazardous risk to fetus. Postpartum woman who has demonstrated negative rubella titration test is good candidate to receive rubella vaccine, provided she practices some form of contraception for 3 months following injection of live, attenuated vaccine—until she has developed state of immunity to the disease. Client should also sign informed consent before receiving rubella vaccine, to indicate that she is aware of her responsibilities and risks associated with artificially induced active immunity therapy.
Complement (C3, C4) activity (blood test)	Instead of testing for activation of entire complement cascade, usually test is performed for two aspects of cascade sequence, to determine if they have been triggered. In event of immune response, levels of C3 and C4 (2 of 11 proteins involved in cascade) decrease, indicating their having been used.	This is a nonspecific test. It is possible that there may be "normal" test result yet immune response occurring in body. In combination with other tests (e.g., LE [lupus erythematosus] prep, ANA [anti-nuclear antibody] and RF [rheumatoid factor] tests), this test may be used to determine progression of the autoimmune disease processes.
C reactive protein (blood test)	This is a nonspecific test indicative of inflammatory process. It is sometimes used to rule out viral infection because protein is not present in cases of virally-caused inflammation.	Because this test is nonspecific, caution must be used in interpreting results. *It is possible for pregnancy or drug therapy with estrogenic birth control pills to produce false positive test.* Also, test may be positive in other types of inflammatory situations, as during acute myocardial infarction, acute phase of rheumatic disease, or rheumatoid arthritis.

Continued.

Table 1-8, cont'd.   *Using Laboratory Test Data Regarding Activated Immune Defense System to Determine Approach to Health Care*

Test Performed	Purpose of Test	Nursing Care Implications
Culture and sensitivity (C & S)	This test permits identification of type of antigen probably responsible for infectious process. Details about Gram's stain, type of environment (aerobic or anaerobic) that supports growth of antigen, and other characteristics of agent can be determined.	Nurse is responsible for collecting correct amount of specimen for culture, in appropriate type container. It is preferable that specimen is collected before antibiotic therapy is initiated, because this therapy could affect and invalidate test results.
	Once a bacteria, virus, or fungus has been identified, test continues, to evaluate effectiveness (or sensitivity) of variety of antibiotic drugs in inhibiting growth of agent. Occasionally a C & S test is performed during a phase of antibiotic therapy, when client has not shown improvement with prescribed medication.	Once results of test are available, it is imperative that client receive medication to which antigenic organisms are sensitive (and not resistant). If client has been receiving a drug to which organism is resistant, nurse must contact physician and report test result immediately.
Immunoelectrophoresis of serum proteins: IgA, IgD, IgE, IgG, IgM (blood test)	Normally this test is used to detect changes in any of immunoglobulins. *In case of a newborn,* this test may be performed to learn if IgM antibodies are present in the cord blood. (NOTE: These large IgM antibodies do not cross placental barrier.)	*If infant is born with suspicion of intrauterine acquired infection,* nurse should save placenta and cord for laboratory analysis (for IgM antibodies and other tests). A positive IgM cord blood test necessitates contacting physician immediately and initiating protective and supportive care to infected infant.
Immunofluorescent antibody (IFA) tests (blood test)	In *direct* test (searching for *antigen*), a fluorescent-labeled antibody is mixed with sample of blood. If antigen is present, it binds with antibody and can be detected with ultraviolet light microscope. In *indirect* test (searching for *antibody*), known antigen is mixed with blood sample and then fluorescein anti-immunoglobulin antibodies are mixed in. If a fluorescein-bound antibody-antigen complex is seen, no antibodies were present and so there was no exposure to that antigen (supposedly, unless immune system is compromised or defective).	*Two tests of this type have significance for maternity clients:* fluorescent treponemal antibody (FTA-ABS) test for syphilis exposure and IFA test for toxoplasmosis. If congenital syphilis of infant is suspected or confirmed, isolation techniques should be instituted for care of infant until such time that she or he is adjudged noncontagious on basis of drug therapy specific to the spirochete.
Sedimentation (erythrocyte) rate (blood test)	During acute systemic inflammatory process, erythrocytes gain in density and therefore fall or settle more rapidly when placed in test tube with anticoagulant. The more quickly cells settle, the more acute and active inflammatory the process is said to be.	Change in rate of sedimentation should signal need to reevaluate those limitations placed on client. (This is not a reliable test during pregnancy when sedimentation rate is normally elevated.)
White blood cell count (WBC) and differential	Total count of white blood cells indicates number of leukocytes circulating in serum. An increase is expected during infectious and inflammatory processes. Decreases are associated with certain diseases or certain therapies (antineoplastic drugs or radiation). Differences in the percentages of the various types of leukocytes is associated with activation of or disturbances in the immune responsiveness specific to the role of the type of WBC that is altered.	Client with increased levels, indicating active immune response, needs supportive care (adequate rest, fluids, and nutrition) to fight invading organisms successfully. Client with decreased levels or with a number of immature WBCs (on differential assessment) would need protective care, since resistance level (immune responsivity) would be low, and thus client would be prone to overwhelming infection(s). At times, protective or reverse isolation must be practiced, along with blood transfusions and passive artificial immunity therapy. If a client with leukopenia is on drug therapy for any condition, nurse must check to be sure that drug therapy does not coincidentally further deplete number of WBCs (by depressing bone marrow function) as side effect; if it does, conference with phy-

Table 1-8, cont'd. *Using Laboratory Test Data Regarding Activated Immune Defense System to Determine Approach to Health Care*

Test Performed	Purpose of Test	Nursing Care Implications
		sician is indicated for alternate drug therapy or supportive therapy to restore client's immune responsiveness. NOTE: Some elevation of WBC in pregnancy (up to 16,000/cu mm) and during labor and early postpartum period (up to 25,000/cu mm) is normal. Neonates are expected to have high levels of WBCs (18,000-40,000) during first few weeks of extrauterine life. As in children (up to about age 8), lymphocytes in infants become more prevalent than neutrophils. This is probably because of activity of thymus gland in infancy and early childhood. An increase in number of neutrophils is considered a healthy response to invasion, indicating intact and well-functioning immune system. If eosinophil content is increased, nurse should assist in assessment of sources of allergy or possible parasitic infestation. If lymphocyte count is decreased or if the subpopulations of T-helper and T-suppressor cells are reversed, client has compromised or deficient immune responsiveness and is in need of protective, supportive care.

GYNECOLOGIC EXAMINATION

Women's health care needs change with age, developmental level, and role expectations. About 40% of women seeking maternity-gynecologic care are adolescents. However, the number of women in their seventh and eighth decades seeking gynecologic care is increasing as the life span lengthens. The woman's movement of the 1960s and 1970s helped to educate women about their bodies. It has also made the client a more knowledgable and assertive consumer of health care. The nurse can help each woman learn about her body and become an active participant in her health care by being a nonjudgmental, sympathetic educator.

The following section summarizes the various issues addressed during a gynecologic assessment and examination.

Gynecologic Health Assessment

Gynecologic health assessment includes an interview, physical examination, and laboratory tests. This section outlines the assessment process and presents procedures for the pelvic examination and for collection of specimens for the Pap smear. During the examination the nurse must be aware of signs of problems, such as supine hypotension and vasovagal syncope, and be prepared to intervene if these conditions occur.

1. Interview: the history
   a. Identifying information
   b. Source and reliability of information
   c. Chief concern
   d. Present problem or illness
   e. Past medical history
   f. Family history
   g. Social and experiential history
   h. Review of systems
2. Physical examination
3. Laboratory tests
   a. Blood: VDRL or other test for syphilis, complete blood count (CBC) with hematocrit, hemoglobin, and differential values; blood type and Rh; antibody screen (Kell, Duffy, rubella, toxoplasmosis, anti-Rh): sickle cell; level of folacin when indicated
   b. Urine: Clean-catch urine specimen tested for glucose, protein, and acetone; microscopic assessment for pus, red blood cells, and casts; culture and sensitivity as necessary
   c. Skin test: Tine or PPD (purified protein derivative [of tuberculin]) for exposure to tuberculosis
   d. Cervical and vaginal smears for cytologic evaluation and for diagnosis of infections

Table 1-9 *Abdominal Assessment*

Assessment Factor	Possible Clinical Significance	Nursing Actions
Inspection		
Skin	Skin:	Describe
Color	Color:	Color
General	General physical condition: pale	Pattern, if color varies
Hyperpigmentation	Linea nigra	Presence, height
Rashes	Infection, allergy, poor hygiene, drug use, nutritional status	Color, size in centimeters, raised or flat, location, and distribution; use palpation as necessary
Lesions	Spider nevi, infections, infestations, moles	
Scars	May result in adhesion or obstruction	
Striae	Old (silver): obesity, pregnancy; reddish: pregnancy, Cushing's syndrome	Color
Dilated veins	Possible vena cava obstruction	Distribution, amount
Turgor	Nutritional status	Degree of turgor, rule out edema
Texture	Nutritional status	Dry, moist
Hair distribution	Hirsutism (endocrine imbalance)	Pattern, amount if unusual
Umbilicus	Displaced upward: pregnancy	Describe
Color	Discoloration: suspect intraperitoneal bleeding	Refer immediately
Contour	Hernia, pregnancy	Reducible? Tender?
Location	Previous surgery may have caused adhesion or obstruction	Position, length, healing of scar
Signs of inflammation	Current infection, cellulitis	Discharge, odor, color, duration, pain
Contour and symmetry: abdominal, inguinal, femoral regions	Protuberant: adipose, gas distension, tumor, ascites, pregnancy	Record: flat, scaphoid (concave), rounded, protuberant isolated bulges; whether bulges are reducible
	Hernias: umbilical, incisional, diastasis recti hernia over linea alba, ovoid bulge in groin	Possible inguinal hernia; check if reducible
	Bulges: full bladder, pregnancy, masses, enlarged lymph nodes	
Peristalsis	Normally seen in a thin person, may indicate intestinal obstruction	Observe across abdomen—from one side, then from other side; use good lighting
Pulsations	Normally seen in epigastrium	Record location and intensity
Auscultation		
Normal	Normal: clicks, gurgles, "growling" (borborygmi with hyperperistalsis); frequency of sounds: 5 to 34/min	Auscultate all four quadrants and epigastrium
		Perform before percussion and palpation
Increased	Increased: diarrhea, early obstructive process	Listen for 2 minutes or more over suspicious area
Decreased	Decreased or absent: paralytic ileus	
High pitched	High-pitched tinkling with abdominal cramps: possible intestinal obstruction	
Percussion		
Fat	Fat: scattered dullness or tympany; umbilicus sunken	Unless pregnancy is far advanced, percuss all four quadrants first, then liver, spleen, stomach, and bowel; or percuss all areas, then percuss and palpate each organ before proceeding to the next; note distribution or absence of sounds
Tympany	Tympany: normally predominates over abdomen; stomach: left lower anterior rib cage; gaseous distension: generalized tympany	
Dullness	Dullness:	Have woman void to facilitate examination
	Supra pubic: full bladder	Note level of lower border in midclavicular line; note upper border; measure boundaries if enlarged
	Liver:	
	Obscured upper border: right pleural effusion	
	Obscured lower border: gas in colon	Describe boundaries; refer

Continued.

Table 1-9, cont'd. *Abdominal Assessment*

Assessment Factor	Possible Clinical Significance	Nursing Actions

Dullness—cont'd	Solid tumor (ovarian): dullness over symphysis pubis, tympany around dullness: umbilicus not displaced upward
	Ascites
	  Supine: dullness down both flanks, meeting over symphysis pubis surrounding tympanic area over umbilicus
	  Left lateral: dullness on dependent half, tympany over superior half
		Describe pattern with woman in supine and left lateral position; refer

Palpation		

Irregular uterine contours
Adnexa
	Uterine anomaly, myomata
	Adnexa
	  Fullness, unilateral pelvic pain over mass, possible left shoulder pain: probable ectopic pregnancy
	  Mass: possible ovarian cyst, tumor
		Describe size, location, and consistency; refer
		Adnexa
		  Describe size in centimeters; characteristics—smooth, irregular, nodular, hard, soft, fluctuant, motility, tenderness, pulsating or not. Rebound tenderness? Ballotable? Refer

Guarding of abdomen caused by pain over McBurney's point	Possible appendicitis	Assess vital signs, describe responses, submit ordered laboratory tests

Procedure 1-1

PELVIC EXAMINATION

DEFINITION

Inspection and palpation of the internal and external structures comprising the female reproductive system. Examination may be done manually or with aid of instrumentation.

PURPOSE

To provide a data base for medical diagnoses, medical therapy, nursing diagnoses, and nursing care. To involve the woman as an active participant in her own health supervision, maintenance, and care.

EQUIPMENT

To obtain specimens for screening potential problems. Gynecologic table and drapes.
Supplies as neccessary.

NURSING ACTIONS	RATIONALE
Wash hands. Ask client to empty her bladder before the examination.	To minimize chance for nosocomial infection. To increase woman's comfort and facilitate accurate assessment.
Instruct woman to remove her clothing (from the waist down if only the pelvic examination is to be done) and put on a cover gown; provide privacy for this.	To provide adequate exposure for thorough gynecologic examination.
Explain purpose of the procedure and how it is done. Describe sensations to expect. Inform the client who will do the procedure, and about how long it will take. Ask her if she wishes a mirror to watch.	To show respect. To reduce anxiety related to knowledge deficit. To provide woman with chance to have more control over situation and to learn more about her body.
Assist the woman into the lithotomy postion (the woman's hips and knees are flexed with the buttocks at the edge of the table with her feet supported by heel or knee stirrups), and drape appropriately.	To increase her comfort and facilitate examination; however, other positions can be used. To meet her need for modesty and provide warmth.

Continued.

Procedure 1-1—cont'd

Adjust pillow under client's head.	To increase her comfort and help relax her abdominal musculature.
Lubricate examiner's fingers with water or water-soluble lubricant before bimanual examination.	To reduce friction and discomfort and to avoid other types of lubricant that can distort findings.
Warm speculum in warm water.	To increase client's comfort since warm metal is less shocking to the mucous membrane.
	To reduce her anxiety by keeping her informed.
During the examination, support client. Explain the procedure during inspection of external genitals, insertion of speculum for examination of vagina and cervix, and bimanual examination of internal organs.	To increase her knowledge about her body.
Refrain from questioning the woman extensively. Hold question until she is sitting up and at eye level with the examiner.	To prevent tension that can develop if she is questioned, especially if she cannot see the questioner's eyes.
Assist with relaxation techniques. Have the woman place her hands on her chest at about the level of the diaphragm, breathe deeply and slowly (in through her mouth and out through her O-shaped mouth), concentrate on the rhythm of breathing, and relax all body muscles with each exhalation (Malasanos et al., 1986).	To decrease common feeling of vulnerability and strangeness when in lithotomy position.
	To help her relax perineum during the examination. NOTE: This breathing technique is particularly helpful for the adolescent or the woman whose introitus may be especially tight. Others for whom the experience may be new or tension provoking can also benefit from using this technique.
Encourage woman to become involved with the examination if she shows interest. For example, a mirror can be placed so that the area being examined can be seen by the woman.	To assist the interested woman and to motive other women to be participants in their own care.
	To provide health teaching.
Distract the attention of the tense woman by placing interesting mobiles or pictures on the ceiling or wall near her head.	To provide distraction that is an effective method of reducing tension.
Remind the woman not to squeeze her eyes closed, clench her fists, or squeeze the nurse's hand.	To help her relax her perineum, since tightening these muscles encourages tightening of the perineal muscles.
Assess woman for and treat imminent untoward responses (see Emergency Procedures, "Vasovagal Syncope," p. 16, and "Supine Hypotension," p. 17).	To ensure the safety and health of the woman.
Instruct woman to bear down when speculum is being inserted.	To open the vaginal introitus and relax perineal muscles for easier insertion of the speculum.
Apply gloves and assist examiner with collection of specimens for cytology such as Papanicolaou smear (see Procedure 1-2). After handling specimens, remove gloves and wash hands.	To implement universal precautions when handling body fluids.
	To reduce possibility of contamination of specimens.
	To minimize nosocomial infections.
Assist woman at completion of examination to a sitting position and then a standing position.	To attain a sitting position comfortably without strain.
	To reduce possibility of transient or orthostatic hypotension that may occur if position is changed rapidly.
Provide tissues to wipe lubricant from perineum.	To provide comfort and promote cleanliness.
Provide privacy for woman while she is dressing.	To show respect and to promote feelings of security and worth.
Inform woman as to the next step in the assessment protocol.	To supply information to reduce tension that arises from facing the unknown.
Record findings on the appropriate forms.	To provide permanent record of data base to foster continuity of care.

Procedure 1-2

PAPANICOLAOU SMEAR (PAP SMEAR, PAP TEST)

DEFINITION

A laboratory technique of cytologic examination.

PURPOSE

To detect abnormalities of cell growth. During gynecologic examination cells from the squamocolumnar junction, the cervix, and the vagina are examined. Identification of endometrial or ovarian cancer *cannot* be obtained with this test.

EQUIPMENT

Speculum
Sterile glove or gloves
Glass slides
Cytologic fixative
Wooden or plastic spatula
Pencil or grease crayon (for putting patient's name on slides)

NURSING ACTIONS	RATIONALE
Instruct the woman that optimum time for test is near the time of ovulation in her menstrual cycle.	To facilitate specimen collection, since cervical os is somewhat open, mucus is plentiful, and menstrual flow does not distort findings.
Instruct woman not to douche, use vaginal medications, or engage in intercourse at least 24 hours before the procedure.	To avoid altering findings that can lead to misdiagnosis. To prevent discomfort, since douching removes vaginal secretions that provide lubrication.
Explain to client the purpose of the test and what sensations she will feel as the specimen is obtained (i.e., pressure, not pain). Inform her of who will perform the test.	To reduce tension that develops when people face the unknown.
Wash hands and apply gloves.	To prevent contamination of slides from other sources, and after slides are prepared to implement universal precautions when handling body fluids.
Assist examiner with test. The cytologic specimen is obtained before any digital examination of the vagina is made, or endocervical bacteriological specimens are taken with cotton swabbing of the cervix.	To prevent cell distortion by lubricant.
Instruct woman to fold her hands over her midriff and breathe as described in Procedure 1-2.	To promote comfort and reduce tension through relaxation and distraction.
Explain to woman that the specimen is taken by placing the S-shaped end of cervical spatula just within the cervical canal at the external os. The blade is rotated 360 degrees so that the surface at the squamocolumnar junction is firmly scraped. If the junction is inside the cervical canal, a swab may be used to obtain cells. If gross exudate is present, the excess is gently pushed away from the os with the end of the spatula.	To obtain cells from the squamocolumnar junction, the most common site of dysplasia and neoplasia.
Explain to woman that the specimen is spread on a slide without rubbing or drying, sprayed lightly with fixative, and allowed to dry.	To prepare the first slide, which contains mainly cells from the endocervix and ectocervix.
Explain to woman that some mucus is obtained from the posterior fornix (vaginal pool) with the rounded end of the spatula, spread on another slide, sprayed, and dried.	To prepare the second slide with mucus that may contain cells from the endometrium, endocervix, and vagina.
Label the slides with the woman's name and site. Include on the form to accompany the slides the woman's name, age, parity, and chief complaint or reason for taking the cytologic specimens. Place slides in carrying container, remove gloves, and wash hands.	To minimize chance of loss or mismatching specimens.
Send the specimens to the pathology laboratory promptly for staining, evaluation, and a written report, with special reference to abnormal elements, including cancer cells.	To prevent cross-contamination. To prevent delay that may cause change in specimen and a false report.
Advise the woman that repeat smears may be necessary if specimen is not adequate.	To reduce anxiety if asked to return.
Instruct the woman concerning routine checkups for cervical or vaginal cancer.	To provide health maintenance information as part of procedure to reach as many people as possible.
Record the examination, date, and any untoward reactions on the woman's prenatal record.	To maintain concise, complete recording for providing care for clients.

EMERGENCY PROCEDURE

VASOVAGAL SYNCOPE

DEFINITION

Transient loss of consciousness resulting from a sudden fall in blood pressure caused by decreased peripheral resistance, decreased cardiac output, reduced venous return, and slowing of the heart. Occurs suddenly.

PURPOSE

To prevent death.

EQUIPMENT

Crash cart (emergency cart).

NURSING ACTIONS	RATIONALE
Alert physician.	To provide essential immediate care.
Assess for signs of shock; decreased blood pressure and increased pulse; apprehension; pallor; diaphoresis; generalized weakness; lightheadedness; vertigo.	To determine the extent of shock response.
Assess level of consciousness: partial to total loss of consciousness, seizures and vomiting, and incontinence of bowel or bladder.	To determine client's state of consciousness and related responses that may place client at additional risk (e.g., vomiting).
Ensure adequate airway:	To permit oxygenation.
Extend head or use jaw-thrust maneuver.	
Suction as required.	To keep airway unobstructed.
Provide oxygen when airway is clear.	To increase tissue perfusion and prevent cellular death.
Begin seizure precautions.	To protect client from injury.
Assist with cardiopulmonary resuscitation (CPR):	To prevent death.
Airway.	To identify and remove obstruction.
Breathing: mouth to mouth or artificial intermittent pressure breathing with oxygen (1:5 compressions with help; 2:15 compressions when alone):	To verify need for and provide external respiratory assistance to maintain oxygenation.
Circulation: external cardiac compression 60 to 80 per minute.	To verify need for and assist with external support to perfuse tissues.
Assist with drugs:	
Atropine sulphate, 0.4 to 1.0 mg, intravenously.	To reduce cardiac vagal tone, increase rate of sinus and atrial pacemakers, and improve atrioventricular conduction.
Epinephrine HCl, 0.5 to 1.0 mg (5 to 10 ml of a 1:10,000 solution) intravenously (USP-DI, 1986); or 1 mg (10 ml of a 1:10,000 solution) endotracheally.	To stimulate alpha and beta receptors; for example, to increase heart rate, force of myocardial contractions, and peripheral vascular resistance.
Assist with direct current defibrillation, 200 to 400 J (Phipps, Long, and Woods, 1987).	To restore normal cardiac rhythm.

EMERGENCY PROCEDURE

SUPINE HYPOTENSION

DEFINITION

While lying in lithotomy position, weight of abdominal contents may compress the vena cava and aorta. Compression of these major vessels results in a drop in blood pressure, pallor, breathlessness, clammy skin, and other signs of shock.

PURPOSE

Reduce compression of the large vessels to allow the woman's symptoms to abate and to bring all body functions back into homeostasis.

EQUIPMENT

None.

NURSING ACTIONS

Remove woman from lithotomy position, and position her on her side until signs and symptoms abate.
Provide the woman with a frank explanation.

RATIONALE

To take the weight of the abdominal contents off of the vena cava and aorta.
To provide knowledge that reduces fear of the unknown and forms basis for self-care.

Client Teaching

The gynecologic examination provides the nurse with an excellent opportunity to educate the woman and encourage her participation in her own health care. Two important areas for client teaching at this time are breast self-examination (BSE) and prevention of urinary tract infection.

Guidelines For Client Teaching

BREAST SELF-EXAMINATION

ASSESSMENT

Woman states she does not know how to examine her breasts.
Woman has potential risk for developing breast lumps and cancer because of history.

NURSING DIAGNOSIS

Knowledge deficit related to self-care: breast self-examination (BSE).

GOALS

Short-term

Woman will verbalize reasons why BSE is important.
Woman will verbalize steps of BSE and rationale for each step.
Woman will demonstrate BSE procedure correctly.

Intermediate (By first postpartum check-up or by next gynecologic examination)

Woman verbalizes steps of BSE and rationale.
Woman states she has examined her breasts once.
After weaning: woman will be familiar with the normal feel and appearance of her breasts.

Long-term

Woman performs BSE every month.

References and teaching aids.

American Cancer Society's pamphlet, *How to examine your breasts.*
Mirror.
Model for practicing palpation and recognition of masses.

Continued.

Guidelines For Client Teaching—cont'd

CONTENT/RATIONALE	TEACHING ACTION
To provide content and rationale for BSE during the menstrual cycle.	Encourage questions to uncover anxieties, concerns, and knowledge gaps about BSE. Review content and rationale, as needed. Encourage questions. Demonstrate for woman.
To perform observation: Woman sits in front of mirror and observes her breasts while assuming four positions.	Assist woman to assume postures correctly.
1. Arms relaxed at her sides 2. Hands pressed against her waist 3. Arms over head 4. Leaning forward Review normal and suspicious characteristics.	Review, compare with woman's breasts and with pamphlet. Assist woman with verbalization of her observations of herself.
To perform palpation: Palpation is performed with the woman in the supine position and a pillow under the shoulder on the side of the breast to be examined.	Using a teaching model or illustration, demonstrate methods of systematic breast palpation.
Examination is performed in a systematic manner and includes the nipple. Palpation of axillary lymph nodes is most easily done by the practitioner. However, the woman can learn too.	Demonstrate palpation on model and on woman's breast; observe return demonstration. Assist woman to supine position with pillow under shoulder on side to be examined. Assist woman through self-examination and verbal description of her findings. Encourage and answer questions.
To know how to report findings: Findings are described by their characteristics (e.g., color, discharge) and by their location.	Review characteristics while referring to pamphlet or other printed matter.
When woman notes reportable signs or symptoms, she needs to note the phase of her menstrual cycle (if she is still cycling).	Using an illustration, show woman how to locate lesion.

EVALUATION Teaching of the cognitive and motor aspects of BSE is considered effective when the woman verbalizes and demonstrates the steps of the procedure. Teaching related to the affective/psychologic aspect of BSE may be considered effective if the woman performs BSE routinely *and* reports any findings immediately.

Guidelines For Client Teaching

PREVENTION OF URINARY TRACT INFECTION

ASSESSMENT

Woman is unaware of self-care measures to prevent urinary tract infection (UTI).

Woman may be pregnant, which predisposes her to UTI, and UTI may be a factor in preterm labor.

Woman may be experiencing postmenopausal urinary tract changes that predispose her to UTI.

NURSING DIAGNOSES

Potential for injury related to UTI urinary elimination, potential for altered patterns related to UTI.

Potential for pain related to UTI.

Knowledge deficit related to preventive actions.

GOALS

Short-term

Woman will be able to verbalize preventive methods.

Woman will learn preventive method.

Intermediate

Woman will routinely incorporate preventive methods in ADL.

Long-term

Woman will prevent UTI and the complications that may arise from it.

Guidelines for Client Teaching—cont'd

References and teaching aids
Texts.
Hospital- or clinic-prepared instructions.
Illustrations.

CONTENT/RATIONALE	TEACHING ACTION
Teach the woman general hygiene measures: Always wipe front to back after urinating or moving bowels. Use a clean piece of toilet paper for each front to back wipe. Wiping in the opposite way, from back to front, may carry bacteria from the rectal area (anus) to the urethral opening and increase risk of infection. Use soft, absorbent toilet tissue, preferably white and unscented. Harsh, scented, or printed toilet paper may cause irritation.	Using an illustration, show woman locations of urinary meatus, vagina, and anus. Provide explanation and rationale for action.
Change tampons, panty shields, or sanitary napkins often. Bacteria can multiply in menstrual blood or on soiled panty shields.	Encourage discussion about perineal hygiene, for example, feelings regarding odors, vaginal discharges, stress incontinence, touching oneself.
Wear underpants and panty hose with a cotton crotch. Avoid wearing tight-fitting slacks or panty shields for long periods. A build up of heat and moisture in the genital area may contribute to the growth of bacteria.	Explain how nylon and synthetic fibers retain heat and moisture.
Explain to the woman proper fluid and food intake: Drink 2 to 3 quarts (8 to 12 glasses) of liquid a day; 8 to 10 ounces of cranberry juice a day may be included, since cranberry juice is more acidic than other fluids and can lower the pH of the urinary tract. A more acidic urinary tract is a less hospitable medium to developing bacteria.	Elicit feelings or ideas concerning cultural, ethnic, religious, or other factors affecting food and fluid intake. Discuss rationale. Discuss fluid intake if woman is edematous, has PIH, or has difficulty sleeping at night as a result of nocturia.
Include lactobacilli in diet. Yogurt that contains the live culture and acidophilus milk may help prevent UTI, as well as vaginal infections. Lactobacilli, which are normally found in the vagina and the urinary tract, maintain the normal pH balance.	Provide rationale for including these foods in the woman's diet. Discuss food preferences.
Teach woman proper urination practices: Urinate frequently. Maintain fluid intake to ensure urination; do not limit fluids to reduce frequency of urination. Do not ignore signals that indicate the need to use the bathroom. Holding urine increases the time bacteria are in the bladder and allows them to multiply. Plan ahead when in situations where you will be unable to urinate for a long period of time, for example, before a long car ride, try to urinate in advance. Always urinate before going to bed at night.	Elicit information about daily schedule, for example, if working, can she get to the bathroom often. Provide rationale.
Urinate before and after intercourse, then drink a large glass of water to urinate again. This helps eliminate a medium for bacteria that are introduced during intercourse.	Provide an explanation concerning the introduction of bacteria during intercourse. Discuss rationale.
Postclimacterium counseling.	

EVALUATION The nurse can be reasonably assured that care was effective if the woman does not develop an UTI.

Summary of Nursing Actions

NURSING CARE FOR GYNECOLOGIC EXAMINATION

I. Goals
  A. Woman is psychologically and emotionally ready for the examination.
  B. Woman's anxiety, embarrassment, and feelings of vulnerability are minimized.
  C. Woman's self-esteem is enhanced.
  D. Woman is physiologically prepared for the examination.
  E. Woman's personal motivation and goals in relation to health maintenance and promotion are heightened.
  F. Any preexisting, hereditary, or genetic problems are identified.
  G. Any adverse sequelae, such as vasovagal syncope, are prevented.
II. Priorities
  A. Establish woman's readiness by assessing maturity beforehand.
  B. Explain procedures thoroughly.
  C. Maintain eye contact when speaking to her.
  D. Keep woman covered and draped at all times.
  E. Encourage self-care.
  F. Identify and initiate treatment promptly.
  G. Encourage participation and dialogue during examination.
III. Assessment
  A. Interview
    1. See "Gynecologic Health Assessment," p. 11.
  B. Physical examination
    1. Breast self-examination see Guidelines for Client Teaching, "Breast Self-Examination," pp. 17-18.
    2. Abdominal assessment, see Table 1-9.
    3. Pelvic examination, see Procedure 1-1, pp. 13-14.
    4. PAP smear (PAP test), see Procedure 1-2, p. 15.
    5. Review of the systems
      a. General symptoms
      b. Skin
      c. Musculoskeletal
      d. Head, eyes, ears, nose, throat (HEENT)
      e. Endocrine-thyroid, menses, pregnancies, breasts
      f. Respiratory
      g. Cardiovascular
      h. Hematologic
      i. Immune
      j. Gastrointestinal
      k. Genitourinary
      l. Neurologic
      m. Psychiatric
  C. Laboratory tests
    1. See "Gynecologic Health Assessment," p. 11.
IV. Potential nursing diagnoses
  A. Knowledge deficit
  B. Potential for injury
  C. Noncompliance
  D. Fear
  E. Pain
  F. Anxiety
  G. Ineffective individual coping
  H. Body image disturbance
  I. Self-esteem disturbance: situational low self-esteem
  J. Impaired verbal communication
  K. Altered health maintenance
V. Plan/implementation
  A. History
    1. Information regarding possible family problems, such as diethylstilbesterol (DES) exposure, breast cancer in female relatives, or other pelvic diseases gathered and recorded for future reference.
  B. Physical examination
    1. Any preexisting disease is treated.
    2. Woman is educated to her body and its function to prevent gynecologic disease.
    3. Promotion of self-care.
  C. Laboratory profile
    1. Information is obtained for prevention and therapy.
VI. Evaluation
  A. Complete history will be taken.
  B. Complete physical will be administered.
  C. Laboratory profile is done.
  D. Woman is prepared for the examination both physically and mentally.
    1. Promotion of self-care accomplished through motivation and education.

References

Malasanos I et al: Health assessment, ed 3, St Louis, 1986, The CV Mosby Co.

Phipps WJ, Long BC, and Woods NF: Medical-surgical nursing: concepts and clinical practice, ed 3, St Louis, 1987, The CV Mosby Co.

United States Pharmacopeia Dispensing Information, St Louis, 1986, The CV Mosby Co.

UNIT

2

Normal Pregnancy

Pregnancy is a time of anxiety, excitement, fear, anticipation, and wonder for the woman and her family. It is a developmental crisis in their lives that necessitates changes in outlook, role responsibilities, and everyday living.

Adaptation to pregnancy involves all of a woman's body systems as the fetoplacental maternal unit becomes an efficient and functional system unto itself.

Each trimester brings new feelings and changes in the woman and her family. This unit addresses those changes: the pregnancy tests and physiologic adaptations of the first trimester; the assessment of fetal well-being and counseling for self-care in the second trimester; and the discomforts and anticipation of labor in the third trimester.

Each section focuses on the changes and needs of that particular trimester. Nutritional requirements for a healthy pregnancy are presented in the beginning because they are so important throughout the pregnancy. Sample nursing care plans and summaries of nursing actions can be found at the ends of each section to tie all the information together.

FIRST TRIMESTER

The prenatal period is a preparation, both physically, in terms of fetal growth and maternal adaptations, and psychologically, in terms of anticipation of parenthood. Pregnancy is unique during a woman's life because only then does the healthy woman seek ongoing health care. It is the responsibility of the nurse and other health care professionals to keep the pregnant woman informed of her progress, teach her self-care strategies, and warn her of impending danger to her and her fetus.

The first trimester sets the tone for her care. Often the diagnosis of pregnancy is a surprise. Whether expected or unexpected, this is a time of rapid change and adjustment. The nurse plays a major role in this adjustment.

The diagnosis of pregnancy is not definitive but takes into account a myriad of objective and subjective signs and symptoms, including blood and/or urine tests that show the presence of increasing levels of human chorionic gonadotropin (HCG).

Positive signs of pregnancy are (1) demonstration of a fetal heart distinct from that of the mother, (2) fetal movement felt by someone other than the mother, and (3) visualization of the fetus with a technique such as ultrasound (Danforth and Scott, 1986).

Terminology Describing the Pregnant Woman

gravida A woman who is pregnant.
parturient A woman in labor.
gravidity Pregnancy without regard to the outcome.
parity The number of *pregnancies* in which the fetus or fetuses have reached viability, not the number of fetuses delivered. Whether the fetus is born alive or its stillborn after viability is reached does not affect parity.
nulligravida A woman who has never been pregnant.
primigravida A woman who is pregnant for the first time.
multigravida A woman who has had two or more pregnancies.
nullipara A woman who has *not* completed a pregnancy with a fetus or fetuses who have reached the stage of fetal viability (legal definition of fetal viability: 22 to 23 weeks of gestational age).
primipara A woman who has completed one pregnancy with a fetus or fetuses who have reached the stage of fetal viability.
multipara A woman who has completed two or more pregnancies to the stage of fetal viability.

Table 2-1 *Gravidity and Parity Using Five-Digit and Two-Digit Systems**

Condition	Five-digit System G T P A L	Two-digit System G/P
judith is pregnant for the first time.	1 - 0 - 0 - 0 - 0	i/0
She carries the pregnancy to term and the neonate survives.	1 - 1 - 0 - 0 - 1	i/i
She is pregnant again.	2 - 1 - 0 - 0 - 1	ii/i
Her second pregnancy ends in abortion.	2 - 1 - 0 - 1 - 1	ii/i
During her third pregnancy, she delivers viable twins.	3 - 2 - 0 - 1 - 3	iii/ii

*G, Times uterus has been pregnant; T, number of term deliveries, P, number of premature births; A, number of abortions (spontaneous or elective); L, number of living children.

Confirming the Pregnancy

An accurate diagnosis of pregnancy requires knowledge of the different pregnancy tests available and how to interpret their results. The nurst must also understand the tremendous part played by hormones in the development of the products of conception and the mother's body responses. Finally, the nurse must be able to assess and diagnose the various signs and symptoms of pregnancy.

Pregnancy Tests

Latex Agglutination Inhibition (LAI)—Gravidex slide, Pregnosticon slide, UGC Beta slide

1. Easy to do
2. Results in 2 minutes
3. Accurate from 4 to 10 days following missed menses

Hemaglutination Inhibition (HAI)—E.P.T. (Home pregnancy test)

1. Easy to do; done in privacy of own home
2. Accurate from 4 days following missed menses
3. Results in 1 to 2 hours
4. One brand, Neocept, gives results at or before missed menses

Radioreceptor Assay (Biocept G)

1. Newest category of tests
2. 1-hour serum test
3. Accurate at time of missed menses

Radioimmunoassay (RIA)

1. Must be performed done by a laboratory
2. Most sensitive test performed
3. Pregnancy diagnosed 8 days after ovulation or 6 days before missed menses
4. Gives results in 1 to 48 hours depending on sensitivity

Direct Agglutination—ELISA

1. Accurate results at or before missed menstruation

Enzyme Immunoassay—Confidot (Home pregnancy test)

1. Easy-to-read results (visible color change)
2. Confirms pregnancy 10 days after fertilization or 4 days before missed menstruation

Table 2-2 *Hormonal Factors in Pregnancy*

Hormone and Source	Principal Effects	Clinical Significance
Fetoplacental Unit Estrogen: produced by ovary and adrenal cortex as in prepregnant state; however, principal source is placenta; synthesized from precursors from fetal liver and adrenals; increase in level of E_3 (estriol) by end of fourth week, by end of pregnancy, 300 × normal; however, low potency of E_3 means estrogenic activity only 30 × normal	Level of circulating estriol rises in pregnancy and so increases in urine and amniotic fluid	Urinary excretion of 30-40 mg/24 hr of estriol by end of pregnancy—an indication of fetal well-being (must be repeated, i.e., serial): Significant decrease indicates fetus in jeopardy (or fetal death) Excessive increase may indicate multiple pregnancy, erythroblastosis fetalis

Table 2-2, cont'd.   Hormonal Factors in Pregnancy

Hormone and Source	Principal Effects	Clinical Significance

Estrogen—cont'd.	Enlargement of uterus:
	  Hypertrophy of musculature
	  Proliferation of endometrium
	  Increase in blood supply
		Probable sign of pregnancy
		Continued growth indicates pregnancy advancing

	Enlargement of breast Growth of glandular tissue ducts, alveoli, nipples Deposition of fat	Breast tenderness
	Enlargement of genitals	Growth of vagina permits passage of infant

	Nutrient metabolism altered:
	  Increases elastic properties of connective tissue (relaxation of pubic joints and pelvic ligaments; cervix enlarges, softens, is stretchable [theory])
		Softening of connective tissue:
		  Backache, tenderness over pubic area, flank pain
		  Cervical dilation

	Decreased secretion of HCl, pepsin	Digestive upsets, nausea, decreased absorption of fat
	Affects thyroid function: thyroxine production increases, but so does production of thyroxine-binding globulin	No major increase in free thyroxine (BMR rises primarily as result of increased oxygen consumption with growth of uterus, fetus, placenta)
	Interferes with folic acid metabolism Increase in total body proteins	Positive nitrogen balance: protein available for fetal growth
	Sodium and water retention by kidney tubules	Increased plasma volume and interstitial fluid volume→edema, fluid reserve

	Hematologic changes:
	  Hypercoagulability of blood
	  Decrease in fibrinolytic activity
	  Increase in sedimentation rate (SR)
		Safety mechanism vs. hemorrhage
		  Tendency for thrombosis to occur (legs)
		  Affects use in clinical diagnosis using SR tests (no diagnostic value)

	Vascular changes:
	  Telangiectasias (spider nevi)
	  Palmar erythema
		No clinical significance; changes usually disappear after pregnancy

	Stimulation of production of melanin-stimulating hormone	Hyperpigmentation (chloasma, linea nigra, areolar tissue, genitals)
Progesterone: produced by corpus luteum for 2 months and by placental trophoblastic cells from about 8-10 days after conception; rises steadily through pregnancy	Promotes development of decidual (secretory) cells in endometrium	Glycogen deposits support nutrition of embryo
	Decreases contractility of gravid uterus	Prevents uterine contractions from causing spontaneous abortion
	Promotes development of secretory portions of lobular-alveolar system	Prepares breasts for lactation

	Nutrient effects:
	  Favors maternal fat deposition
		Nutritional significance:
		  Energy available for maternal and fetal needs

	Reduced gastric motility, sphincters relaxed	Regurgitation (heartburn); small, frequent feedings tolerated
	Increases sodium excretion	Hyponatremia may develop
	Increases sensitivity of respiratory center to CO_2	Respiratory rate increases; decreased alveolar and arterial Pco_2 (feeling of breathlessness)
	Reduces tone of smooth muscle	Colonic activity diminishes (constipation) Reduced tone of bladder and ureters (distension, urinary stasis, urinary tract infections) Vascular tone decreases (venous dilation; stasis in lower limbs with edema, varicosities)

Continued.

Table 2-2, cont'd.   Hormonal Factors in Pregnancy

Hormone and Source	Principal Effects	Clinical Significance
Progesterone: cont'd.		Decreased tone in gallbladder: reduced motility; incidence of gallbladder disease increases
	Raises body temperature 0.5° C	Feelings of warmth, perspiration increases
Human chorionic gonadotropin (hCG): produced by syncytiotrophoblast; peak level by day 60-70 of gestation, levels fall after fourth month, disappear 2 weeks after pregnancy ends	Maintenance of corpus luteum in early pregnancy	Corpus luteum not necessary after first few weeks—placenta produces sufficient hormones
	Exerts interstitial cell–stimulating effect on testes of male fetus	Testosterone levels in male fetus rise
	May have immunologic properties	May inhibit lymphocyte response to foreign protein, the fetal portion of placenta
	May cause allergic response	May be cause of hyperemesis gravidarum
		Diagnostic value:
		Persistence of hCG after spontaneous abortion symptomatic of hydatidiform mole or choriocarcinoma
		Basis for hormone test for pregnancy
		Decreased level in threatened abortion
		Increased level with multiple pregnancies
Human placental lactogen (hPL) or chorionic growth hormone (CGH) (also called human chorionic somatomammotropic hormone [hCS]) produced by syncytiotrophoblast; detectable by week 5 or 6; rises steadily, disappears 2 weeks after delivery	Similar action to pituitary growth hormone:	Glucose metabolism changes result in:
	Glucose metabolism:	Glucose available for fetal energy needs (only energy source for fetus)
	Decreases use of glucose for energy by maternal organism by increasing lipolysis to make fatty acids available for energy (carbohydrate sparer)	
	Glycogen deposition increased, cells saturated (inhibits glyconeogenesis), causing blood glucose levels to rise	Diabetogenic effect in mother (increased blood glucose levels stimulate beta cells of islets of Langerhans to produce more insulin)—may "burn out," producing diabetes mellitus
	Carbohydrates and insulin required for hormone activity	Fetal pancreas produces insulin by week 12; maternal insulin does not cross placenta; fetal pancreas may overproduce if continuous hyperglycemic stimulus is present; at birth infant becomes hypoglycemic and brain growth is endangered
	Protein metabolism:	Protein metabolism:
	Increases protein synthesis	Protein available for fetal and maternal growth needs
	Decreases breakdown and utilization of protein for energy (mobilizes free fatty acids; if excessive, may cause ketosis)	
	Acts synergistically with hydrocortisone and insulin in development of alveoli of breast (lactogenic effect)	Preparation of breasts for lactation
	Amount secreted depends on size of placenta	Research to determine whether level of circulating hPL (hCS, CGH) an indicator of normal pregnancy

Table 2-2, cont'd.   Hormonal Factors in Pregnancy

Hormone and Source	Principal Effects	Clinical Significance
Origin: Multiple Organs		
Prostaglandins: widely distributed in human body, including seminal fluid, brain, nerves, most endocrine organs, endometrium, decidua, and amniotic fluid	Reproductive system: play a role in erection, ejaculation, ovulation, formation of corpus luteum, uterine motility, parturition, and milk ejection Cardiovascular system: play a role in platelet aggregation, blood pressure increase	Prostaglandins are used to induce labor in second-trimester abortions; may be used (research in progress) for induction of labor at term
Ovary, Corpus Luteum		
Relaxin	Present in many mammalian species and may serve to: Promote cervical softening Remodel collagen	Same as principal effects
Pituitary		
Pituitary growth hormone: produced by anterior pituitary	Decreases markedly during pregnancy and rises slowly to prepregnancy level 6-8 weeks after delivery	May be reason why insulin requirements decrease after delivery (hPL ↓ with delivery of placenta)
Follicle-stimulating hormone (FSH): produced by anterior pituitary	Decreases markedly during pregnancy; remains low for 10-12 days after delivery Increases then to follicular-phase concentrations during third week after delivery	Ovulation ceases during pregnancy
Prolactin (PRL): produced by anterior pituitary	Lactation: stimulates production of fat, lactose, and casein by mammary glandular cells after placenta is delivered May play role in regulation of fluid exchange across fetal membranes, lung maturation, and pregnancy maintenance	Milk not produced prenatally despite high levels because high levels of estrogen have a local inhibitory effect on mammary gland
Melanocyte-stimulating hormone: produced by anterior pituitary	Causes darkening of integument and nevi: chloasma; linea nigra; darkening of nipples, areolae, and vulva	Pigmentation changes are objective, presumptive signs of pregnancy; usually fade after delivery
Beta-endorphins and encephalins: produced by middle lobe of pituitary	Display analgesic properties	Discomfort is lessened or made more tolerable
Oxytocin: produced by *posterior* pituitary	Causes uterus to contract Action suppressed by action of progesterone until production of oxytocin exceeds that of progesterone Stimulates myoepithelial cells in mammary glands to eject milk	May be used to induce or augment labor Spurt of oxytocin during expulsive phase of labor to ensure efficient muscle contraction during and immediately after birth Sensory receptors in nipple stimulate release of oxytocin via reflex arc. During lactation oxytocin stimulates myoepithelial cells in the mammary gland to eject milk
Thyroid Gland		
Thyroxine: produced by thyroid gland with stimulation from anterior pituitary	Gland enlargement with 20% increase in function: BMR increased to 25% near term; BMR returns to nonpregnant level within 1 week after delivery; return to normal size, within 6 weeks	Woman may experience palpitations, tachycardia, emotional lability, heat intolerance, fatigability, and increased perspiration

Table 2-3   *Signs and Symptoms of Pregnancy in Order of Appearance**

Presumptive	Probable	Positive
Subjective Symptoms		
Amenorrhea (4 weeks)† Nausea, vomiting (4 weeks) Breast sensitivity (6 weeks) Urinary symptoms (6 weeks) Lassitude/fatigue Constipation Weight gain Fingernail changes Quickening (16-20 weeks) Mood swings	Same as presumptive symptoms; when combined with probable signs, strong suspicion of pregnancy	No symptoms positively diagnostic of pregnancy
Objective Signs		

Elevation of BBT
 Integumentary changes
   Pigmentation
   Striae gravidarum
   Telangiectases (spider nevi)
   Acne, hirsutism
   Epulis
 Breast changes (8 weeks)
   Enlargement
   Secondary areolae
   Montgomery's tubercles
   Precolostrum (16 weeks)
 Abdominal enlargement
 Pelvic changes
   Vagina (Chadwick's sign; leukorrhea) (8 weeks)
   Cervix (softening; Goodell's sign; dried mucus in granular pattern) (6-8 weeks)
   Uterine softening (Hegar's sign) (6 weeks)
   Relaxation of bony pelvic joints and ligaments
   Vulval varicosities (10 weeks)
	Uterine enlargement:
	   Size of large hen's egg (7 weeks)
	   Size of an orange (10 weeks)
	   Size of a grapefruit; uterus becomes an abdominal organ (12 weeks)
	 Uterine contractions (Braxton Hicks' sign) (20 weeks)
	 External ballottement (24 weeks)
	 Internal ballottement (14 weeks)
	 Uterine souffle
	 Laboratory tests (except radioimmunoassay of beta subunit of hCG‡; this endocrine test provides definitive results)
		FHT‡
		   Echocardiography (5 weeks)
		   Real-time ultrasound imaging (heart motion can be visualized at 7 weeks)
		   Electronic device (8-12 weeks)
		   Electrocardiogram (12 weeks)
		   Auscultation of fetal heart (17-18 weeks)
		 Palpation of fetal movement (about 20 weeks)
		 Ultrasonographic (echographic) evidence of gestational sac confirms presence of intrauterine gestation (6 weeks); fetal breathing movements can be visualized by 11 weeks; detection of FHT (8-12 weeks); by week 14 the fetal head and thorax can be visualized, and subsequently the placenta can be localized
		 Laboratory tests
		   Immunologic (6 weeks)
		   Radioimmunoassay (can diagnose pregnancy as early as 23 days after first day of last menstrual period, about 5 days before next menstrual period would have been due)
		   Home pregnancy test (9 days after end of missed period)
		   Clinical test
		   Progesterone withdrawal

*Clinical diagnosis of pregnancy depends on the ability to interpret presumptive, probable, and positive physical signs and symptoms.
†Time of appearance of symptoms is provided when predictable.
‡FHT, Fetal heart tones; hCG, human chorionic gonadotropin.

Table 2-4   *Differential Assessment of Signs and Symptoms of Pregnancy*

Symptoms	Possible Causes of Diagnostic Error
Abdominal enlargement	Obesity, abdominal muscle relaxation, tumors, ascites, ventral abdominal hernia
Amenorrhea	Emotional factors: severe emotional shock, tension, fear of or strong desire for pregnancy Endocrine factors: adrenal or ovarian neoplasms, thyroid or pituitary disorders, lactation, menopause Metabolic factors: anemia, malnutrition, diabetes mellitus, degenerative disorders Systemic disease: acute or chronic infection (tuberculosis, brucellosis) or malignancy Local causes (cervical obstruction; jogging)
Braxton Hicks' contractions	Contractions of muscles of abdominal wall

Table 2-4, cont'd.   *Differential Assessment of Signs and Symptoms of Pregnancy*

Symptoms	Possible Causes of Diagnostic Error
Breast sensitivity (mastalgia; mastodynia)	Infectious processes: mastitis, cystic mastitis, premenstrual tension
	Pseudocyesis (false pregnancy)
	Estrogen excess associated with anovulatory periods or ovarian tumors
Cervical and uterine changes in shape, size, consistency	Tumors, adenomyosis, cervical stenosis with hematometra or pyometra, tubo-ovarian cysts
	Normal-size uterus displaced by a pelvic tumor (fibroid or myoma)
Clinical and laboratory findings	Poor thermometer, faulty use of thermometer, inaccurate recording
Elevation of BBT	Corpus luteum cyst
Pregnancy tests	Drug ingestion: progesterone
	False results, incorrect interpretation of results
	Elevation of hCG levels for a few days after spontaneous abortion
	Elevation of hCG: hydatidiform mole, choriocarcinoma
Lassitude and fatigue	Psychologic: emotional disorders
	Pathologic: anemia, infection, malignant disease
Epulis	Infection, dental calculus, vitamin C deficiency
Hyperpigmentation of skin	Local causes (excessive sunlight, tanning)
	System diseases (Addison's disease)
	Use of oral contraceptives
Leukorrhea	Infections: vaginal, cervical
	Tumors
Nausea or vomiting	Emotional factors: anxiety, pseudocyesis, anorexia nervosa
	Gastrointestinal disorders: hiatal hernia, ulcers, enteritis, appendicitis
	Systemic disease: acute infection—influenza, encephalitis
	Allergies
Nipple discharge (milklike)	Drug ingestion: oral contraceptives, psychotropic drugs
	Tumors
	Syndromes (also associated with amenorrhea): hypothalamic or anterior pituitary disorders
Pseudocyesis	Emotional factors
	Pituitary tumor
Quickening	Peristalsis; "gas"
Souffle	Heard over vascular tumors or aneurysms or in thin women; may be abdominal aortic pulsation

Estimated Date of Delivery

Following the diagnosis of pregnancy the woman's first question usually concerns when she will deliver. This date has traditionally been termed the *estimated date of confinement* (EDC). To promote a more positive perception of both pregnancy and delivery, however, the term *estimated date of delivery* (EDD) is usually used. Nägele's rule is as follows: add 7 days to the first day of the LMP, subtract 3 months, and add 1 year. The formula becomes EDD + ([LMP + 7 days] − 3 months) + 1 year. For example, if the first day of the LMP was July 10, 1989, the EDD is April 17, 1990. In simple terms, add 7 days to the LMP and count forward 9 months.

Nägele's rule assumes that the woman has a 28-day cycle and that the pregnancy occurred on the fourteenth day. An adjustment is in order if the cycle is longer or shorter than 28 days. With the use of Nägele's rule, only about 4% to 10% of gravidas will deliver spontaneously on the EDD. Most women will deliver during the period extending from 7 days before to 7 days after the EDD.

FETAL DEVELOPMENT AT 13 WEEKS

1. Differentiation of tissues complete as period of organogenesis ends
2. Human appearance
3. Sex distinguishable
4. Skeleton ossifying
5. Tooth buds forming
6. Respiratory activity evident
7. Insulin secreted (since eighth week)
8. Kidneys secreting
9. Intestine returns to abdomen
10. Head is one-third of total length
11. Length: 9 cm (3½ in)
12. Weight: 15 g (½ oz)
13. Fetus less susceptible to malformation from teratogenic agents

Routine Prenatal Screening

After the pregnancy has been confirmed, the physician orders routine screening tests to set up a data base and identify high-risk pregnancies at the outset. Table 2-5 discusses the description, purpose, and normal values of these tests.

Table 2-5 *Routine Prenatal Screening Tests*

Description and Purpose	Normal Values
Complete Blood Count (CBC) Performed to detect anemia A series of tests done on whole blood to determine various cell counts Performed routinely for baseline information and serially for comparison Contains white cell count and differential, homoglobin, hemtocrit, and red cell indices Repeated in last trimester	RBCs 4.0-5.3 million/mm^3 MCH 27-33 pg (picograms) MCHC 32-36% (g/100 mL) MCV 86-98 mcg^3 WBCs 4300-10,800 mm^3 Basophils (0.4%-1.0% (40-100/cu^3) Eosinophils 1%-3% (50-300/cu^3) Lymphocytes 25%-40% (100-4500/ mm^3) Monocytes 2%-8% (100-800/mm^3) Neutrophils 54%-75% (3000-7500/ mm^3) Hemoglobin 12-16g/100 mL Hematocrit 37%-48% (37-48/100 mL) Platelets 150,000-350,000/mm^3
RH Typing/RH Antibody Titer To identify fetuses at risk for developing erythroblastosis fetalis or hyperbilirubinemia in neonatal period Performed on whole bood of pregnant woman to determine need for Rh immunoglobulins if she is Rh negative and her partner is Rh positive Rh antibody titer also done to determine antibody level produced by Rh positive fetus, which may warrant exchange transfusion of infant at birth	Rh positive (+) Rh negative (−) Negative (0): no antibodies present Titer >1:64 indicates possible exchange transfusion
Blood Type/Cross-Matching To identify fetuses at risk for developing erythroblastosis fetalis or ABO incompatibility problems Performed on whole blood to determine blood type before giving a transfusion Performed on pregnant woman for baseline data	Typing: O, A, B, AB Cross-matching: no agglutination, hemolysis
Rubella Antibody Titer To determine immunity to rubella Performed on blood serum to determine antibody production against rubella virus and susceptibility to rubella (German measles) Virus is teratogenic to fetus when contracted by pregnant woman	1:8 titer or less: rubella susceptibility 1:8-1:32 titer: rubella exposure or vaccination immunity 1:32-1:64 titer: immunity to rubella
Sickle Cell Screen To identify women carrying the trait who thereby put the fetus at risk for sickle cell anemia To identify women with sickle cell anemia Performed on whole blood to determine presence of hemoglobin S (HgS), a particular type of hemoglobin characteristic in RBCs that have the sickle cell trait Performed routinely on black pregnant woman; if trait is present, partner is also tested Trait is recessive hereditary blood abnormality; when both parents have trait, infant may be born with sickle cell anemia	Negative: no sickling of RBCs HgS: 0%

Table 2-5, cont'd.   *Routine Prenatal Screening Tests*

Description and Purpose	Normal Values

Hepatitis Virus Screen
  To identify women with active disease or in carrier state
  Performed on blood serum to determine presence of hepatitis A or B antigens and/or hepatitis A or   Negative
    B antibodies
  May test for surface antigen/antibody or core antigen/antibody

Fasting Blood Glucose (FBG) Test
  To identify women with hypoglycemia or hyperglyecemia (diabetes mellitus or gestational diabetes)
  Performed on serum, plasma, or whole blood to determine levels of glucose   70-110 mg/100 mL (serum or
  1- or 3-hour test may be ordered in second trimester   plasma)
                                                          Chemstrip test: negative

Human T-Cell Lymphocyte Virus No. 3 (HTLV-3, HIV test)
  To identify HIV-positive women
  To screen high-risk populations
  Performed on high-risk populations only   Negative
  Performed on blood that identifies antibodies produced by the HTLV-3 virus
  Shows exposure to, not presence of, AIDS
  Permission must be obtained to perform this test; counseling must be provided if results are positive

VDRL, RPR
  To identify women with untreated syphilis
  Performed on serum to determine presence of *Treponema pallidum,* which causes syphilis   Negative, non-reactive

Tuberculin Skin Test (Tine Test)
  To screen high-risk populations
  Performed by pressing a four-pronged disk impregnated with PPD-t into the superficial layers of the   Negative: no raised area of skin or
    skin on the volar or dorsal aspect of the arm   a zone <5 mm in diameter
  Results evaluated in 48-72 hours

Blood Urea Nitrogen (BUN) Test
  To evaluate renal function
  Performed on blood serum to determine concentration of urea excreted by kidneys   8-20 mg/100 mL

Creatinine Test
  To evaluate renal function
  Performed on blood serum to determine level of creatinine excreted by glomeruli of kidneys   0.6-1.5 mg/100 mL

Electrolyte Test
  To evaluate level of possible renal compromise in women with history of diabetes, hypertension, or
    renal disease
  Performed on blood serum, plasma, or 24-hour urine to determine levels of charged particles (cat-   *Serum:*
    ions and anions) that influence acid-base balance of body CO_2: 24-30 mEq/L
                                                                Chloride: 100-106 mEq/L
                                                                Calcium: 4.3-5.5 mEq/L
                                                                Magnesium: 1.5-2.0 mEq/L or
                                                                  1.8-3.0 mg/100 mL
                                                                Potassium: 3.5-5.0 mEq/L
                                                                Phosphorus: 1.8-2.6 mEq/L or
                                                                  3.0-4.5 mg/100 mL
                                                                Sodium: 135-145 mEq/L
                                                              Urine:
                                                                Chloride: 110-254 mEq/L
                                                                Calcium: 300 mg/24 hr or less/
                                                                  diet
                                                                Magnesium: 6.0-9.0 mEq/24 hr
                                                                Potassium: 25-100 mEq/24 hr

Continued.

Table 2-5, cont'd.   *Routine Prenatal Screening Tests*

Description and Purpose	Normal Values
Electrolyte Test—cont'd.	Phosphorus: 0.2-0.6 mEq/L or mg/day/intake Sodium: 50-220 mEq/24 hr
Creatinine Clearance Test To evaluate renal function Performed on urine to determine levels of creatinine excreted by kidneys	104-125 mL/min
Urinalysis To identify women with unsuspected diabetes mellitus, renal disease, hypertensive disease of pregnancy, or infection Performed on random urine specimen to determine gross and microscopic characteristics of urine Repeated periodically	Color: straw/yellow Odor: aromatic Turbidity: clear pH: 4.6-8.0 Specific gravity: 1.010-1.025 Protein: negative Glucose: negative Ketones: negative Blood: negative Bile/bilirubin: negative RBC: 0-1 or rare WBC: 0-4 or rare Bacteria: negative Casts: rare hyaline Crystals: few Epithelial cells: few
Urine Culture To identify women with asymptomatic bacteremia Performed on clean-catch voided urine or catheter specimens to detect presence of infection within urinary system Repeated periodically	No growth, or 10,000 organisms/mL or less
Gentourinary Culture To screen high-risk populations for asymptomatic infection Microscopic examination of secretions obtained from cervix, urethra, vagina, vulva, or anus to determine presence of pathogenic organisms that have been transmitted sexually Pathogenic organisms identified in these cultures include: *Chlamydia vaginalis, Escherichia coli, Neisseria gonorrhoeae, Candida albicans,* herpes, *Trichomonas* spp. Repeated in third trimester	Negative for pathogenic organisms Presence of normal organisms
Papanicolaou Smear (Pap Smear) To screen for cervical intraepithelial neoplasia and herpes symplex type 2 Cells are obtained from cervix and vaginal pool for cytologic examination	Negative: no atypical cells
Electrocardiogram (EKG, or ECG) To evaluate cardiac function in women with history of hypertension or cardiac disease Noninvasive procedure in which electrical impulses of resting heart are recorded	Normal tracing of complexes and intervals: P-wave, QRS complex, T-wave Pulse 60-100, regular in rhythm and volume Normal sinus rhythm

DANGER SIGNS

Complications of Pregnancy

1. Visual disturbances—blurring, double vision, or spots
2. Swelling of face, fingers or over sacrum
3. Headaches—severe, frequent, or continuous
4. Muscular irritability or convulsions
5. Epigastric pain (perceived as severe stomach ache)
6. Persistent vomiting—beyond first trimester, severe vomiting at any time
7. Fluid discharge from vagina—bleeding or amniotic fluid (anything other than leukorrhea)
8. Signs of infections—chills, fever, burning on urination, diarrhea
9. Pain in abdomen—severe or unusual
10. Change in fetal movements—absence of fetal movements after quickening, any unusual change in pattern or amount

Physiologic Changes in Pregnancy

A woman's body goes through many changes during pregnancy. All systems change in some way to accomodate the growing fetus and prepare for delivery and lactation. A summary of these changes follows.

Reproductive System

I. Uterus
   A. Weight increased about 20 fold
   B. Capacity increased 1000 fold
   C. Hormonal stimulus: initially from corpus luteum, then by placenta
      1. Estrogen: myometrial growth
      2. Progesterone: early—prepares endometrium for implantation; later—inhibits contractile activity of myometrium
   D. Walls thicker in beginning of pregnancy (after fifth lunar month, muscles stretch and distend, thinning walls)
   E. Braxton Hicks contractions occurring despite progesterone (increases movement of blood through intervillous spaces)
   F. Position changes (lifts out of pelvis and dextrorotates)
   G. Displaces intestine laterally and superiorly
      1. When woman is supine, uterus lies on *vena cava and aorta, causing supine hypotensive syndrome*
      2. Best position for late pregnancy is *left lateral*
II. Cervix: mucosa undergoes changes
   A. Glandular tissue and secretions increase (estrogen-induced)
   B. Endocervical glands secrete thick tenacious mucus; mucous plug forms, seals canal, and is excreted when labor starts (known as bloody show)

C. Increased vascularization causes softening and discoloration (see Table 2-3)

III. Ovaries: cease ovum production; corpus luteum continues to produce progesterone until placenta is established

IV. Vagina: estrogen increases vaginal secretions
   A. Secretion is thick, white, acidic
      1. Fights pathogens
      2. Encourages yeast growth
   B. Smooth muscle hypertrophies; connective tissue relaxes enough to let infant pass at birth
V. Breasts: under influence of both estrogen and progesterone, the following occurs
   A. Breast size increases
   B. Breasts become more nodular
   C. Superficial vessels become prominent
   D. Nipple is erectile and areola is pigmented; hypertrophy of Montgomery's tubercules occurs
   E. Colostrum (first milk) may start at end of third trimester

Respiratory System

   A. Increased tidal volume, oxygen consumption, and vital capacity
   B. Diaphragm elevated, substernal angle increased
   C. Flared rib cage
   D. Changes in breathing from abdominal to thoracic
   E. Possible nasal stuffiness and epistaxis due to estrogen influence

Cardiovascular System

   A. Increased blood volume
   B. More plasma than RBCs (physiologic dilutional anemia)
   C. Decreased normal hemoglobin and hematocrit levels
   D. Increased WBCs
   E. Increased tendency for blood to clot
   F. Heart displaced upward and to right
   G. Increased cardiac output and heart rate
   H. Stagnation of blood in lower extremities—dependent edema, varicose veins, postural hypotension
   I. Blood pressure remaining unaltered: lowest during second trimester, highest during last week
   J. Decreased cerebrospinal fluid space; spinal anesthesia may go to a higher level and with a greater drop in blood pressure

Gastrointestinal System

   A. Nausea and vomiting
   B. Peculiarities of taste and smell
   C. Gum disease
   D. Ptyalism
   E. Decreased gastric acidity
   F. Relaxation of cardiac sphincter of stomach, causing reflux or heartburn
   G. Constipation due to increased levels of proges-

terone, delayed emptying time, and decreased intestinal motility

  H. Hemorrhoids

  I. Possible liver and gall bladder changes

Urinary Tract

  A. Urinary frequency during first and third trimester caused by pressure on bladder from uterus

  B. Greater susceptibility of bladder to infection

  C. Decreased capacity of bladder

  D. Dilation of ureter and kidney, especially on right side

  E. Increased glomerular filtration rate, renal plasma flow urea, and creatinine clearance

  F. Increased renal plasma flow

  G. Glycosuria

Skin

  A. Pigmentation of nipple and areola

  B. Linea nigra and striae gravidarum

  C. Chloasma or mask of pregnancy

  D. Acne

  E. Spider nevi on chest, neck, face, arms, and legs

Skeleton

  A. Absence of bone demineralization

  B. Possible dental caries due to change in saliva pH

  C. Relaxed pelvic joints due to hormone relaxin (gives woman waddling gait)

  D. Postural change: increased lumbosacral curve

  E. Possible shoulder slump

Metabolic System

  A. Most metabolic functions increase

Endocrine System

  A. Possible increase in size and activity of thyroid
    1. BMR increases
    2. Hypothyroid may cause spontaneous abortion

  B. Parathyroid hormone that parallels fetal calcium needs

  C. Anterior pituitary prolongs corpus luteum

Table 2-6   *Discomforts During the First Trimester*

Discomfort	Physiology	Treatment
Breast changes, new sensations: pain, tingling	Hypertrophy of mammary glandular tissue and increased vascularization, pigmentation, and size and prominence of nipples and areolae caused by hormone stimulation	Supportive maternity brassiere with pads to absorb discharge may be worn at night; wash with warm water and keep dry
Urgency and frequency of urination	Vascular engorgement and altered bladder function caused by hormones; bladder capacity reduced by enlarging uterus and fetal presenting part	Kegel's exercises; limit fluid intake before bedtime; reassurance; wear perineal pad; refer to physician for pain or burning sensation
Languor and malaise; fatigue (early pregnancy, usually)	Unexplained, may be due to increasing levels of estrogen, progesterone, and hCG or to elevated BBT; psychologic response to pregnancy and its required physical/psychologic adaptations	Reassurance; rest as needed; well–balanced diet to prevent anemia
Nausea and vomiting, "morning sickness"—occurs in 50% to 75% of pregnant women; starts between first and second missed periods and lasts until about fourth missed period; may occur any time during day; if mother does not have symptoms, expectant father may; may be accompanied by "bad taste" in mouth	Cause unknown (may result from hormonal changes, possibly hCG; may be partly emotional, reflecting pride in, ambivalence about, or rejection of pregnant state)	Avoid empty or overloaded stomach; maintain good posture—give stomach ample room; stop or decrease smoking; eat dry carbohydrate on awakening; remain in bed until feeling subsides, or alternate dry carbohydrate 1 hour with fluids such as hot tea, milk, or clear coffee the next hour until feeling subsides; eat 5 to 6 small meals per day; avoid fried, odorous, spicy, greasy, or gas-forming foods; consult physician if intractable vomiting occurs; reassurance
Ptyalism (excessive saliva)—may occur starting 2 to 3 weeks after first missed period	Elevated estrogen levels (?); may be related to reluctance to swallow because of nausea	Astringent mouth wash; chewing gum; support
Psychosocial dynamics: mood swings, mixed feelings	Hormonal and metabolic adaptations; plus feelings about female role, sexuality, timing of pregnancy, and resultant changes in one's life and life-style	Treatment same as prevention; both partners need reassurance and support; support significant other who can reassure woman about her attractiveness, etc.; improved communication with her partner, family, and others; refer to social worker, if needed, or supportive services (financial assistance, food stamps)

1. Thyrotropin and adenotropin alter metabolism to support pregnancy
2. Prolactin is responsible for initial lactation

D. Posterior pituitary secretes oxytocin, promotes uterine contractility, and stimulates milk ejection
    1. Vasopressin increases blood pressure through vasoconstriction

General Considerations

Pregnancy is a normal condition, not a disease process, and health care professionals should assist the woman in achieving optimal health during this time for the sake of both the woman and her fetus. Although virtually all women experience some discomfort during pregnancy, the nurse who is knowledgeable about these problems can provide support and assistance in understanding and dealing with them. Good nutrition during pregnancy is one of the hallmarks of prenatal care. Research has shown that malnutrition, obesity, anemia, and other vitamin-nutrient deficiencies can cause birth defects and developmental problems in the fetus and newborn. Nurses must teach and counsel women about nutrition throughout their pregnancy. The nurse must also know about medications and immunizations during pregnancy.

The nurse can be very instrumental in assisting the pregnant woman to maintain as normal a lifestyle as possible.

This includes teaching the woman about moderate cise, sexual closeness with her partner, and self-care activities. The nurse should also educate the woman about potentially harmful activities, such as drug use.

Weight Gain During Pregnancy. Optimum weight gain of the mother during pregnancy makes an important contribution to the pregnancy's successful course and outcome. The acceptable weight gain for most healthy women of normal weight for height carrying a single fetus is 12 kg (27 lb) (Naeye, 1979; Dohrmann and Lederman, 1986) with a range of 10 to 14.5 kg (22 to 32 lb). It is recommended that a woman increase her caloric intake 300 calories a day while pregnant and 200 calories a day while lactating.

Products	Weight
Fetus	3400 g (7.5 lb)
Placenta	450 g (1 lb)
Amniotic fluid	900 g (2 lb)
Uterus (weight increase)	1100 g (2.5 lb)
Breast tissue (weight increase)	1400 g (3 lb)
Blood volume (weight increase)	1800 g (4 lb) (1500 ml)
Maternal stores	1800 to 3600 g (4 to 8 lb)
TOTAL	11,000 to 13,000 g (11 to 13 kg; 24 to 28 lb)

Guidelines for Client Teaching

IRON SUPPLEMENTATION

ASSESSMENT

1. Gravida is in her second trimester. She mentions that she has been ingesting dry laundry starch because "all pregnant women crave it."
2. Woman is chewing ice from a paper cup while waiting to be seen by the physician.
3. Laboratory values: hemoglobin 10.2 g/dl; hematocrit, 34%.

NURSING DIAGNOSES

Altered nutrition: less than body requirements related to pica and the ingestion of nonnutritive substances.

Knowledge deficit related to pica and its possible significance.

Knowledge deficit related to proper nutrition, iron deficiency, and its effect on woman and her fetus.

GOALS

Short-term

Gravida starts taking iron supplement, as prescribed, immediately.

Gravida's laboratory data for hemoglobin and hematocrit indicate beginning improvement with the next test.

Gravida stops ingesting dry laundry starch.

Intermediate

Gravida continues to take iron supplements as long as prescribed.

Gravida understands anemia and its potential effects on her and her baby.

Gravida eats foods that are nutritionally sound.

Long-term

Woman and her baby do not suffer any adverse effects of anemia.

REFERENCES AND TEACHING AIDS

Printed instructions for using iron supplements.

Hospital-supplied pamphlets on nutrition, including information on food groups and supplements.

Laboratory slips showing woman's blood values.

Continued.

Guidelines for Client Teaching—cont'd.

CONTENT/RATIONALE	TEACHING ACTIONS
To provide information about pica, share the following: Pica is a learned behavior. Cravings are not uncommon; if diet is well-balanced, occasional indulgence is probably not harmful. Many cultures have specific beliefs about cravings and "making the baby" or ease of delivery. Nonnutritive foods may provide unwanted calories, interfere with the absorption of iron, and contribute to iron-deficiency anemia.	Few women are willing to volunteer information on pica, so sensitive questioning is necessary to uncover the practice. Discuss the reasons for woman's cravings. Provide information on this practice without demeaning the woman's underlying cultural beliefs. Encourage discussion and questions.
To facilitate understanding of woman's condition: Discuss woman's laboratory report. Define hemoglobin, hematocrit, red blood cells, anemia; explain values and normal parameters.	Review, assess woman's level of understanding. Discuss clinical significance of the differences.
To increase woman's knowledge of nutrition: Discuss building blood through diet. Explain types and amounts of bloodforming nutrients. Explain that food sources of nutrients, such as liver and other red meats, dried beans, dried fruit, deep green vegetables, eggs, and enriched cereals, provide sources of iron.	Review; help woman identify food sources of nutrients in her current diet; praise her. Assist with menu selection to meet woman's preferences and her cultural prescriptions and proscriptions. Involve family members in planning dietary intake if possible.
To increase woman's knowledge of medical therapy for iron-deficiency anemia: Discuss building blood through iron supplementation (30 to 60 mg of elemental iron [150 to 300 mg of ferrous sulfate]). Explain that iron is absorbed most readily in the ferrous form in the presence of acid, before meals, but iron tablets on an empty stomach are highly irritating. Explain that enteric forms of iron supplementation are less effective because of poor absorption beyond the duodenum. Identify foods that decrease iron absorption: milk, cereal, and eggs.	Review this information Discuss and plan proper administration: Divide daily dose into 3 equal doses. Take tablets with a citrus fruit juice, which is a good source of vitamin C, or with vitamin C, 500 mg, orally, once daily. Take tablets after eating food that does not include cereal, eggs, or milk. Time medication to fit woman's (family's) mealtime and her convenience. After the first trimester and nausea has subsided, woman may be able to take the tablet with orange juice between meals.
To foster woman's compliance: Discuss side effects of iron supplementation: stools become dark-green to black in appearance; they may become more formed, contributing to constipation, or become loose; and gastric irritation and bad taste may occur. Monitor woman's progress—within 1 week there is an increase in the number of reticulocytes (immature red blood cells) and in the rate of hemoglobin synthesis.	Review side effects sensitively. Review woman's laboratory findings that confirm her improvement and provide her with tangible proof of her success; give appropriate praise.
To protect older children: Review need to secure medications from other children.	Review safety precautions against accidental ingestion of chemicals.

EVALUATION The nurse can be assured that teaching was effective when her laboratory report shows improvement in anemia (e.g., increase in reticulocyte count, mean corpuscular hemoglobin, hemoglobin, and hematocrit). The woman will indicate she has dark stools, can and does choose appropriate foods, and reduces or eliminates pica. The woman verbalizes her understanding of pica and anemia, and their potential effects on her and her fetus.

MEDICATIONS FOR NORMAL PREGNANCY

Ferrous Salts (Over the Counter)

Brand names: Ferrous fumerate, Ferrous gluconate, Ferrous sulfate

Dosage forms: po (tablet or liquid)

Side effects: GI discomforts, nausea, dark stools, constipation, stained teeth (liquid)

Drug interactions: avoid use with antacids and tetracyclines

Patient education: may cause dark stools; should be taken with citrus juice (increases absorption); should not be taken with dairy products

Prenatal Vitamins (Prescription)

Brand names: Stuart Prenatal, Materna, Natabec, Pramilet

Dosage forms: po (tablets)

Side effects: GI discomfort, nausea

Patient education: should not be taken on empty stomach, especially in beginning of pregnancy, when nausea is a problem

Table 2-7 *Immunizations During Pregnancy*

Immunization	Comments
Cholera	Only meet international travel requirements
Hepatitis A	After exposure; newborns of mothers who are incubating or ill should receive 1 dose after birth
Hepatitis B	Hepatitis B hyperimmune globulin to infant soon after delivery, followed by vaccination
Influenza	Evaluate pregnant woman for immunization according to criteria applied to others
Measles	Live virus vaccine contraindicated on theoretic grounds during pregnancy; pooled immune globulins for postexposure prophylaxis
Mumps	Contraindicated on theoretic grounds during pregnancy
Plague	Should be used only if substantial risk of infection
Poliomyelitis	Not recommended routinely for adults but mandatory in epidemics or when traveling to endemic area
Rabies	Same as nonpregnant
Rubella	Contraindicated, although teratogenicity of vaccine appears to be negligible
Tetanus-diphtheria	Give toxoid if no primary series or no booster in 10 years; for postexposure prophylaxis with unvaccinated tetanus immune globulin and toxoid
Typhoid	Recommended if traveling in endemic region
Varicella	Varicella-zoster immune globulin may be given; indicated for newborns whose mothers developed varicella within 4 days before or 2 days after delivery Immunize before travel to high-risk area but postpone travel if possible

Guidelines For Client Teaching

EXERCISE

ASSESSMENT

1. Gravida requests information about relaxation, rest, relief of discomforts (e.g., backache, heartburn, insomnia), and exercises.

NURSING DIAGNOSES

Potential alteration in comfort related to emotional or physical tension.

Knowledge deficit related to exercise in pregnancy.

GOALS

Short-term

Woman increases self-care skills by learning at least two exercises.

Woman relieves a current discomfort.

Woman learns limits of safe exercise for self.

Intermediate

Woman reports positive results from exercises used (e.g., increase in comfort, sense of well-being).

Woman appreciates the role of appropriate exercise in health maintenance.

Long-term

Woman continues to exercise appropriately across the life span as one self-care activity in health maintenance.

REFERENCES AND TEACHING AIDS

Illustrations

Cassettes of "New Age" music (e.g., sounds of waterfalls, birds, ocean waves) or other appropriate music.

Full-length mirror, floor mat or comfortable seats, pillows.

Lay references available at bookstores everywhere.

ACOG Guidelines on Exercise for Pregnant Women

Continued.

Guidelines For Client Teaching—cont'd

CONTENT/RATIONALE	TEACHING ACTION

To identify maternal anatomic and physiologic adaptations since these affect and are affected by exercise:
  Factors to consider:
    Energy level may be low because of poor sleeping and increased energy cost of increase in metabolic rate and weight and emotional adjustment.
    Change in center of gravity, stretching of abdominal muscles, strain on muscles in general, and relaxation of joints.
    Altered coordination, balance, and concentration and occasional faintness.
    Fetal needs for oxygen.
    Prepregnancy established exercise routine and body condition and current state of health.
	Encourage discussion of woman's exercise habits, reasons for and results of exercises she now uses, current discomforts and methods being employed to alleviate them, and exercises she wishes to learn.

To promote sense of well-being:
  Follow the exercise tips for pregnant women found in ACOG guidelines.
  Learn and practice pelvic tilt (rock).
  Use "Flying exercise" for relief of heartburn and dyspnea.
	Encourage woman to listen to her body.
	Assess gravida's ability to assess her pulse.
	Demonstrate.
	Guide gravida through exercise.
	Use illustrations.

EVALUATION The nurse can be reasonably assured that care was effective when goals for care have been met. The woman demonstrates exercises appropriately. Woman states she uses exercises as needed and that doing so relieves her discomfort.

Guidelines For Client Teaching

SEXUAL COUNSELING DURING PREGNANCY

ASSESSMENT
1. Woman experiencing adaptations to pregnancy (fatigue, nausea).
2. Woman indicates breasts hurt when touched.
3. Woman and husband request information.
4. This is woman's first pregnancy, with no history of vaginal bleeding or uterine cramping.

NURSING DIAGNOSES
Knowledge deficit, alternative positions.
Sexuality, altered patterns.
Potential for anxiety if reactions are perceived as abnormal.
Potential for ineffective individual coping.

GOALS
Short-term
To validate and ensure the universality of their responses.
To meet information needs.
To problem-solve regarding solutions and needed changes.

Intermediate
To continue to make adjustments regarding sexuality throughout pregnancy.
To verbalize mutual satisfaction with their choices.

Long-term
To continue to make mutually acceptable adjustments regarding sexuality across the life span.

REFERENCES AND TEACHING AIDS
Bing E and Colman L: Making love during pregnancy, New York, 1982, FA Davis Co.
Rakowitz E and Rubin GS: Lovemaking in pregnancy. Lamaze Parents' Magazine, 1985 edition, ASPO Lamaze, 55 Northern Blvd, Greenvale, LI, NY, 11548-1390.
Plastic learning models, illustrations.

Guidelines For Client Teaching—cont'd

CONTENT/RATIONALE	TEACHING ACTION
To broaden knowledge base regarding sexuality and sexual expression during pregnancy: Discuss maternal physiologic adaptations to pregnancy: breasts, nausea, fatigue, abdominal changes, perineal enlargement, leukorrhea, pelvic vasocongestion, and orgasmic responses. Discuss maternal and paternal responses to pregnancy. Identify clients' cultural prescriptions and proscriptions. Discuss responses to interview questions. Inform couple that, although her libido may be depressed during first trimester, it increases during the second and third trimesters. In subsequent visits and postpartum, discuss: 1. Breast-feeding; father's responses, mother's fantasies and sexual feelings during breast-feeding, milk spurt during orgasm. 2. Resumption of sexual relationship after delivery.	Provide a safe, open, nonjudgmental atmosphere. Remain alert to personal beliefs and values to avoid decreasing one's effectiveness in providing sexual counseling. Validate feelings, give permission. Ask about things they have heard, read; what they want to discuss. Time the discussions to clients' phase in childbearing cycle and readiness to learn.
To encourage problem-solving and experimentation in mutual sexual gratification: Discuss: 1. Alternative behaviors (e.g., mutual masturbation, foot massage, cuddling). 2. Alternative positions (e.g., female-superior, side-lying).	Provide comfortable environment, offer alternatives, show illustrations.

To prevent potential intrauterine infection and reduce anxiety of injury to fetus:
1. Inform that intercourse is safe as long as it is not uncomfortable for the woman and the membranes have not ruptured.
2. Review signs of ruptured membranes.
  a. Nitragine test tape turns blue or blue-green.
  b. A positive ferning on a slide.
  c. Nile blue stain shows some yellow squamous cells, some blue squamous cells, and hair.
3. Caution against use of hot tubbing. Extreme temperatures that increase maternal temperature can compromise fetal well-being.
4. Discuss cultural prescriptions and proscriptions unique to their situation.
	Show illustrations of fetus in utero with closed cervix and intact membranes.

PRECAUTIONS FOR DRUG USE DURING PREGNANCY

ASSESSMENT

1. Woman expresses/demonstrates knowledge deficit regarding hazards of substance abuse, including smoking and ingestion of alcohol during pregnancy.
2. Woman states she sees no harm in over-the-counter (OTC) drugs or vitamins.

NURSING DIAGNOSES

Knowledge deficit related to drug use or abuse during pregnancy, including OTC medications, alcohol, and cigarette smoking.

Potential for fetal injury related to exposure to hazardous chemicals.

Potential for altered fetal growth and development related to exposure to hazardous chemicals.

Potential for altered nutrition related to drug-abuse.

GOALS

Short-term

Gravida will discuss the use of *any* drug with her physician beforehand.

Woman states she is aware that even OTC medications can be harmful to her pregnancy and fetus.

Woman indicates she knows the hazards of alcohol and cigarettes during her pregnancy.

Intermediate

Woman states she understands the reasons for not using any drug that was not prescribed by her physician at this time (even OTC medications).

Woman is educated about teratogenesis.

Woman reduces or stops smoking and alcohol consumption during pregnancy.

Woman adjusts dietary intake to supply appropriate amounts of nutrients.

Long-term

Woman understands consequences of drug, alcohol, and cigarette use.

Woman does not self-medicate.

REFERENCES AND TEACHING AIDS

Printed instructions prepared by nurses, physicians, or others.

Charts and pamphlets showing the development of the fetus at various times.

Pamphlets from the March of Dimes discussing drug, alcohol, and cigarette use and abuse during pregnancy.

CONTENT/RATIONALE	TEACHING ACTION
To provide information about fetal development: Pregnancy is divided into trimesters of 3 months each. During these first months (the period of organogenesis) human development goes from ovum to embryo to fetus. This period of life is characterized by rapid cell division. All principle organ systems are being established at this time and are extremely vulnerable to the effects of chemical teratogens.	Using charts and visual aids show client how the baby is formed at this time. Discuss the rapid cell division and growth that is going on inside of her.
Interference at this time can result in major congenital malformations or abnormalities.	Discuss how environmental agents such as drugs, alcohol and smoking can interrupt normal development of the organs. Allow woman time to ask questions. Use simple, easy-to-understand language. Provide basic information.
To provide information about the use of prescription drugs: Information concerns the subject of self-medication with OTC drugs that are usually seen as harmless. Combinations of drugs may cause problems too.	Inform the woman that her physician is aware of the consequences of drug use at this time, therefore, physician would not prescribe any medication that would harm her baby or her pregnancy. Discuss how OTC drugs either alone or in combination could be troublesome. Caution the woman strongly about taking any drug without first checking with her doctor.
To alert woman to hazards of alcohol and smoking: No safe level of alcohol consumption has yet been established. The period of greatest susceptibility and dose-response relationship are not known.	Discuss the prudence of alcohol consumption at this time. Explain this is still an area of questionable unknowns.
Cigarette smoking or second-hand smoking (exposure to smoke-filled rooms) is associated with fetal growth retardation, decreased placental perfusion, and possible decrease in milk production. Harmful substances from cigarette smoking are transferred in breast milk to baby and inhaled by baby.	Discuss how smoking can effect the woman's fetus and pregnancy. If the woman is a smoker, discuss the options she has on ways to stop. If she is resistant to stop, then try to offer ways in which she can cut down.

EVALUATION The nurse may be reassured that teaching was effective if the woman does not use OTC drugs, alcohol, other drugs of abuse, or smoke during pregnancy. She is able to verbalize understanding that these chemicals are harmful to her and her fetus.

*Sample Nursing Care Plan**

INITIAL PRENATAL VISIT

ASSESSMENT	NURSING DIAGNOSIS (ND)/ PLAN (P)/GOAL (G)	RATIONALE/ IMPLEMENTATION	EVALUATION
Woman suspects pregnancy; needs confirmation of diagnosis. Sexual intercourse without contraception. Missed menstrual period(s).	ND: Knowledge deficit related to diagnosis of pregnancy. P: Meet woman's knowledge needs. G: The woman will become knowledgeable about diagnosis of pregnancy and her status (pregnant or not).	*To confirm the diagnosis the nurse will:* Establish a client data base. Take a nursing history. Do a preliminary health history. Obtain laboratory data as deemed necessary by physician. Provide time to discuss physician's diagnosis and explanations.	Woman verbalizes understanding of diagnostic measures. Woman learns whether she is pregnant.
Woman asks when she will have the baby.	ND: Knowledge deficit related to estimated date of delivery (EDD). P: Meet woman's knowledge needs. G: The woman will become knowledgeable about her EDD.	*To determine the EDD the physician and nurse will:* Calculate EDD based on: Information from the client data base. Information from nursing history. Naegle's rule. Ultrasound. Fundal height measurements.	Woman verbalizes understanding of the EDD and asks relevant questions.
		To inform the woman the nurse will: Explain how the EDD is determined. Reinforce physician's explanation that it is not 100% accurate.	Woman understands that she may give birth just before or after the EDD.
Woman needs a schedule for subsequent prenatal visits.	ND: Knowledge deficit related to schedule of prenatal visits throughout pregnancy. P: Meet woman's knowledge needs. G: The woman will schedule appointments throughout pregnancy G: The woman will keep scheduled appointments. G: The woman understands the importance of regular visits.	*To educate the woman the nurse will:* Inform the woman of the schedule for prenatal visits. Discuss the importance of adhering to the schedule unless otherwise informed.	Woman schedules appointments as per plan. Woman keeps scheduled appointments. Woman understands and verbalizes rationale of appointment schedule.

*Also see Summary of Nursing Actions, Nursing Care During First and Second Trimester of Pregnancy, pp. 41-43 and 53-55.

Continued.

Sample Nursing Care Plan—cont'd

INITIAL PRENATAL VISIT

ASSESSMENT	NURSING DIAGNOSIS (ND)/ PLAN (P)/GOAL (G)	RATIONALE/ IMPLEMENTATION	EVALUATION
Woman asks what she should do differently and how her body will change now that she's pregnant.	ND: Knowledge deficit related to the psychologic and physiologic adaptations to pregnancy. ND: Knowledge deficit related to self-care behavior. P: Meet woman's knowledge needs. G: The woman will be able to identify her body's physiologic and psychologic adaptations to pregnancy. G: The woman will use self-care behaviors to maintain an optimum level of wellness for herself and the fetus.	*To determine the woman's present level of health the nurse will:* Interview woman and gain the information for the prenatal health assessment. *To teach the woman about changes resulting from pregnancy the nurse will:* Explain normal psychologic and physiologic adaptations to pregnancy. *To teach the woman how to care for herself properly the nurse will:* Inform the woman of self-care techniques. Explain the purpose and importance of each technique.	Woman verbalizes understanding of physiologic and psychologic adaptations to pregnancy. Woman asks appropriate questions regarding physiologic and psychologic adaptations to pregnancy. Woman verbalizes that she feels well. Physical assessment confirms that woman and fetus are healthy.
Woman says that making love has become uncomfortable.	ND: Altered sexuality patterns related to discomforts of early pregnancy. P: Meet woman's knowledge needs. G: Woman will understand how physiology of pregnancy affects intercourse.	*To teach about physiological affects of pregnancy on intercourse the nurse will:* Discuss sexuality and sexual behaviors during pregnancy. Discuss those symptoms the woman is experiencing that affect intercourse and foreplay.	The woman will ask appropriate questions and verbalize understanding of information discussed.
Woman indicates she is unaware of signs and symptoms that could signal danger to her and her fetus during pregnancy.	ND: Knowledge deficit of signs and symptoms, potential for danger to mother and fetus. P: Meet woman's knowledge needs. G: The woman will gain knowledge about danger signs during pregnancy.	*To determine possible medical implications the nurse will:* Obtain information about preexisting or concurrent medical conditions. *To teach the woman about possible danger signs the nurse will:* Discuss danger signs with the woman. Inform the woman of signs and symptoms she should consider abnormal. Provide the woman with a printed paper with danger signs of pregnancy and phone number of physician, hospital, and clinic.	The woman verbalizes understanding of problems or danger signs that should be reported.

Summary of Nursing Actions

NURSING CARE RELATED TO MATERNAL AND FETAL NUTRITION

I. Goals
   A. For the mother: to consume adequate amounts of required nutrients each day
   B. For the unborn baby: to have adequate nutrients and a healthy maternal-placental unit
   C. For the family: to increase the family's knowledge of adequate nutrition within their cultural-ethnic context

II. Priorities
   A. Pregnancy reaches term with both mother and newborn in optimum nutritional state
   B. Mother's and family's knowledge needs regarding nutrition are met
   C. Family is able to purchase, store, and prepare needed foods

III. Assessment
   A. Interview
      1. Health history
      2. Psychosocial history: background data and dietary assessment
      3. Review of woman's physical systems
   B. Physical examination
   C. Laboratory tests
      1. See Table 2-5 ("Routine Prenatal Screening Tests")

IV. Potential nursing diagnostic categories
   A. Potential for injury
   B. Altered nutrition: less or more than body requirements
   C. Impaired verbal communication
   D. Family coping: potential for growth
   E. Ineffective individual coping
   F. Altered health maintenance
   G. Noncompliance to sound nutrition
   H. Spiritual distress
   I. Knowledge deficit
   J. Diarrhea
   K. Constipation
   L. Altered oral mucous membrane
   M. Altered growth and development
   N. Fatigue
   O. Potential for infection

V. Plan/implementation
   A. Support person
      1. Greet woman and family by name
      2. Provide privacy as needed
      3. Obtain translator, if necessary
      4. Acknowledge effort woman makes in altering or maintaining diet; use praise when appropriate.
      5. Refer woman (and family) to appropriate community agencies for additional assistance (school, welfare, public health nurse).
   B. Teacher/counselor/advocate
      1. Make woman participate in her own care
      2. Refer woman to physician and registered dietitian for special dietary and pharmaceutic prescriptions for unique circumstances (e.g., diabetes, anemia, hypertension, malnutrition, obesity).

Confer with these people regularly to ensure team approach to care.
      3. After analyzing woman's understanding of nutrition and food preparation, briefly discuss physiologic demands and needs (maternal and fetal) on body stores and daily intake. See Guidelines for Client Teaching, "Iron Supplementation" (pp. 33-34).
      4. Share results with woman, and reinforce laboratory results, weight gain, and blood pressure. Discuss how nutritional status fits in.
      5. Discuss nutrition and related folklore and myths with woman.
         a. Utilize openings gained for identifying myths, explore realities, and clarify or correct misinformation.
         b. If some beliefs are firmly held, discuss alternative food sources for needed nutrients.
      6. Check to see how woman is managing her iron, vitamin, and mineral supplements. Use teaching tool for iron supplementation as necessary.
      7. Discuss discomforts of pregnancy that can be managed by means of foods and fluids (see Table 2-6, "Discomforts During the First Trimester").
   C. Technician
      1. Obtain weight.
      2. Obtain blood pressure.
      3. Test urine specimens for glucose, protein, and acetone (ketones).
      4. Obtain blood specimens to send to laboratory.
      5. Record all data.

VI. Evaluation
   A. By end of second prenatal visit
      1. Gravida is assessed for nutritional status.
      2. Nutrition risk factors are identified.
      3. Nutrition care plans are developed and initiated (e.g., education, vitamin, mineral supplementation).
   B. Throughout pregnancy
      1. Pregnant woman's dietary intake is maintained at appropriate levels for calories and all needed nutrients.
      2. Woman's pattern of weight gain is within normal limits; gravida gains approximately 454g (1 lb) per month during first trimester, and 425g (15 oz) per week during last two trimesters.
      3. Gravida's hemoglobin and hematocrit remain at or above minimal values (sea level):

	HGB	HCT
first trimester	11 g/dl	37%
second trimester	10.5 g/dl	35%
third trimester	10 g/dl	33%

      4. Interuterine fetal growth remains appropriate for gestational age.
      5. Gravida's urine remains negative for glucose and ketones.

Continued.

Summary of Nursing Actions—cont'd

6. Referrals are made to community resources as necessary for acquisition of necessary food.
C. By end of pregnancy
1. Gravida has gained appropriate amount of weight.
2. Woman is knowledgeable regarding nutrition: calories, nutrients, and food preparation.
3. Gravida is knowledgeable regarding effects of drugs, alcohol, and tobacco on nutrition and fetal growth: pica; malnutrition, obesity, underweight; special needs for adolescents (when appropri-

ate); nutrition-related conditions (phenyketonuria [PKU], diabetes if appropriate).
4. Woman has opportunity to explore choices for feeding for newborn (breast, bottle).
D. Pregnancy outcome
1. Pregnancy reaches term.
2. Mother suffers no adverse sequelae.
3. Newborn's weight and condition are within normal limits.
4. Newborn is well developed and suffers no adverse sequelae from poor nutrition of mother, drugs, alcohol, or tobacco.

Summary of Nursing Actions

NURSING CARE DURING INITIAL VISIT

I. Goals
  A. For the mother: to have a physically safe and emotionally satisfying pregnancy
  B. For the unborn child: to have an uncomplicated intrauterine existence
  C. For the family: to have an experience that promotes loving and concerned parenting for the child and enhances the personal growth of all individuals involved
II. Priorities
  A. Establish plan of care related to woman's EDC and family circumstances.
  B. Monitor woman, fetus, and family for normal adaptations to pregnancy.
  C. Initiate remedial therapy for abnormal adaptations to pregnancy.
  D. Promote client recognition of normal and abnormal adaptations to pregnancy.
  E. Promote client and family participation in care.
  F. Provide supportive care to client and family.
III. Assessment
  A. First visit (protocol remains the same no matter when it occurs in pregnancy)
    1. Interview
      a. Health history
        (1) Family history
        (2) Medical history
        (3) Sexual history
        (4) Obstetric history
        (5) Present pregnancy
      b. Psychosocial history
        (1) Identifying data
        (2) Perception
        (3) Support systems
          (a) Family
          (b) Community
        (4) Coping mechanisms
        (5) Parenting potential

      C. Review of woman's physical systems
    2. Physical examination
      a. Vital signs, blood pressure, weight
      b. Head
      c. Neck
      d. Thorax
      e. Abdomen
      f. Extremities
      g. Pelvic examination
    3. Laboratory tests
      a. See box, "Pregnancy Tests," p. 22.
      b. See Table 2-5, "Routine Prenatal Screening Tests"
IV. Potential nursing diagnoses
  A. Potential for injury
  B. Anxiety
  C. Impaired verbal communication
  D. Ineffective family coping: compromised
  E. Ineffective individual coping
  F. Knowledge deficit
  G. Potential alteration in family processes
  H. Self esteem disturbance: situational low self esteem
  I. Personal identity disturbance
  J. Altered role performance
  K. Potential spiritual distress
  L. Powerlessness
  M. Fatigue
  N. Potential impaired adjustment
V. Plan/implementation
  A. Support person
    1. Client
      a. Establish rapport and caring relationship with woman (or couple).
      b. Orient to initial visit.
      c. Encourage woman to express her likes and dislikes.
    2. Maternal emotional health
      a. Listen to description of emotional responses

Summary of Nursing Actions—cont'd

to pregnancy (e.g., words, tone of voice, affect).

    b. Observe body language (e.g., tension, eyes averted).

  3. Client and family

    a. Encourage partner to accompany woman on prenatal visits.

    b. Include partner in discussion of maternal and fetal well-being.

B. Teacher/counselor/advocate

  1. Establish plan of care based on EDC (EDD).

    a. Develop plan of care for continuing assessment of fetal well-being.

    b. Schedule regular office or clinic visits every 4 weeks for 32 weeks, every 2 weeks until week 36, and weekly until term or until labor begins.

    c. Review plan of care with woman and family.

      (1) Schedule when convenient for woman, provide written copy for patient

      (2) Check for woman's understanding of reasons for periodic reevaluation.

      (3) Physical examinations: describe routine physical examinations, including instructions for obtaining clean-catch urine specimens for routine analysis.

  2. Provide written list of danger signals and written directions for obtaining medical care if abnormal symptoms occur.

  3. Instruct woman on general health care:

    a. Personal hygiene

    b. Diet

    c. Rest and exercise

    d. Dental care

    e. Use of medications

    f. Sexual counseling

  4. Instruct woman to avoid supine position. Provide

information concerning physiologic basis, prevention, and treatment of physical symptoms woman may be experiencing (e.g., urgency and frequency of urination, languor and malaise, and nausea and vomiting).

C. Technician

  1. Maternal

    a. Inquire as to general health of client.

    b. Note appearance, grooming, energy level.

    c. Assist with examinations.

  2. Fetal

    a. Check FHR and other systems if appropriate to gestational age.

VI. Evaluation

A. Emotional support

  1. Nurse and client

    a. Client and family respond positively to personnel.

    b. Anxiety appears lessened. Client is able to question nurse regarding learning needs.

    c. Client is able to work with nurse to plan care appropriate to her needs.

  2. Maternal emotional health

    a. Client is able to express feelings openly (i.e., pleasure, dismay, anger, anxiety, fear).

  3. Client and family

    a. Client expresses feelings of support from family and friends.

B. Knowledge and skills

  1. Client able to describe plan of care.

  2. Client verbalizes understanding of danger signals and to whom to report problems.

  3. Client asks questions freely about anticipated problems.

  4. Client verbalizes understanding of physiologic basis, prevention, and treatment of common discomforts.

SECOND TRIMESTER

By the second trimester the pregnancy usually has been positively diagnosed. The woman and her family have had time to adjust to the pregnancy, and the initial visit or two have been completed. For many women, dicomforts common to the first trimester are resolving. The reality of the baby begins to excite her as she feels it kick and she is allowed to hear the heartbeat during subsequent visits to the physician or clinic.

Adaptation to pregnancy is as much physical as emotional. The following pages provide information for the nurse to assist the woman to feel physically and emotionally safe and comfortable during the second trimester. A sample nursing care plan for subsequent prenatal visits and a summary of nursing actions for care during the first and second trimester are also included.

FETAL DEVELOPMENT AT 26 WEEKS

1. Viable at week 24
2. Fetal movements obvious
3. FHR readily heard
4. Scalp hair, eyebrows, eyelashes, fine downy lanugo and vernix cover the skin
5. Eyelids still fused
6. Skin is red, shiny, and thin
7. Face is wrinkled, giving an "old man appearance"
8. Length is 30 cm (12 in)
9. Weight is 600 g (1¼ lb)
10. Uterus at or just above level of umbilicus

Table 2-8   *Problems Related to Maternal Adaptations to Pregnancy*

Discomfort	Physiology	Prevention/Treatment
Pigmentation deepens (striae gravidarum, chloasma, linea nigra, fingernails, hair, nipples and areolae); acne, oily skin	Melanocyte-stimulating hormone (from anterior pituitary)	Not preventable; usually resolved during puerperium; reassurance given to women and their families about these manifestations of pregnant state
Spider nevi (telangiectasias)—appear during trimesters 2 or 3 over neck, thorax, face, and arms (in that order) in two thirds of women	Focal networks of dilated arterioles (end-arteries) from increased concentration of estrogens	Not preventable; reassurance that they fade slowly during late puerperium; rarely disappear completely
Palmar erythema occurs in 50% of pregnant women; may accompany spider nevi	Diffuse reddish mottling over palms and suffused skin over thenar eminences and fingertips may be caused by genetic predisposition or hyperestrogenism	Not preventable; reassurance that condition will fade within 1 wk after giving birth
Pruritus (noninflammatory)	Unknown cause; various types as follows:	Keep fingernails short and clean; refer to physician for diagnosis of cause
	Nonpapular	Not preventable; symptomatic: Keri baths; mild sedation
	Closely aggregated pruritic papules	Not preventable; as for nonpapular type
	Increased excretory function of skin and stretching of skin possible factors	Distraction; tepid (not hot) baths with sodium bicarbonate or oatmeal added to water; lotions and oils; change of soaps or reduction in use of soap; loose clothing
Palpitations	Unknown; should not be accompanied by persistent cardiac irregularity	Not preventable; reassurance; refer to physician if accompanied by symptoms of cardiac decompensation
Supine hypotension (vena cava syndrome) and bradycardia	Posture induced by pressure of gravid uterus on ascending vena cava when woman is supine; reduces uterine-placental and renal perfusion	Side-lying position or semi-sitting posture, with knees slightly flexed
Faintness and, rarely, syncope (orthostatic hypotension): may persist throughout pregnancy	Vasomotor lability or postural hypotension from hormones; in late pregnancy may be caused by venous stasis in lower extremities	Moderate exercise, deep breathing, vigorous leg movement; avoid sudden changes in position and warm crowded areas*; move slowly and deliberately; keep environment cool; avoid hypoglycemia by eating 5 to 6 small meals per day; elastic hose; sit down as necessary; if symptoms are serious, refer to physician
Food cravings	Cause unknown; cravings determined by culture or geographic area	Not preventable; satisfy craving unless it interferes with well-balanced diet; report unusual cravings (e.g., pica: laundry starch, clay, dirt) to physician
Heartburn (pyrosis, or acid indigestion): burning sensation in lower chest or upper abdomen, occasionally with burping and raising of a little sour-tasting fluid; may also occur in first trimester	Progesterone slows GI tract motility and digestion, reverses peristalsis, relaxes cardiac sphincter, and delays emptying time of stomach; stomach displaced upward and compressed by enlarging uterus	Limit or avoid gas-producing or fatty foods and large meals; maintain good posture; keep torso upright; bend down at knees to reach below the waist; sips of milk for temporary relief; hot tea, chewing gum; physician may prescribe antacid between meals (NOTE: *Do not* use baking soda or Alka-Seltzer or patent medicines); flying exercise; refer to physician for persistent symptoms
Constipation	GI tract motility slowed because of progesterone, resulting in increased resorption of water and drying of stool; intestines	Six glasses of water per day; roughage in diet; moderate exercise; maintain regular schedule for bowel move-

*Caution woman to rise slowly and sit on edge of bed or to assume hands-and-knees posture before rising, and to get up slowly after sitting or squatting.

Table 2-8, cont'd. *Problems Related to Maternal Adaptations to Pregnancy*

Discomfort	Physiology	Prevention/Treatment
	compressed by enlarging uterus; predisposition to constipation because of oral iron supplementation	ments; use relaxation techniques and deep breathing; *do not* take stool softener, laxatives, other drugs, or enemas without first consulting physician; *never* ingest mineral oil, since this inhibits absorption of fat-soluble vitamins
Flatulence with bloating and belching	Reduced GI motility because of hormones, allowing time for bacterial action that produces gas; swallowing air	Chew solid foods slowly and thoroughly; avoid gas-producing foods, fatty foods, large meals; exercise; regular bowel habits
Varicose veins (large distended, tortuous, superficial veins); may be associated with aching legs and tenderness; may be present in legs and vulva; hemorrhoids (piles) are varicosities in the perianal area	Hereditary predisposition; relaxation of smooth muscle walls of veins because of hormones, causing pelvic vasocongestion; condition aggravated by enlarging uterus, gravity, and bearing down for bowel movements; thrombi from leg varices rare but may be produced by hemorrhoids	Avoidance of obesity, lengthy standing or sitting, constrictive clothing, and constipation and bearing down with bowel movements; moderate exercises; rest with legs and hips elevated; support stockings applied before rising; thrombosed hemorrhoid may be evacuated; relieve swelling and pain with hot sitz baths, local application of astringent compresses
Leukorrhea: often noted throughout pregnancy	Hormonally stimulated cervix becomes hypertrophic and hyperactive, producing abundant amount of mucus	Not preventable; *do not douche;* hygiene; perineal pads; reassurance; refer to physician if accompanied by pruritis, foul odor, or change in character or color
Headaches (through week 26)	Emotional tension (more common than vascular migraine headache); eye strain (refractory errors); vascular engorgement and congestion of sinuses from hormone stimulation	Emotional support; prenatal teaching; conscious relaxation; refer to physician for constant "splitting" headache, after assessing for pregnancy-induced hypertension (PIH)
Carpal tunnel syndrome (involves thumb, second and third fingers, lateral side of little finger)	Compression of median nerve from changes in surrounding tissues: pain, numbness, tingling, burning; loss of skilled movements (typing); dropping of objects	Not preventable; elevation of affected arms, splinting of affected hand may help; surgery is curative
Periodic numbness, tingling of fingers (acrodysesthesia): occurs in 5% of pregnant women	Brachial plexus traction syndrome from drooping of shoulders during pregnancy (occurs especially at night and early morning)	Maintain good posture; wear good supportive maternity brassiere; reassurance that condition will disappear if lifting and carrying baby does not aggravate it
Round ligament pain (tenderness)	Stretching of ligament caused by enlarging uterus	Not preventable; reassurance, rest, good body mechanics to prevent overstretching ligament; relieve cramping by squatting or bringing knees to chest
Joint pain, backache, and pelvic pressure; hypermobility of joints	Relaxation of symphyseal and sacroiliac joints because of hormones, resulting in unstable pelvis; exaggerated lumbar and cervico-thoracic curves caused by change in center of gravity from enlarging abdomen	Maternity girdle; good posture and body mechanics; avoid fatigue; wear low-heeled shoes; conscious relaxation; firm mattress; local heat and back rubs; pelvic rock exercise; rest; reassure that condition will disappear 6-8 wk after delivery

Guidelines For Client Teaching

BODY MECHANICS DURING PREGNANCY

ASSESSMENT

1. Pregnant woman's center of gravity changes.
2. Woman has poor posture resulting in frequent backaches.
3. Woman needs instruction on proper body mechanics to perform activities of daily living (ADL) comfortably and safely.

NURSING DIAGNOSES

Alteration in comfort: backache, related to poor posture and body mechanics.
Knowledge deficit related to self care.
Potential for injury related to poor body mechanics.

GOALS

Short-term

Woman will identify potential sources of backaches.
Woman will learn and use good posture.

Intermediate

Woman will learn and use proper body mechanics.

Long-term

Woman will continue to use good posture and proper body mechanics throughout pregnancy.

REFERENCES AND TEACHING AIDS

Printed instructions and diagrams.
Full-length mirror, floor mat, straight-backed chair.
Many references available for lay people such as Marshall C: From here to maternity, Citrus Heights, Calif, 1986, Conmar Publishing Co (PO Box 641, 95610).

CONTENT/RATIONALE	TEACHING ACTION
To understand maternal adaptations that could predispose to backache:	
Softening and relaxation of pelvic joints occur in response to circulating steroid hormones.	Use illustrations to describe maternal adaptations, and correct/incorrect body alignment and center of gravity.
Abdominal muscles are stretched and weakened and the anterior portion of pelvis gradually tilts downward as the uterus increases in size and weight.	Use illustration to describe change in abdominal musculature.
Curvature of lumbarsacral vertebras increases as woman leans backward to maintain her balance.	
Shortening of and strain on back muscles and ligaments results in backache if the woman does not learn to correct this curvature.	
An improperly fitted maternity bra that provides inadequate support to the enlarging breasts and poor posture adds to the strain on muscles and ligaments high in the back, thus aggravating backache.	Use illustration of breast changes to emphasize increase in size and weight.
To develop a kinesthetic sense for good body alignment during pregnancy, practice the following:	
Pelvic tilt (rock) in standing position against a wall, or lying on floor. Using a solid surface makes it easier to feel lumbar curve.	In front of mirror, demonstrate pelvic tilt exercise and good posture.
Pelvic tilt (rock) on hands and knees, and while sitting in straight-back chair.	In front of mirror, guide woman through exercise and aligning body into good posture. Emphasize *feel* of movements and posture by voice and touch.
Abdominal muscle contractions during pelvic tilt while standing, lying, or sitting helps strengthen rectus abdominis.	
Good posture to restore proper body alignment—head, shoulders, lumbarsacral curve, knees, and feet placement.	Use illustrations as needed.
To learn good body mechanics, practice the following:	
Leg muscles are used to reach objects on or near floor. Bend at the knees, not the back. The back is kept straight. Knees are bent to lower body to squatting position. Feet are kept 12 to 18 inches apart for a solid base to maintain balance.	Use illustrations, demonstrate and evaluate return demonstration.

Guidelines For Client Teaching—cont'd

CONTENT/RATIONALE	TEACHING ACTION
Lift with the legs. To lift heavy object (young child), one foot is placed slightly in front of the other and kept flat as woman lowers herself on one knee. She lifts the weight holding it close to her body, and never higher than chest high. To stand up or sit down, one leg is placed slightly behind the other as she raises or lowers herself.	
To prevent round ligament pain and strain on abdominal muscles, use correct posture.	Provide anticipatory guidance on several discomforts of pregnancy.
Squat or taylor sit to stretch ligaments.	
Lift objects by squatting and standing with object in hand, straight back; this way lifting is with knees.	
To learn self-care techniques to prevent and/or relieve backache:	Discuss with woman and her family.
Several comfort measures provide comfort directly and by reducing tension:	Review comfort measures and discuss which would work for her.
Warm showers.	
Heating pad.	
Rest as needed.*	
Massage, vibrator.	
NOTE: Avoid hot-tubbing	
Reduce lumbar curve with any of the following:	Encourage and answer questions.
Correct posture	Practice sitting, pelvic rock and abdominal contraction.
Maternity girdle to support weak abdominal muscles	
For prolonged standing (e.g., ironing, out-of-home employment), place one foot on low footstool or box; change positions often.	
Move car seat forward so that knees are bent and higher than hips. If needed, use a small pillow to support low back area.	
Sit in chairs low enough to allow both feet on floor and preferably with knees higher than hips.	
Practice pelvic tilt and abdominal contraction.	
Wear sturdy, supportive, low-heeled (no more than 1 inch) shoes.	
Ensure a good night's sleep. Use a firm mattress, or if preferred, a water bed. Sleep in side-lying position, supported by pillows, as needed (e.g., under abdomen, between knees).	Discuss which method woman can implement.

EVALUATION Teaching has been effective when all goals have been attained. Woman uses good posture and body mechanics on subsequent visits. Woman wears appropriate clothing and shoes. Woman verbalizes the self-care measures she continues to use. Woman states she no longer has backache or other muscle strain.

*It is recommended that employers have a place where women can lie down during their breaks.

Guidelines For Client Teaching

RELAXATION

ASSESSMENT
1. Gravida states she "just can't relax."
2. Gravida asks for information.
3. Gravida appears tired or tense.

NURSING DIAGNOSES

Potential alteration in comfort related to emotional or physical tension.

Knowledge deficit related to self care through relaxation techniques.

GOALS

Short-term

Woman learns sources of tension.

Woman increases self-care skills by learning at least two methods of relaxation.

Intermediate

Woman reports success with methods learned.

Woman expands self-care skills by learning additional relaxation measures to prevent or reduce stress.

Long-term

Woman utilizes and reports success with relaxation measures in labor and postpartum.

Woman continues to use and expand skills with relaxation within her family, across the life span.

REFERENCES AND TEACHING AIDS

Illustrations

Cassettes of "New Age" music and nature soundtracks (e.g., sounds of waterfalls, birds, ocean waves).

Full-length mirror, floor mat or comfortable seats, pillows.

Many lay references available at bookstores everywhere.

Preparation for parenthood classes.

CONTENT/RATIONALE	TEACHING ACTION
To identify sources of tension:	Validate the universality of tension and need for active relaxation.
Maternal adaptation to pregnancy underlies many discomforts.	Utilize gravida's readiness to learn to teach self-care skills that could last a lifetime for her and, if she teaches it, for her family.
The change in center of gravity, increase in weight and metabolic rate, and awkwardness increase tension on muscles and ligaments. Fetal activity interrupts rest.	
Psychosocial adaptations require energy.	
The combined sources often interrupt sleep and rest. Decreased resilience throughout pregnancy is characteristic.	
To present a variety of methods from which gavida can choose the most appropriate for her:	
Conscious relaxation with active imagery.	Keep abreast of a variety of methods.
Learning to relax.	Present each without imposing own preferences.
Exercises are relaxing for many people, see Guidelines for Client Teaching, "Exercises," pp. 35-36.	Use illustrations.
Use of good body mechanics aids relaxation.	Play cassettes.
Knowledge of common discomforts and self-care measures can contribute to relaxation.	Demonstrate.
	Assist woman through practice.
Exercises to stretch and rest back muscles at home or at work:	Refer clients to classes for therapeutic touch, acupressure and massage, yoga, and hypnosis per client requests.
Stand behind a chair. Support and balance self using the back of the chair. Squat for 30 seconds; stand for 15 seconds. Repeat 6 times, several times per day, as needed.	Alert clients that if unable to relax because of persistent physical or emotional discomfort, that physician must be notified.
While sitting in chair, lower head to knees for 30 seconds. Raise up. Repeat 6 times, several times per day, as needed.	

EVALUATION Nurse can be reasonably reassured that teaching was effective when the goals for care are met. Woman demonstrates relaxation techniques appropriately. Woman states she uses the techniques and feels that they bring her relief.

Guidelines For Client Teaching

SAFETY

ASSESSMENT

1. Woman is pregnant.
2. Pregnant woman works within the home, in the yard, drives or rides in a car, and works as a hairdresser.

NURSING DIAGNOSES

Knowledge deficit related to source of safety hazards.
Knowledge deficit related to safety measures.
Potential for injury to mother and fetus related to possible hazards in the environment and workplace.

GOALS

Short-term

Woman is alerted to sources of safety hazards.
Woman is alerted to self-care related to safety measures.
Woman will use car safety belt and head rest consistently.
Woman will verbalize rationale for and consistently use gloves and good ventilation when using any chemicals, or avoid their use.

Intermediate

Woman will eliminate exposure to chemicals and fumes.

Long-term

Woman will persist in use of safety measures throughout life span.

REFERENCES AND TEACHING AIDS

Printed instructions and information from sources such as clinic, doctor, safety councils.
Copy of "Standards for Maternity Care and Employment" (U. S. Children's Bureau).

CONTENT/RATIONALE	TEACHING ACTION
To identify factors that make safety awareness and measures critical during pregnancy:	
Maternal adaptations to pregnancy involve relaxation of joints, alteration in center of gravity, and neurologic changes responsible for faintness and discomforts. Problems with coordination and balance are common.	Encourage and answer questions regarding maternal changes.
Embryonic and fetal development is vulnerable to environmental teratogens.	Exercise caution to avoid causing anxiety.
To explore sources of safety hazards:	Review Guidelines for Client Teaching, "Precautions for drug use," p. 38.
Many potentially dangerous chemicals are present in the home and yard. These include cleaning agents, paints, a variety of sprays, herbicides, and pesticides. The soil and water supply may be unsafe in some places.	Learn status of local area from community health agencies.
The work place often contain obvious and hidden hazards.	Review standards of maternity care and employment.
Recent legislation specifies appropriate use of vehicular seat belts, but some people ignore it.	
Recreation requiring coordination and balance is best deferred.	Encourage and answer questions regarding which changes woman is able to implement.
High altitudes (not in pressurized aircraft) could jeopardize oxygen intake.	
Spouse's exhaled breath and clothes may contain contaminants.	
To increase self-care through consistent use of safety measures:	Present alternatives and problem-solve solutions together.
Read all labels for ingredients and proper use of product.	Explore with woman what she does during the course of a typical day. Make a list of potential/actual hazards and mutually problem-solve solutions (e.g., avoid use, provide substitutions, ensure ventilation and proper dis-
Ensure adequate ventilation with "clean" air.	
Dispose of wastes appropriately.	

Continued.

Guidelines For Client Teaching—cont'd

Wear gloves when handling chemicals.
Change job assignments or work-place as necessary.
Use good body mechanics.
Use safety features on tools/vehicles; wear goggles, helmets, as specified.
Avoid activities requiring coordination, balance, and concentration.
Take rest periods, reschedule daily activities to meet rest and relaxation needs.
While traveling, use safety seat belts and head rests.

posal, use safety equipment, make changes in sports and recreation, and schedule rest periods).

Show illustration of how to wear a safety belt and discuss.

EVALUATION Nurse will know that teaching has been effective when all goals have been achieved. Woman can verbalize knowledge of hazards and problem-solve solutions. Woman consistently implements self-care safety measures. She and fetus experience no harm from safety-related causes.

Guidelines For Client Teaching

NIPPLE PREPARATION FOR BREAST-FEEDING

ASSESSMENT
1. Pregnant woman has decided to breast-feed.
2. Woman is motivated to learn about nipple preparation for breast-feeding.
3. Woman is in the sixth month of pregnancy.
4. Woman is not at risk for preterm labor.

NURSING DIAGNOSES
Knowledge deficit related to nipple preparation for breast-feeding.
Potential for nipple injury related to lack of prenatal preparation.

GOALS
Short-term
Woman learns her nipple formation and when to begin preparation techniques.

Intermediate
Woman performs those techniques needed to toughen and prepare her nipples for breast-feeding.

Long-term
Woman will be prepared psychologically for knowing and handling her breasts before initiating breast-feeding.
Woman has prepared her nipples adequately so that breast-feeding occurs with no injury to her nipples.

REFERENCES AND TEACHING AIDS
Books and pamphlets on breast-feeding from La Leche League, clinics.
Illustrations.
Variety of nipple shields.
List of references, or examples:
La Leche League International: The womanly art of breast feeding, Franklin Park, Ill, 1981, The League.
Riordan JM: A practical guide to breast feeding, St Louis, 1983, The CV Mosby Co.

Guidelines For Client Teaching—cont'd

CONTENT/RATIONALE	TEACHING ACTIONS
To determine nipple formation retractile or erectile:	Instruct and demonstrate how to perform the *pinch test.*
Have woman place thumb and forefinger on her areola and press inward gently. This will cause her nipple to stand erect or to retract (invert). Most nipples erect.	Use illustrations as necessary. Guide woman through pinch test. Encourage and answer questions.
Inverted nipples need more preparation time. Nipple preparation for these women can start during the last 2 months of pregnancy.	
To provide information about actual techniques:	Discuss these procedures with the woman and provide time for her questions. Provide a chart to illustrate the anatomy of the breast.
Nipples are cleansed with warm water to prevent blocking of the ducts with dried colostrum. They are dried with a rough towel. Soap is not used because it removes protective oils that keep nipples supple. Soften dried precolostrum secretion with lanolin-based cream (e.g., Masse).	
Breasts are milked to remove colostrum and keep the milk ducts clear.	Demonstrate this procedure to the woman. If necessary ask for a return demonstration. Encourage discussion and questions. Provide pictures.
Western dress precludes natural toughening of nipples. Toughening of nipples can be accomplished in a variety of ways.	Provide options so woman can use method best suited to her, and to her spouse. Demonstrate. Use illustrations.
Following a bath or shower, towel dry nipples well, but not so hard as to cause irritation or soreness.	
Grasp nipple between thumb and forefinger. Roll nipples gently for short time each day. Since this procedure may cause uterine contractions, it may be contraindicated for those women at risk for premature labor.	Demonstrate. Use illustrations. Prepare the woman for and discuss the stimulation of uterine contractions.
Undress to bra, drop flaps over nipples. Expose nipples to air and sunlight for short periods of time each day. Avoid sunburn.	Discuss.
Incorporate oral stimulation of nipples by spouse during sexual intercourse.	Discuss. Recognize that this activity may be unacceptable to some people.
To encourage protraction of inverted nipples:	
Utilize one or more of the methods described above.	
Place forefingers close to inverted nipple, pressing firmly into breast tissue, and gradually pulling away from areola. Massage is done vertically and horizontally, about 5 times. Repeat each day.	Demonstrate. Use illustrations. Provide written instructions.
Obtain nipple cups designed specifically for correcting inverted nipples. Plastic doughnut-shaped cups are available for correcting inversions or retractions. A continuous, gentle pressure exerted around the areola pushes the nipple through a central opening in the inner shield. Nipple cups should be worn during the last 2 trimesters of pregnancy for 1 to 2 hours daily. The time for wearing them should be increased gradually. Brand names for these cups include Woolwich, Netsy, La Leche League Cups, Nurse-Dri, Free and Dry, and Hobbit Shields.	Present displays of nipple cups. Encourage woman to handle cups and try them. Alert her to the fact that these cups can also be worn after childbirth. However, because body warmth can foster rapid bacterial growth and contamination, milk that collects in the cup should be discarded and not fed to the infant (Riordan, 1983).

EVALUATION Nurse will know that teaching was effective when woman correctly performs suggested techniques to prepare her breasts for breast-feeding. Evaluation of the long-term goals must be deferred until the postpartum period.

Sample Nursing Care Plan*

SUBSEQUENT PRENATAL VISITS: SECOND TRIMESTER

ASSESSMENT	NURSING DIAGNOSIS (ND)/PLAN (P)/GOAL (G)	RATIONALE/ IMPLEMENTATION	EVALUATION
Woman making subsequent office or clinic visit.	ND: Knowledge deficit related to second trimester of pregnancy. P: Review schedule for care. G: The woman will become knowledgable about the second trimester of pregnancy.	*To determine woman's general well-being the nurse will*: Interview woman regarding events since previous visit. Inquire about any complaints or problems. Answer any questions woman may have. Identify personal and family needs. Assess learning needs.	Woman understands and verbalizes rationale for sharing any relevant information with the nurse. Woman exhibits a readiness to learn by verbalizing and asking appropriate questions.
Physical evaluation of gravida.	ND: Altered body systems related to second trimester of pregnancy. P: Share findings from examination. G: The woman will maintain physical well-being during pregnancy by gaining knowledge about normal physical alterations during this time.	*To determine woman's physical well-being the nurse will*: Monitor the gravida's weight gain and blood pressure. Measure fundal height. Listen to fetal heart tones. Test urine for sugar and protein.	Woman understands and verbalizes rationale for observation of these parameters. Woman cooperates by bringing urine specimen with her.
Gravida needs education regarding self-care activities.	ND: Knowledge deficit related to self care activities during second trimester of pregnancy. P: Review self-care activities. G: Woman will learn self-care activities.	*To educate the woman the nurse will*: Discuss importance of keeping scheduled appointments. Discuss good nutrition, eating habits, and a favorable weight gain. Explain importance of maintaining an exercise program. Discuss safety hazards relevant to work and travel. Explain importance of wearing nonrestrictive and flattering clothes to help woman with her self-image.	Woman keeps scheduled appointments. Woman reports eating habits and maintains a favorable weight gain. Woman verbalizes an understanding of a safe exercise program and safety hazards associated with work and travel. Woman refrains from wearing regular girdles, garters, or other restrictive clothes.
Lack of knowledge regarding danger signs.	ND: Knowledge deficit related to danger signs during second trimester. P: Teach danger signs. G: Woman will learn to recognize those signs and symptoms that signal danger for her and her fetus.	*To educate woman the nurse will discuss the following signs and symptoms with the client*: Absence of fetal movement or change in pattern of fetal movement. Swollen feet, ankles, hands, puffy eyes. Rapid gain in weight.	Woman verbalizes understanding of these danger signs and asks relevant questions. Woman knows where to call if she should experience any of these signs or symptoms.

*Also see Summary of Nursing Actions for Nursing Care During First and Second Trimester of Pregnancy, pp. 41-43 and 53-55.

Sample Nursing Care Plan—cont'd

SUBSEQUENT PRENATAL VISITS: SECOND TRIMESTER

ASSESSMENT	NURSING DIAGNOSIS (ND)/PLAN (P)/GOAL (G)	RATIONALE/ IMPLEMENTATION	EVALUATION
		Headaches, blurred vision, dizziness. Premature rupture of membranes. Vaginal bleeding. Sudden, sharp pains in abdomen. Provide gravida with phone numbers of doctor or hospital.	

Summary of Nursing Actions

NURSING CARE DURING FIRST AND SECOND TRIMESTER

I. Goals
  A. For the mother: to have a physically safe and emotionally satisfying pregnancy.
  B. For the unborn child: to have a uncomplicated intrauterine existence.
  C. For the family: to have an experience that promotes loving and concerned parenting for the child and enhances the personal growth of all individuals involved.

II. Priorities
  A. Establish plan of care related to woman's EDC and family circumstances.
  B. Monitor woman, fetus, and family for normal adaptations to pregnancy.
  C. Initiate remedial therapy for abnormal adaptation to pregnancy.
  D. Promote client recognition of normal and abnormal adaptations to pregnancy.
  E. Promote client and family participation in care.
  F. Provide supportive care to client and family.

III. Assessment
  A. Interview
    1. Health history
      a. Current family happenings and their effect on woman
      b. Problems she may be experiencing
      c. Knowledge and understanding of danger signals and to whom to report
      d. Knowledge of diet
      e. Amount of participation woman (or couple) desires in childbirth and whether classes are appropriate
      f. Woman's knowledge of infant care, including methods of feeding
    2. Psychosocial history
      a. Reactions to pregnancy

      b. Understanding of sexual responses
      c. Self-image
      d. Understanding of plan of care
      e. Awareness of fetal movements
    3. Review of woman's physical systems
  B. Physical examination
    1. Temperature, pulse, respiration (TPR), blood pressure: (BP), and weight
    2. Fundal height and gestational age
    3. Fetal heart rate and fetal activity
    4. Edema
    5. Skin
    6. Pelvic examination (as necessary)
      a. Vagina
      b. Cervix
      c. Uterus
    7. Breasts (as necessary)
  C. Laboratory tests
    1. See Table 2-5, "Routine Prenatal Screening Tests"
    2. Other tests (as necessary)
      a. Blood
      b. Urine
      c. Identification of infection or risk factors

IV. Potential nursing diagnoses
  A. Ineffective family coping: compromised
  B. Ineffective individual coping
  C. Altered health maintenance
  D. Knowledge deficit
  E. Altered nutrition: more or less than body requirements
  F. Body image disturbance
  G. Self esteem disturbance: situational low self esteem
  H. Fatigue
  I. Fear
  J. Altered role performance

Summary of Nursing Actions—cont'd

K. Altered family processes
L. Powerlessness
M. Noncompliance (specify)
N. Altered tissue perfusion (renal, cerebral, cardiopulmonary, gastrointestinal, peripheral)
O. Diarrhea
P. Constipation
Q. Altered patterns of urinary elimination
R. Fluid volume excess (edema)
S. Potential for injury
T. Impaired skin integrity

V. Plan/implementation
  A. Support person
    1. Nurse with client
      a. Use appropriate interview techniques
        (1) Greet by name in unhurried manner.
        (2) Provide a relaxed and trusting atmosphere.
        (3) Provide privacy.
        (4) Validate normalcy of their responses (if they fall within normal limits).
        (5) Provide information as needed.
        (6) Respect cultural, ethnic, religious, or other responses.
        (7) Ensure confidentiality.
      b. Review protocol for schedule and care.
        (1) Set next appointment time.
        (2) Inquire as to convenience of appointments.
      C. Discuss problems, work mutually toward solutions.
        (1) Review problems associated with noncompliance.
    2. Maternal emotional health
      a. Provide information and support related to emotional responses or problems (e.g., mood swings, relationships with family members, feelings towards fetus).
      b. Initiate discussions related to the woman's self-concept (i.e., body image, self-esteem, ambivalence, happiness or depression, anxiety, fear or anger).
    3. Client and family
      a. Promote partner's participation in routine visits and parent-preparation classes.
      b. Assist mother in broadening her network of support people.
      c. Listen and counsel on husband-wife relationship:
        (1) Discuss alternatives in sexual expression.
      d. Encourage sibling participation in routine visits
        (1) See Guidelines for Client Teaching, "Sibling Preparation," p. 60.
      e. See Guidelines for Client Teaching, "Grandparent Preparation," p. 59.
  B. Teacher/counselor/advocate
    1. Review danger signals of complications of pregnancy.
      a. Vaginal bleeding
      b. Burning or pain on urination

      c. Chills or elevated temperature
      d. Exposure to communicable disease (e.g., rubella)
      e. Nausea and vomiting beyond week 12 or persistent or severe vomiting anytime
      f. Abdominal pain or cramping
      g. Reduction in or absence of fetal movement (after quickening)
      h. Woman reports abnormal symptoms promptly
    2. Review changes common to first and second trimester, physiologic basis, prevention, and treatment.
      a. *First trimester*
        (1) Pain and tingling in the breasts
        (2) Urgency and frequency of urination
        (3) Languor and malaise (fatigue)
        (4) Nausea and vomiting (morning sickness)
      b. *Second trimester*
        (1) Constipation
        (2) Heartburn
        (3) Increased pigmentation
        (4) Leg cramps
        (5) Pica
        (6) Food cravings and food avoidances
        (7) Leukorrhea
        (8) Round ligament plan
    3. Provide answers to common questions relating to:
      a. Clothing
      b. Bathing and swimming
      c. Employment
      d. Travel
      e. Physical activity
      f. Dental problems
      g. Immunization
      h. Drugs
      i. Substance abuse
      j. Radiation
      k. Resources available
        (1) Education
        (2) Dental evaluation
        (3) Medical service
        (4) Social service
        (5) Emergency room
    4. Instruct woman and family concerning fetal development, maternal adaptations, maternal and fetal symptomatology and significance. (This is a gradual process and may take weeks to complete.)
    5. Instruct woman and family concerning maternal and fetal needs (e.g., care during travel, continuity of care).
    6. Provide nutritional guidance.
      a. Weight gain
      b. Balanced diet
      c. Special nutritional needs: iron supplements
    7. Comment on appearance and energy level.
    8. Instruct on choices for infant feeding.
    9. Instruct regarding choices in prenatal education classes.
  C. Technician

Summary of Nursing Actions—cont'd

1. Implement appropriate techniques for physical assessment and analyze findings. Share findings with woman or couple as appropriate.
2. Comment in positive manner about her appearance; inquire about energy level. Review exercise and relaxation techniques, see Guidelines for Client Teaching, "Exercise," pp. 35-36.
3. Share findings prn.
4. Instruct woman regarding significance of findings. Review resting positions.
5. Review significance of findings.
6. Review anticipated changes.
7. Review method of counting fetal movement and procedure for reporting any changes.
8. Review significance of ultrasound (sonography), urine estriol tests, NST, and CST.

VI. Evaluation
  A. Emotional support
    1. Client and family participate in interview
    2. Client verbalizes understanding of schedule and need for continuity of care, physical examination, reporting of abnormal symptoms.
    3. Client complies with plan of care.
    4. Client follows diet plan, takes only prescribed medications, refrains from smoking tobacco and drinking alcohol, exercises regularly.
  B. Maternal emotional health
    1. Reactions indicative of positive psychologic response to pregnancy, including birth process and parenthood:
      a. During second trimester, woman usually is reasonably free of symptoms; she is more tranquil and at ease; reality of child is now recognized, and most women come to accept their pregnant state; however, feelings of ambivalence come and go.
      b. Negative feelings about self-image are recognized as temporary; expresses pride or pleasure about being pregnant.
  C. Client and family
    1. Partner's expresses commitment to pregnancy (e.g., observer, style, ethnic expression).
    2. Couple verbalizes understanding of sexual responses and reports that sexual relationships are mutually accepted and serve as a means of communication.
    3. Sibling begins to accept idea of new brother or sister.
    4. Grandparents act as an important part of support network.
  D. Knowledge and skills
    1. Woman or couple verbalize understanding of physiologic basis, need for immediate treatment, and how to obtain necessary care for complications of pregnancy.
    2. Women or couple verbalize understanding of physiologic basis for, and prevention and treat-

ment of, problems common to first and second trimesters.
    3. Woman and family verbalize understanding of rationale for answers to common questions.
    4. Woman and family verbalize understanding of fetal development, FHR, and fetal movement, adaptation, and status and understanding of fetal and maternal needs during pregnancy.
    5. Woman and family verbalize understanding of maternal and fetal nutritional needs.
      a. Physical response indicates compliance with nutritional counsel.
      b. Woman verbalizes understanding of choices regarding infant feeding.
    6. Woman verbalizes understanding of choices and availability of prenatal education classes.
    7. Woman seeks assistance for problems such as infections (cold), allergies, or substance abuse (smoking, drinking).
  E. Physical care—maternal
    1. Findings from physical assessment are within normal limits.
    2. Appearance is healthy, grooming is adequate, energy level is normal.
    3. Temperature, pulse, respiration, blood pressure, and weight
      a. Temperature, normal range
      b. Pulse, normal range
      c. Respiration, 18-20/min
      d. Blood pressure, normal range of less than +30 systolic and +15 diastolic over baseline; may decrease slightly in midpregnancy
      e. Weight gain
        (1) Weeks 1-13: about 3-4 lb (1.4 to 1.8 kg)
        (2) Weeks 12-26: about 12-14 lb (5.6-6.3 kg)
        (3) Weeks 27-40: approximately 0.5 lb (0.23 kg) per week.
    4. Edema, dependent edema not yet apparent.
    5. Abdomen, gradual enlargement, see height of fundus
    6. Uterus
      a. Progressive enlargement to accommodate growing products of conception.
      b. Fundal height
        (1) 12-13 weeks: felt just above pubic symphysis;
        (2) 16 weeks: felt 3-4 cm above pubic symphysis;
        (3) 20 weeks: felt 2-3 cm below umbilicus
        (4) 24 weeks: felt at umbilicus
    7. Skin, changes not noticeable.
  F. Fetal
    1. Fetal heart rate (FHR) heard by Doppler principle (Dopptone) at 8-12 weeks, by fetoscope at 17-18 weeks
    2. Fetal movements felt at 17-19 weeks (quickening)
    3. Fetal breathing movements detected by sonography by 18½ weeks

THIRD TRIMESTER

During the last trimester, discomforts associated with advancing pregnancy and concerns about the approaching labor preoccupy expectant families. In addition to individual counseling, preparation for childbirth classes are available to assist expectant parents as they prepare for transition into parenthood. Expectant families approaching childbirth have many needs. Siblings and grandparents must be considered, too. Clearly the nurse is in a pivotal position within the team of health care providers to assist parents with these needs during the third trimester of pregnancy.

Adaptations to pregnancy go into the third trimester and continue through labor readiness. Table 2-9 discusses this subject, some of the problems the woman may experience, and suggested treatments. The nurse must be sure the gravida can recognize preterm as well as normal labor. Preparation for childbirth teaching should also include grandparents and siblings. This section ends with a sample nursing care plan and summary of nursing action for care during the third trimester.

FETAL DEVELOPMENT AT 40 WEEKS

1. Nutrients and maternal immunoglobulins are stored
2. Subcutaneous fat deposited
3. Dramatic storage of iron, nitrogen, and calcium
4. In male, testes are within well-wrinkled scrotum
5. In female, labia are well-developed and cover vestibule
6. Lanugo shed, except for shoulders, generally
7. Body contours plump
8. Decreased vernix
9. Scalp hair 2 to 3 cm (1 in) long
10. Cartilage in nose and ears well developed
11. 45 to 55 cm (18 to 22 in) in length
12. Weighs 3400 g (7½ lb) (average)
13. Fundal height below xiphoid after lightening

Table 2-9   *Problems Related to Maternal Adaptations During the Third Trimester*

Problem	Physiology	Treatment
Shortness of breath and dyspnea—occur in 60% of pregnant women	Expansion of diaphragm limited by enlarging uterus; diaphragm is elevated about 4 cm (1½ in); some relief after lightening	Good posture; flying exercise; sleep with extra pillows; avoid overloading stomach; stop smoking; refer to physician if symptoms worsen to rule out anemia, emphysema, and asthma
Insomnia (later weeks of pregnancy)	Fetal movements, muscular cramping, urinary frequency, shortness of breath, or other discomforts	Reassurance; conscious relaxation; back massage or effleurage; support of body parts with pillows; warm milk or warm shower before retiring
Psychosocial responses: mood swings, mixed feelings, increased anxiety	Hormonal and metabolic adaptations; feelings about impending labor, delivery, and parenthood	Reassurance and support from significant other and nurse; improved communication with partner, family, and others
Gingivitis and epulis (hyperemia, hypertrophy, bleeding, tenderness): condition will disappear spontaneously 1 to 2 months after delivery	Increased vascularity and proliferation of connective tissue from estrogen stimulation	Well-balanced diet with adequate protein and fresh fruits and vegetables; gentle brushing and good dental hygiene; avoid infection
Urinary frequency and urgency returns	Vascular engorgement and altered bladder function caused by hormones; bladder capacity reduced by enlarging uterus and fetal presenting part	Kegel's exercises; limit fluid intake before bedtime; reassurance; wear perineal pad; refer to physician for pain or burning sensation
Perineal discomfort and pressure	Pressure from enlarging uterus, especially when standing or walking; multiple gestation	Rest, conscious relaxation and good posture; maternity girdle; refer to physician for assessment and treatment if pain is present; rule out labor
Braxton Hicks' contractions	Intensification of uterine contractions in preparation for work of labor	Reassurance; rest; change of position; practice breathing techniques when contractions are bothersome; effleurage; rule out labor
Leg cramps (gastrocnemius spasm)—especially when reclining	Compression of nerves supplying lower extremities because of enlarging uterus; reduced level of diffusible serum calcium or elevation of serum phosphorus; aggravating factors: fatigue, poor peripheral circu-	Rule out blood clot by checking for Homans' sign; use massage and heat over affected muscle; stretch affected muscle until spasm relaxes; stand on cold surface; oral supplementation with calcium carbonate or cal-

Table 2-9, cont'd. *Problems Related to Maternal Adaptations During the Third Trimester*

Problem	Physiology	Treatment
	lation, pointing toes when stretching legs or when walking, drinking more than 1 L (1 qt) of milk per day	cium lactate tablets; aluminum hydroxide gel, 1 oz, with each meal removes phosphorus by absorbing it
Ankle edema (nonpitting) to lower extremities	Edema aggravated by prolonged standing, sitting, poor posture, lack of exercise, constrictive clothing (e.g., garters), or by hot weather	Ample fluid intake for "natural" diuretic effect; put on support stockings before arising; rest periodically with legs and hips elevated, exercise moderately; refer to physician if generalized edema develops; *diuretics are contraindicated*

Guidelines For Client Teaching

PRETERM LABOR RECOGNITION

ASSESSMENT

1. Pregnancy after the twentieth week but before the thirty-seventh week.
2. Gravida has no signs or symptoms of preterm labor at present.

NURSING DIAGNOSES

Knowledge deficit related to the warning signs of preterm labor.
Potential for injury to fetus related to preterm birth.
Potential for body image disturbance: situational low self-esteem related to preterm delivery.
Potential for spiritual distress related to preterm labor.

GOALS
Short-term

Woman begins to learn the warning signs and symptoms of preterm labor.

Intermediate

Woman remains alert for preterm labor without undue anxiety.
Woman definitely recognizes warning signs and symptoms and can detect uterine contractions herself.

Long-term

Woman knows what to do if she should exhibit any of the warning signs and symptoms of preterm labor.
Regardless of outcome of pregnancy, woman will maintain or enhance her self-concept and supportive family processes, and spiritual distress is avoided or minimized.

REFERENCES AND TEACHING AIDS

Printed instructions outlining warning signs and symptoms, steps to take if woman has problems, and the doctor's phone number.
Illustrations or charts.

CONTENT/RATIONALE	TEACHING ACTIONS
To understand the definition: Premature labor occurs after the twentieth week but before the thirty-seventh week of pregnancy. It is a condition in which uterine contractions (tightenings of the womb) cause the cervix (mouth of the womb) to open earlier than normal. It could result in the birth of a preterm baby. Babies born before 37 weeks may have problems breathing, eating, and keeping warm.	Read through pamphlet with woman or group of women. Women can use group for support.
To understand the cause: Although certain factors or reasons may increase a woman's chances of having preterm labor, such as carrying twins, the specific cause or causes of preterm labor are not known. Sometimes a woman may have preterm labor for no apparent reason.	Encourage discussion of this information and clarify or answer any questions woman may have. Discuss the woman's risk factors, if she has any.

Continued.

Guidelines For Client Teaching—cont'd

CONTENT/RATIONALE	TEACHING ACTION
To understand need for early recognition: It may be possible to prevent a preterm birth by knowing the warning signs and symptoms of preterm labor and by seeking care early if warning signs and symptoms should occur.	Reassure woman that she is not responsible if preterm labor proceeds despite her efforts.
To understand the difference between normal and preterm labor uterine contractions: It is *normal* to have some uterine contractions throughout the day. They usually occur when a woman changes positions, such as from sitting to lying down. These usually irregular and mild contractions are called Braxton Hicks' contractions. They help with uterine tone and uteroplacental perfusion. It is *not normal* to have frequent uterine contractions (every 10 minutes or more often for one hour). Contractions of labor are regular, frequent, and hard. They may also be felt as a tightening of the abdomen or a backache. This type of contraction causes the cervix to efface and dilate.	Instruct woman in self-detection of uterine contractions: Since the onset of premature labor is subtle and often hard to recognize, it is important to know how to feel your abdomen for uterine contractions. You can feel for contractions this way: While lying down, place your fingertips on the top of your uterus. A contraction is the periodic "tightening" or "hardening" of your uterus. If your uterus is contracting, you will actually feel your abdomen get tight or hard, and then feel it relax or soften when the contraction is over. Discuss and answer questions. Demonstrate. Watch return demonstration. Praise accomplishments appropriately.
Warning signs and symptoms include: Uterine contractions that occur every 10 minutes or more with or without other signs. Menstrual-like cramps felt in lower abdomen constantly or intermittently. Low dull backache felt below the waistline constantly or intermittently. Pelvic pressure that feels like baby is pushing down constantly or intermittently. Abdominal cramping with or without diarrhea. Increase or change in vaginal discharge; more than usual or change in consistency or color.	Read through warning signs and symptoms with the client. Instruct the woman to begin assessment as follows: If you think you are having uterine contractions or any of the other signs and symptoms of premature labor: Lie down tilted toward your side. Place a pillow at your back for support. Sometimes lying down for an hour may slow down or stop the signs and symptoms. Do not lie flat on your back, because lying flat may cause contractions to occur more often or may result in supine hypotension syndrome. Do not turn completely on your side because you may not be able to feel the contractions. Check for contractions for 1 hour.
To foster compliance and assist with decision-making: It is often difficult to identify preterm labor. Accurate diagnosis requires assessment by the care provider usually in the hospital or clinic.	To tell how often contractions are occurring, check the minutes that elapse from the beginning of one contraction to the beginning of the next. Discuss and answer questions. Demonstrate positions. Suggest posting these instructions where they can be seen by everyone. Assist the woman with decision-making by providing written instructions such as the following: Call your doctor, clinic, or delivery room, or go to the hospital if: You have uterine contractions every 10 minutes or more often for 1 hour (more than 5 contractions in 1 hour) *or* You have any of the other signs and symptoms for 1 hour *or* You have any spotting or leaking of fluid from your vagina.

EVALUATION Teaching has been effective when all goals have been met. Woman verbalizes knowledge of the warning signs and symptoms and knows how to contact her physician. If preterm labor occurs, she recognizes it and informs her physician immediately. Regardless of the outcome of pregnancy, woman will maintain or enhance her self-concept and supportive family processes, and spiritual distress is avoided or minimized.

Guidelines For Client Teaching

GRANDPARENT PREPARATION

ASSESSMENT

1. Expectant parents voice concerns about role of grandparents and request assistance (depends on grandparent's readiness to learn).
2. Expectant grandparents request information about hospital policies and procedures, modern childbirth methods, new parents' needs, and their own roles.
3. Expectant grandparents would like to provide support to expectant parents before and after the birth of the baby.

NURSING DIAGNOSES

Knowledge deficit related to hospital policies, childbirth methods, and how to provide support to expectant parents.

Altered family processes related to addition of a new family member.

Potential for ineffective individual coping related to need for role change.

GOALS

Short-term

Grandparents are oriented to hospital routines and policies.

Grandparents are oriented to childbirth method and experience expected by their children.

Grandparents learn current techniques of infant care.

Intermediate

Grandparents prepare for role change from parents to grandparents.

Grandparents begin to define mutually acceptable role-relationship with their children.

Grandparents relive and come to terms with own childbirth experience.

Long-term

Grandparents develop and maintain mutually satisfying role-relationship with children and new grandchild.

Grandparents become effective and supportive grandparents and parents.

REFERENCES AND TEACHING AIDS

Audiovisual materials: films, slides, charts.

List of references available to the general public.

Tour of maternity unit; introduction to gowns, shoe covers, and caps.

Values clarification or attitude awareness exercise (Horn and Manion, 1985).

CONTENT/RATIONALE	TEACHING ACTION
To explore values and attitudes: Values-clarification, attitude awareness exercise: When I think about myself as a grandparent, I feel _____. Children bring a couple _____. Breast feeding is _____. Pacifiers are _____. Labor is _____. During their child's labor and delivery, grandparents should _____. The happiest (most satisfying) memory of my (my wife's) labor and childbirth was _____. The unhappiest (least satisfying) memory of my (my wife's) labor and childbirth was _____.	Develop and administer values and attitudes exercise. Use exercise as a basis for starting small-group discussion. Encourage members of group to compare and contrast own experiences, values, and attitudes.
To explore knowledge base of science and technology concerning the birth process: Conduct grandparents class. Use prioritized list of topics they wish to discuss as focus. *To expand learning and orient to environment of maternity area, provide:* Tour of unit. Hands-on experience with equipment and supplies. Introduction of personnel. Description of personnel's services and responsibilities. *To bring closure to class:* Review the grandparent's questions. Discuss their comparisons. Summarize the experience.	Elicit topics the grandparents wish to discuss, write on a chalkboard, and ask group to prioritize list; encourage questions. Use appropriate audiovisual materials: charts, films, slides. Offer or conduct a tour of the maternity area including restrooms, waiting room, telephones, cafeteria, and selected supplies (gowns, shoe-covers) and equipment (fetoscope). Introduce the grandparents to available personnel and review their roles. Return group to classroom. Encourage questions. Encourage the grandparent's to compare and contrast their own experiences with the class content. Provide printed material. Thank the group for their interest.

EVALUATION Teaching has been effective when grandparents develop and maintain a mutually satisfying role-relationship with their children and grandchildren. Goals have been met when grandparents become effective and supportive to their children and grandchildren.

SIBLING PREPARATION

ASSESSMENT

1. Couple expecting second child in 3 months. Four-year-old son asking many questions about the baby in "mommy's tummy". Child resistant to living at aunt's house during mother's hospitalization.
2. Parents express desire for preparation of older sibling.

NURSING DIAGNOSES

Knowledge deficit related to older sibling's capabilities and needs.

Impaired verbal communication related to older child's development level.

Altered family process related to addition of new family member.

GOALS

Short-term

Child and parents feel less anxious about the mother's impending hospitalization.

Child begins to develop realistic expectations of newborn.

Parents begin to develop strategies to prepare the older child for the mother's hospitalization and newborn sibling.

Intermediate

Child begins to prepare for role transition to be brother.

Parents begin to develop strategies for caring for older sibling and new child.

Parents begin to prepare for role transition necessitated by addition of new member to family.

Long-term

Child develops realistic expectations of newborn.

Child and parents learn new coping skills.

Parents successfully make role transition necessitated by addition of new member to the family.

REFERENCES AND TEACHING AIDS

Audiovisual materials: films, slides, doll, cassette recordings, materials with which to draw pictures.

See bibliography for list of references available to parents and small children.

Enroll and attend a sibling class.

Sibling visitation while mother is hospitalized.

CONTENT/RATIONALE	TEACHING ACTION
To allay anxiety related to an unknown environment (Johnsen and Gaspard, 1985):	Prepare a room to convey warmth and friendliness.
Have older sibling:	Explain hospital clothing, then change to scrub outfit worn by fathers and nurses.
Visit hospital classroom.	Help child try on hospital gowns, masks, and caps.
Dress up in hospital clothing.	During tour, answer questions and expect child to abide by hospital "rules."
Learn hospital "rules," such as walk slowly, and talk quietly.	
Tour maternity area, see and touch telephone that he can use to talk to his mother.	
See naked newborn.	
To help child form realistic expectations of the newborn:	Read stories and employ role-playing.
Have older sibling practice in new role:	Ask open-ended or leading questions.
By listening to stories about what newborns can do and how older children react to new born babies.	Help child with holding the doll.
By holding a doll with care to support the head.	Demonstrate ways to console a crying baby, such as singing and talking.
By exploring what he can do when the baby cries. Hear sound of newborn cries and cooing as they vary with hunger, contentment, desire for company, and complaining about a dirty or wet diaper.	Caution against picking up baby.
	Caution against touching the baby's head.
	Play cassette of baby sounds and encourage questions and discussion.
To help child substitute acceptable behavior for unacceptable behavior with the newborn:	
Have older sibling practice through role-playing:	Role-play situation demonstrating positive responses to newborn in selected situations.
When newborn gets a present and older child does not.	Involve older child with problem-solving in selected situations.
When parent spends time with the newborn.	
When the child gets angry with the newborn.	
To help child recognize his feelings:	
Have older sibling:	Show film and encourage discussion.
Watch a film depicting jealousy, anger, and being left out (Johnsen and Gaspard, 1985).	
Participate in discussion of film and how to ask for help when needed.	Lead discussion; encourage comments.
Participate in drawing a picture to show how he feels and what he understands of his mother's pregnancy and the coming baby.	Provide equipment, space and directions for drawing, such as "draw a picture of your family."
	Ask child to tell a story about his picture.

EVALUATION The nurse can be reasonably assured that the teaching plan has been effective when all goals have been met. Older sibling demonstrates realistic expectations of the newborn and remains reassured about parental love. Child and parents learn new coping skills. Parents and sibling successfully make the role transition necessitated by addition of a new family member.

*Sample Nursing Care Plan**

THIRD TRIMESTER

ASSESSMENT	NURSING DIAGNOSIS (ND)/PLAN (P)/GOAL (G)	RATIONALE/ IMPLEMENTATION	EVALUATION
Woman in third trimester. Teaching needs: danger signs recognition of preterm labor.	ND: Knowledge deficit related to signs and symptoms of preterm labor. P: Provide information; discuss. G: Woman will learn signs and symptoms of preterm labor.	*To introduce the definition of preterm labor the nurse will*: Provide written materials defining signs and symptoms of preterm labor; nurse will read through this information with woman.	Woman verbalizes understanding of signs and symptoms of preterm labor.
	ND: Anxiety related to development of preterm labor. P: Provide information: discuss. G: Woman will remain calm and alert and report signs and symptoms promptly if they occur.	*To convey the need for early recognition the nurse will*: Discuss the causes of preterm labor. Inform gravida of warning signs and symptoms. Reassure woman. *To help gravida understand difference between normal and preterm uterine contractions the nurse will*:	Woman verbalizes understanding and asks appropriate questions.
	ND: Potential for injury to woman and fetus, related to preterm birth. P: Provide information: discuss. G: Injury to fetus and gravida will be averted	Discuss the differences. Supervise practice timing frequency of contractions.	Woman gives return demonstration.
Premature rupture of membranes (PROM).	ND: Potential for injury to fetus, related to PROM. P: Provide information; discuss. G: Injury to fetus from prolapsed cord or sepsis will be prevented or decreased.	*To teach woman how to recognize PROM the nurse will*: Describe rupture of membranes: a gush or trickle of clear watery discharge that seems to come from vagina. Tell woman that a positive diagnosis of PROM must be made at clinic or hospital.	Woman verbalizes understanding of information. Woman knows where to go if symptoms appear.
Absence or change in fetal movements.	ND: Knowledge deficit related to assessment of fetal movement, its change in character, or its absence. P: Provide information; discuss. G: Woman will learn to assess the character and frequency of fetal movement.	*To teach woman about fetal movement the nurse will*: Discuss fetal movements she is experiencing. Provide information on fetal activity. Discuss cessation, diminution, and acceleration of fetal movement.	Woman verbalizes understanding of information. Woman reports any change in fetal activity.
Teaching needs: discomforts. Diminished tolerance to activities of daily living (ADL).	ND: Activity intolerance related to maternal adaptations. P: Provide information; discuss.	*To help woman conserve energy the nurse will*: Discuss the importance of frequent rest periods during the day.	Woman (couple) verbalizes understanding of information.

*Also see Summary of Nursing Actions, Nursing Care of During Third Trimester of Pregnancy, pp. 64-67.

Continued.

Sample Nursing Care Plan—cont'd

ASSESSMENT	NURSING DIAGNOSIS (ND)/PLAN (P)/GOAL (G)	RATIONALE/ IMPLEMENTATION	EVALUATION
	G: Woman (couple) will learn ways of conserving her energy.	Aid the woman in forming strategies to help her relax while on the job. Discuss ways in which the woman's partner can help her with household duties.	Woman (couple) verbalizes understanding of information.
Diminished sexual activity.	ND: Altered sexuality patterns related to discomforts of third trimester of pregnancy. P: Provide information; discuss. G: Woman (couple) will learn alternate ways of achieving sexual satisfaction during this time.	*To help the woman (couple) identify and accept changes in sexuality the nurse will*: Assess couple's sexual relationship. Encourage open discussion. Supply information on alternative methods, positions, etc. Encourage verbalization of fears and anxieties.	Sexual needs are met and are mutually satisfying. Couple verbalizes understanding and accepts changes in sexual patterns.
Problems sleeping.	ND: Sleep pattern disturbance related to late pregnancy. P: Provide information; discuss. G: Woman will learn ways to adjust sleep schedule and positions to aid in sleeping.	*To help woman develop strategies to rest and sleep the nurse will*: Assess the woman's "normal" requirement of sleep. Assess woman's level of fatigue and her response to decreased amount of sleep (decreased coping mechanisms, etc.) Suggest strategies such as relaxation techniques, warm bath/shower, reading, warm milk before bed, back rub. Suggest alternate positions for sleeping using more pillows.	Woman reports increased sleep/rest. Woman's fatigue reduced, coping mechanism increased.
Constipation.	ND: Constipation related to late pregnancy. P: Provide information; discuss. G: Woman will continue to eat fresh fruits, vegetables, and whole grain products and drink plenty of water to aid in bowel regularity.	*To help woman minimize problem the nurse will*: Dicuss high fiber diet. Discuss fluid intake. Discourage use of laxatives and cathartics: may cause premature labor. Discuss exercise.	Woman verbalizes understanding of information.
Urinary frequency.	ND: Altered patterns of urinary elimination related to late pregnancy. P: Provide information; discuss; review client teaching: prevention of urinary tract infection (UTI). G: Woman understands information and infection does not occur.	*To teach woman about return of urinary frequency and edema the nurse will*: Provide information about third trimester physiologic changes. Advise woman to lie in left lateral position. Discuss adequate fluid intake. Discourage use of diuretics.	Woman verbalizes understanding of information.

Sample Nursing Care Plan—cont'd

ASSESSMENT	NURSING DIAGNOSIS (ND)/PLAN (P)/GOAL (G)	RATIONALE/ IMPLEMENTATION	EVALUATION
		Discourage sodium restriction in diet. Discuss ways to prevent UTI which is one of the leading causes of premature labor. Discourage long periods of standing or sitting. Suggest use of support hose.	Woman knows signs and symptoms of UTI to report to physician.
Expressed emotional anxiety.	ND: Ineffective family/individual coping, related to adaptations to pregnancy. P: Provide information; discuss. G: Woman (couple) will learn and demonstrate positive coping techniques.	*To help woman (couple) minimize anxiety and develop coping strategies the nurse will*: Assess level of anxiety Discuss those areas and situations that cause woman's (couple's) anxiety. Strongly suggest childbirth education classes (prenatal classes). Give reassurance	Resolution of problems through open discussion. Couple attends classes and works through those anxieties related to labor and delivery.
Backache.	ND: Pain: backache related to postural changes and relaxed joints. P: Provide information; discuss; demonstrate and observe return demonstration. Review client teaching: exercise, body mechanics, and relaxation. G: Woman reports greater comfort.	*To help woman minimize discomfort of backache the nurse will*: Discuss causes. Teach woman relaxation techniques and exercises. Teach woman about proper body mechanics and good posture. Supply written materials on the above for woman's future reference. Discuss types of shoes and types of heels woman should be wearing.	Woman verbalizes understanding of information. Woman uses proper body mechanics and demonstrates good posture.
Shortness of breath.	ND: Ineffective breathing pattern related to limited diaphragmatic excursion in late pregnancy. P: Provide information; discuss. G: Woman will learn ways to cope with shortness of breath until lightening occurs.	*To teach woman ways of coping with shortness of breath the nurse will*: Discuss posture and exercises. Discuss positioning body for sleep with extra pillows. Strongly suggest cessation of smoking. Discuss overeating.	Woman accepts information and utilizes suggestions given by nurse.
Leg cramps. Varicose veins.	ND: Pain related to maternal adaptations. P: Provide information, discuss, and demonstrate. G: Woman will learn self-care strategies to diminish discomfort.	*To minimize discomfort from leg cramps and varicose veins the nurse will*: Discuss diminution of fatigue, amount of milk ingested per day, and adequate calcium intake. Discuss use of maternity support hose. Suggest frequent rest periods and elevation of legs.	Woman verbalizes understanding of information given. Woman asks appropriate questions.

Summary of Nursing Actions

NURSING CARE DURING THIRD TRIMESTER

I. Goals
  A. For the mother: to have a physically safe and emotionally satisfying pregnancy
  B. For the unborn child: to have an uncomplicated intrauterine existence
  C. For the family: to have an experience that promotes loving and concerned parenting for the child and enhances the personal growth of all individuals involved

II. Priorities
  A. Establish plan of care related to woman's EDD and family circumstances.
  B. Monitor woman, fetus, and family for normal adaptations to pregnancy.
  C. Initiate remedial therapy for abnormal adaptations to pregnancy.
  D. Promote client recognition of normal and abnormal adaptations to pregnancy.
  E. Promote client and family participation in care.
  F. Provide supportive care to client and family.
  G. Educate woman and family to danger sign of early labor.
  H. Educate woman and family to normal signs of labor.

III. Assessment
  A. Interview
    1. Health history
      a. Current family happenings and their effect on woman
      b. Problems she may be experiencing
      c. Knowledge and understanding of danger signals
      d. Preparation for emergency arrangements
      e. Knowledge and understanding of labor process and of symptoms of beginning labor
      f. Understanding of responsibilities related to preparing for hospital or home delivery.
    2. Psychosocial history
      a. Emotional status (e.g., anxiety about labor and control of pain).
      b. Client and family responses to unborn child
      c. Sibling and grandparent response to coming birth of child
      d. Preparation for care of family at home during woman's absence
      e. Plans for postdelivery care of infant and understanding of infant's needs
      f. Anticipatory worry concerning new parenting responsibilities, sibling rivalry, recuperation from pregnancy and birth, and family planning
      g. Knowledge of diet
      h. Knowledge of fetal movements
      i. Knowledge of positions for rest and relaxation
    3. Review of woman's physical systems
  B. Physical examination
    1. Temperature-pulse-respiration, blood pressure, weight

    2. Fundal height and gestational age
      a. Fetal heart rate (FHR) and fetal activity
      b. Additional measures other than palpation may be employed to determine presentation, position, and size of infant (e.g., ultrasonography and area of maximum density of fetal heartbeat).
      c. Precise calculations of fetal age may be made with use of various techniques.
    3. Edema
    4. Skin
    5. Pelvic examination is made on weekly visits from week 38 to term to permit evaluation of amount of cervical softening, effacement, and dilatation, and station of presenting part
    6. Breasts
  C. Laboratory tests
    1. Blood
    2. Urine
    3. Cervical and vaginal smears for gonorrhea (repeated at 36 weeks).

IV. Potential nursing diagnoses
  A. Potential for injury
  B. Anxiety
  C. Constipation
  D. Diarrhea
  E. Altered health maintenance
  F. Knowledge deficit
  G. Noncompliance (specify)
  H. Alteration in nutrition: more or less than body requirements
  I. Sleep pattern disturbance
  J. Altered tissue perfusion: cerebral, cardiovascular, renal, gastrointestinal, peripheral
  K. Altered patterns of urinary elimination
  L. Altered family processes
  M. Potential altered parenting
  N. Body image disturbance
  O. Self-esteem disturbance: situational low self-esteem
  P. Altered sexuality patterns
  Q. Powerlessness
  R. Sleep pattern disturbance
  S. Ineffective family coping: compromised
  T. Pain
  U. Potential activity intolerance
  V. Fatigue
  W. Fear
  X. Stress incontinence
  Y. Potential for trauma
  Z. Altered role performance

V. Plan/implementation
  A. Support person
    1. Nurse and client
      a. Use appropriate interview techniques.
        (1) Greet by name in unhurried manner.
        (2) Provide a relaxed and trusting atmosphere.
        (3) Provide privacy.

Summary of Nursing Actions—cont'd

(4) Validate normalcy of their responses (if they fall within normal limits).

(5) Provide information as needed.

(6) Respect cultural, ethnic, religious, or other responses.

(7) Ensure confidentiality.

b. Review protocol for schedule and care.

(1) Set next appointment time. Medical and nursing care is increased to permit detection of any abnormal maternal or fetal response: woman is examined every 2 weeks between 32 and 36 weeks every week between 36 and 40 weeks; if indicated plan of care is modified.

c. Inquire as to convenience of appointment.

(1) Discuss problems: work mutually toward solutions.

(2) Review problems associated with non-compliance.

2. Discuss physiologic basis, prevention, and treatment for changes common in the third trimester (discomforts):

a. Hemorrhoids, vulvar varicosities

b. Varicosities

c. Leg cramps, ache, or edema

d. Hypermobility of joints

e. Backache

f. Return of urinary frequency

g. Shortness of breath

h. Round ligament pain

i. Discomfort from Braxton Hicks contractions and differentiation from "false labor"

k. Emotional changes

l. Sexual needs and changes; intercourse

3. Provide answers to common questions relating to:

a. Clothing

b. Bathing and swimming

c. Employment

d. Travel

e. Physical activity

f. Dental problems

g. Immunization

h. Drugs

i. Substance abuse

j. Radiation

k. Resources available

(1) Education

(2) Dental evaluation

(3) Medical service

(4) Social service

(5) Emergency room

4. Instruct woman and family

a. Concerning fetal development, maternal adaptations, maternal and fetal symptomatology and significance. (This is a gradual process. It may take weeks to complete).

b. Concerning maternal and fetal needs (e.g., care during travel, continuity of care).

5. Comment on appearance, energy level; instruct regarding choices in infant feeding; and provide nutritional guidance:

a. Weight gain

b. Balanced diet

c. Special nutritional needs

d. Supplements

6. Instruct regarding choices in prenatal education classes.

7. Instruct regarding effects on woman or unborn child of such problems; suggest or institute remedial care.

8. Encourage client and family to discuss feelings.

9. Discuss preparation for labor.

a. Symptoms of impending labor and what information to report

b. Breathing and relaxation techniques

c. Involvement of husband or significant other

d. Provision for needs of other children

e. Plans to get to hospital

10. Maternal emotional health

a. Discuss parental awareness of unborn child's reponse to stimuli, such as light, sound, maternal posture or tension, and patterns of sleeping and waking

b. Discuss woman's feeling relating to her self-concept (i.e., self-image self-esteem, sense of power and being in control).

c. Discuss mother and daughter relationships: acceptance and use of mother as role model.

d. Provide opportunities for discussion of probable emotional tensions related to:

(1) Childbirth experience such as fear of pain, loss of control, and possible delivery of child before reaching hospital.

(2) Responsibilities and tasks of parenthood

(3) Mutual parental concerns arising from anxiety for safety of mother and unborn child.

(4) Mutual parental concerns related to siblings and their acceptance of new baby.

(5) Mutual parental concerns about social and economic responsibilities.

(6) Mutual parental concerns for cognitive dissonance arising from conflicts in cultural, religious, or personal value systems.

e. Provide opportunities for discussion of mother's awareness of her body's responses such as "this pregnancy feels O.K." or "something is wrong" and provide acknowledgement of mother's ability.

11. Client and family

a. Discuss husband and wife's relationships; partner's commitment to pregnancy, and coping with ambivalence and mood changes.

b. Discuss the growing relationship between mother and unborn child and other family members.

c. Discuss sexual relationships if parners wish

Continued.

Summary of Nursing Actions—cont'd

to do so. Instruct as to techniques for sexual expression.

B. Teacher/counselor/advocate
1. Review prenatal danger signals and instruct woman to report the following signs and symptoms immediately:
   a. *Vaginal bleeding.* Rule out brownish spotting occurring 48 h after vaginal examination. Rule out "show" of pinkish mucus. Woman is to come to hospital's emergency area immediately for diagnosis and treatment if bleeding is other than one of preceding types.
   b. Symptoms of preeclampsia-eclampsia.
   c. Cessation, noticeable diminution, or acceleration in amount of fetal movement: woman is to come to clinic or physician's office for evaluation.
   d. Rupture of membranes: woman is to come to clinic or physician's office for evaluation.
   e. Burning or pain on urination: woman is to come to clinic or physician's office for evaluation and to bring urine sample for analysis.
   f. Chills or elevated temperature.
   g. Abdominal pain.
   h. Persistent nausea and vomiting.
   i. Signs and symptoms of premature labor: woman is to come to labor unit for evaluation.
   j. Modify original plan of care if maternal or fetal complications are detected. Institute specific remedial intervention.
2. Review plans of labor, terminology, and what care to expect.
3. Discuss preparation for baby.

C. Technician
1. Maternal
   a. Comments in positive manner about her appearance. Inquire about energy level. Review rest and relaxation techniques.
   b. Shares findings prn.
   c. Instruct woman regarding significance of findings.
   d. Review resting position.
   e. Review significance of findings.
   f. Let woman and family listen to FHR. Review significance of findings.
   G. Review physiologic basis for skin changes, varicosities.
   h. Instruct regarding posture and resting.
   i. Begin preparation of breasts for breast feedings.
   j. Review necessity for repetition of tests as necessary.
   k. Review prevention and treatment of anemia.

VI. Evaluation
A. Emotional support
1. Client and family participate in interview.
2. Client verbalizes understanding of schedule, need for continuity of care, physical examination to be done, reporting of abnormal symptoms.
3. Client complies with plan of care: client follows diet plan, takes only prescribed medications, refrains from smoking, drinking alcoholic beverages, and exercises.
4. Client verbalizes acceptance of pregnancy and unborn child. Ambivalent feelings lessen. Mother expresses feelings of closeness to her unborn child and assigns personal characteristics.
5. Client expresses satisfaction with herself, her relationships, her feelings of competence.
6. Client expresses feelings of closeness to her own mother or accepts feelings of distance.
7. Client verbalizes feeling of tension arising from fears or anxieties pertaining to labor, parental responsibilities, safety of mother and child, and relationships with significant others.
8. Mother expresses confidence in her knowledge of her own body.
9. Husband and wife express feelings of acceptance of husband and wife's choice of role in pregnancy and in labor.
10. Mother, father, and siblings talk about unborn child as part of the family.
11. Woman and partner verbalize understanding of various modes of sexual expression (which are safe, which to avoid) and of medical acceptance of sexual intercourse with penile penetration until rupture of membrane; feelings of frustration and resentment over abstinence expressed early in third trimester and acceptance expressed toward end of third trimester.

B. Knowledge and skills
1. Woman or couple verbalizes understanding of physiologic basis, need for immediate treatment, and how to obtain necessary care for complications of pregnancy.
2. Woman or couple verbalizes understanding of physiologic basis, prevention, and treatment of problems common to third trimester.
3. Woman and family verbalize understanding of rationale for answers to common questions.
4. Woman and family verbalize
   a. Understanding of fetal development, fetal heart rate, and fetal movements, and maternal adaptation and status.
   b. Understanding of fetal and maternal needs during pregnancy.
5. Woman and family verbalize understanding of maternal and fetal nutritional needs.
   a. Physical response indicates compliance with nutritional counsel.
   b. Verbalizes understanding of choices regarding infant feeding.
6. Verbalizes understanding of choices and availability of prenatal education classes.
7. Woman seeks assistance for problems such as

Summary of Nursing Actions—cont'd

infections, colds, allergies, and substance abuse (smoking or drinking).

8. Verbalizes readiness for labor.
   a. Expresses eagerness to be done with pregnancy; complaints about awkwardness, annoyance about symptoms (shortness of breath and backache) expressed; questions asked about how soon appearance will be back to "normal."
   b. Interest centered around preparing for labor and delivery.
   c. Expresses anxiety over pain in labor, behavior during labor, care of other children.
9. Verbalizes understanding of preparation for delivery; symptoms of impending labor (i.e., uterine contractions, rupture of membranes, bloody "show"), what to report, and where to go for delivery.
10. Verbalizes understanding of delivery process.
11. Requests information about care for new baby:
    a. Plans for care of newborn; help at home; preparation of siblings.

C. Physical care
   1. Maternal
      a. Appearance is healthy, grooming adequate, energy level normal.
      b. Temperature-pulse-respiration, blood pressure, weight
         (1) Temperature, normal range
         (2) Pulse, gradual rise of +8 to +10 by thirty-fifth week
         (3) Respirations, 18-20/min; occasional shortness of breath and sighing breaths may be troublesome at times.
         (4) Blood pressure, systolic no greater than +30 and diastolic no greater than +15 over baseline, which is normally higher (+6 to +10) as term approaches.
         (5) Weight gain, week 27 to term: no more than 1 lb. (0.45 kg) per week; approximately 27 ± 4 lb (11 kg) gain over prepregnancy weight (less than 20 lb [9 kg] puts fetus at risk).
         (6) Edema, dependent edema of lower legs, ankles, and feet.
      c. Abdomen, enlargement continues: see fundal height. Near end of pregnancy striae gravidarum may occur; in multipara glistening silvery striae from earlier pregnancies may be seen. Linea nigra at midline of abdomen.

d. Uterus, continued progressive enlargement of uterus.
   (1) Fundal height at 36 weeks: almost to xiphoid process; 40 weeks; 2 cm below caused by "lightening."
   (2) Readiness for labor: Braxton Hicks contractions may be felt.
e. Fetus, FHR, and rhythm are normal (120-160 beats/min) and regular; will be less if fetus is asleep and greater with fetal movement.
   (1) Fetal movements increase with maternal movements, may lessen during fetal sleep, same pattern of movements every 24 hours.
   (2) Fundal heights, abdominal growth and estimation of weight within normal limits for the estimated gestational age; presentation, size of infant and maternal pelvic configuration permit vaginal delivery.
   (3) Engagement occurs about 2 weeks before term in nullipara; may not occur until labor is well established in parous woman.
f. Skin, may develop chloasma (mask of pregnancy), vascular spiders, palmar erythema (red palms).
g. Varicose veins may appear in lower legs and vulva.
h. Pelvic examination, findings are within normal limits.
   (1) Vagina, highly distensible. Leukorrhea persists.
   (2) Cervix, readiness for labor: Cervix becomes more softened as term approaches. In parous women, external os of cervix may be about 3 cm dilated by week 35.
   (3) Pelvis, pelvic measurements adequate in relation to size of fetus (reexamined near term).
i. Breasts, striations may appear if increase in size of breasts is extensive.
   (1) Areola become larger and more deeply pigmented and glands of Montgomery's appear.
   (2) Lactogenesis begins with secretion of colostrum; may be expressed by gentle massage.
   (3) Preparation of breasts for breast feeding begins.
D. Laboratory tests; see Table 2-5.

References

Danforth DN and Scott JR, editors: Obstetrics and gynecology, ed 5, Philadelphia, 1986, JB Lippincott Co.

Dohrmann KR and Lederman SA: JOGN Nurs 15(6):446, 1986.

Horn M and Manion J: Creative grandparents: bonding the generations, JOGN Nurs 14:233, May/June 1985.

Johnsen NM and Gaspard ME: Theoretical foundations of a prepared sibling class, JOGN Nurs 14:237, May/June 1985.

Naeye RL: Weight gain and the outcome of pregnancy, Am J Obstet Gynecol 135:3, 1979.

Riordan JM: A practical guide to breastfeeding, 1983, The CV Mosby Co.

Waller, MM: Siblings in the childbearing experience, NAACOG Update Series 1: lesson 17, 1984.

UNIT

3

Normal Labor and Delivery

Labor and delivery is the culmination of months of waiting and anticipation. How a woman and her family come through it depends on preparation, maturity, past experiences, and the actions of health care professionals.

Nursing care of the woman during this time is challenging. The nurse has not one client to care for but two: the mother and the fetus. Nurses must have a firm grasp of the essential factors, processes in labor, and maternal and fetal adaptations as well as the effects of anesthesia and analgesia on both.

Correct assessment and skillful management of all the stages of labor are essential for the woman and her family to have a successful and safe outcome. Fetal monitoring is so important that standards of care have been set for it.

This unit includes important information about each stage of labor, including fetal monitoring, emergency procedures, danger signs, and client teaching. Sample nursing care plans and summaries of nursing action are found at the end of each section.

ESSENTIAL FACTORS AND PROCESSES AND MATERNAL/FETAL ADAPTATIONS

During pregnancy, the mother and the fetus prepare to accomodate themselves to each other during the labor process. The fetal-placental unit has grown and developed in preparation for extrauterine life. The mother has undergone various physiologic adaptations during the period of gestation that prepare her for the birth process and role of mother. Labor and delivery is the culmination of the childbearing cycle; it is an intense period during which the products of conception are expelled from the uterus. To implement nursing care in labor the nurse must use the nursing process. The essential factors and processes of labor must be understood along with the maternal and fetal adaptations to labor.

THE 5*ps*

Passage (Birth Canal)

A. Size of pelvis (diameters of pelvic inlet, midpelvis, outlet)
B. Types of pelvis (see Table 3-3, "Comparison of Pelvic Types")
    1. Gynecoid—classic female pelvis; favorable influence on labor
    2. Android—resembles male pelvis; unfavorable influence on labor
    3. Anthropoid—resembles pelvis of anthropoid apes; favorable influence on labor
    4. Platypelloid—flat pelvis; unfavorable influence on labor
C. Cervical dilation; distensibility of lower uterine segment; capacity for distension of pelvic floor, vaginal canal, and introitus

Passenger (see Table 3-1, "Fetal Lie, Presentation and Position")

A. Size of the fetal presenting part
B. Fetal attitude (flexion or extension)
C. Fetal lie (longitudinal or transverse)
D. Fetal presentation (part entering pelvis)
E. Fetal position (relationship of presenting part to the pelvis)
F. Number of fetuses
G. Placenta: type, sufficiency of, and site of insertion

Powers

A. Primary powers: intensity, duration, and frequency of uterine contractions
B. Secondary powers: bearing-down efforts

Psyche or Psychologic Response

1. Physical preparation for childbirth
2. Racial and sociocultural heritage
3. Previous experiences
4. Support systems
5. Emotional readiness, maturity, emotional integrity
6. Environment

Position of Mother

1. Standing
2. Walking
3. Side-lying
4. Squatting
5. Hands and Knees
6. Birthing chair

    The progress of labor depends on the interaction of the above 5 factors.

Adaptation to Labor

    The position of the fetus in utero, obstetric measurements, and the woman's pelvic type all affect the progress and character of labor. The nurse needs to understand these factors and how they affect the woman's labor. It is also important for the nurse to be aware of the adaptations made by the mother's body during the process of labor.

Table 3-1   *Fetal Lie, Presentation, and Position*

	Presenting Part	Example of Position
Longitudinal Lie		
Cephalic		
Vertex	Occiput	Left occipito-transverse (LOT)
Brow	Brow	Left brow anterior (LBA)
Face (chin) (rare)	Mentum	Right mento-posterior (RMP)
Pelvic		
Breech	Sacrum	Right sacro-anterior (RSA)
Transverse Lie		
Shoulder	Scapula	Right scapulo-anterior (RScA)

Table 3-2   *Obstetric Measurements*

Plane of inlet (superior strait). The principal pelvic diameters of the plane of the inlet are as follows:

Conjugates		
Diagonal	12.5-13 cm	From *inferior border* of symphysis pubis to sacral promontory
Obstetric: measurement that determines whether presenting part can engage or enter superior strait	1.5-2 cm less than diagonal (radiographic)	From *posterior surface* of symphysis pubis to sacral promontory (normally ≥10 cm)
True (vera) (anteroposterior)	≥11 cm (12.5) (radiographic)	From *upper margin* of symphysis pubis to sacral promontory
Transverse diameter	≥13 cm	Usually colon obscures this by filling left pelvis
Oblique diameter (R or L)	≥12.75 cm	From sacroiliac joint on one side to opposite iliopectineal prominence

Midplane of pelvis. The midplane of the pelvis normally is its largest plane and the one of greatest diameter.

Anteroposterior diameter	≥11.5 cm	From midsymphysis to sacrum (at fused second and third sacral vertebrae)
Transverse diameter (interspinous diameter)	10.5 cm	Narrowest transverse diameter in the midplane
Posterior sagittal diameter	4.5 cm	Segment of anteroposterior diameter dorsal to line between ischial spines; although midplane is comparatively large, critical shortening of interspinous or posterior sagittal diameter of midplane may cause pelvic dystocia

Plane of pelvic outlet. The outlet presents the smallest plane of the pelvic canal. It encompasses an area including the lower portion of the symphysis pubis, the ischial tuberosities, and the tip of the sacrum. The significant diameters are as follows:

Anteroposterior diameter	11.9 cm	From lower border of symphysis pubis to tip of sacrum; coccyx may be displaced posteriorly during labor and is not considered to be a fixed bone
Transverse diameter (intertuberous diameter)	≥8 cm	From inner border of one ischial tuberosity to other
Posterior sagittal diameter	9 cm	Projected from tip of sacrum to a point in space where intertuberous diameter transects anteroposterior projection

Table 3-3   *Comparison of Pelvic Types*

	Gynecoid (50% of Women)	Android (23% of Women)	Anthropoid (24% of Women)	Platypelloid (3% of Women)
Brim	Slightly ovoid or transversely rounded	Heart shaped, angulated	Oval, wider anteroposteriorly	Flattened anteroposteriorly, wide transversely
Depth	Moderate	Deep	Deep	Shallow
Side walls	Straight	Convergent	Straight	Straight
Ischial spines	Blunt, somewhat widely separated	Prominent, narrow interspinous diameter	Prominent, often with narrow interspinous diameter	Blunted, widely separated
Sacrum	Deep, curved	Slightly curved, terminal portion often beaked	Slightly curved	Slightly curved
Subpubic arch	Wide	Narrow	Narrow	Wide
Usual mode of delivery	Vaginal Spontaneous Occiput anterior position	Cesarean Vaginal Difficult with forceps	Vaginal Forceps/spontaneous occiput posterior or occiput anterior position	Vaginal Spontaneous

Table 3-4 *Maternal Anatomic and Physiologic Adaptation to Labor*

Body System	Normal Adaptation to Labor	Observable Findings
Cardiovascular		
Cardiac output	Increases; during each contraction 400 ml blood is emptied from uterus into maternal vascular system	Pulse slows BP increases No alteration in FHR
WBC	Mechanism unknown; possible WBC level changes secondary to physical/emotional stress	$\geq 25,000/mm^3$
Peripheral vascular system	Response to cervical dilation; compression of vessels by fetus passing through birth canal	Malar flush Hot or cold feet Hemorrhoids
Respiratory		
Rate	Increased physical activity with increased oxygen consumption	Rate increases
Acid/base balance	Hyperventilation may be cause of increased pH early in labor; pH returns to normal by end of first stage	None if hyperventilation is controlled
Renal		
Fluids/electrolytes	Diaphoresis Increased insensible water loss through respirations Occasionally NPO	Possible temperature elevation Thirst
Bladder	Becomes an abdominal organ starting with the second trimester	When filling, palpable above symphysis pubis
	Deterrents to spontaneous voiding: tissue edema secondary to pressure from presenting part, discomfort, sedation, embarrassment	Possible inability to void spontaneously
Urine constituents	Breakdown of muscle tissue from the physical work of labor	1 + proteinuria
Integument	Great distensibility in area of vaginal introitus; degree of distensibility varies with the individual	Minute tears in skin around vagina
Musculoskeletal	Marked increase in muscle activity (in addition to uterine activity)	Diaphoresis Fatigue 1 + proteinuria ? Increased temperature
	Backache and joint ache (unrelated to fetal position) secondary to increased joint laxity at term	Verbal/nonverbal cues indicating back discomfort
	Leg cramps secondary to labor process and pointing of toes	Verbal/nonverbal cues
Neurologic	Sensorium alterations change as woman moves through phases of first stage of labor and as she moves from one stage to the next	Euphoria to increased seriousness to amnesia between contractions to elation or fatigue after delivery
	Discomfort (see discussion on pain during childbirth)	
	Endogenous endorphins and encephalins and physiologic anesthesia of perineal tissues with decreased perception of discomfort	Verbal/nonverbal cues absent or minimal
Gastrointestinal	Mouth breathing, dehydration, emotional response to labor	Verbal/nonverbal cues indicating dry mouth
	Decreased motility and absorption; delayed stomach emptying time	Nausea/vomiting of undigested foods eaten after onset of labor
	Nausea as a reflex response to full cervical dilation	Nausea/vomiting Belching
	History of diarrhea concurrent with onset of labor or	Verbal cue
	Presence of hard or impacted stool in rectum	Palpable on vaginal examination Fecal material extruded during delivery
Endocrine	Level of estrogen decreases; levels of progesterone, prostaglandins, and oxytocin increase	Labor is initiated and maintained
	Metabolism increases	Blood glucose may decrease

FETOPELVIC RELATIONSHIPS

A. Lie—Relationship of fetal long axis to long axis of mother
   1. Longitudinal: axes are parallel
   2. Transverse or oblique: axes are perpendicular
B. Presentation—part of the fetus that lies over the inlet
   1. Cephalic (vertex, sinciput, mentum, face, brow)
   2. Breech—complete or footling
   3. Shoulder
C. Presenting part—leading or most dependent portion of fetus, lying over internal os of cervix
D. Attitude—relation of fetal body parts to each other
   1. Flexion
   2. Extension
E. Position—relation of denominator to front, back, or sides of mother's pelvis
   1. Anterior
   2. Posterior
   3. Transverse
F. Denominator—part of the presentation that indicates or determines position of fetus in utero
   1. Cephalic presentation (occiput)
   2. Breech (sacrum)
   3. Face presentation (mentum)
G. Engagement—largest transverse diameter of presentation has passed through maternal pelvic inlet or brim
H. Station—relationship of presenting part of fetus to maternal ischial spines
I. Synclitism—biparietal dimeter of fetal head parallel to planes of pelvis
J. Asynclitism—nonparallel relationship between biparietal diameter of fetal head and planes of pelvis
K. Molding—ability of fetal head to change shape and adapt to unyielding maternal pelvis

Mechanisms and Stages of Labor

Nurses should be aware of the basics of labor, such as its mechanisms, its stages, and their duration. These subjects are discussed on the following pages.

MECHANISMS OF LABOR

Engagement (when biparietal diameter of fetal head passes the pelvic inlet)

1. Nulliparas: occurs before onset of active labor
2. Multiparas: occurs during active labor due to more relaxed musculature

Descent (refers to progress of presenting part through pelvis)
1. Depends on 3 forces:
   a. Pressure of amniotic fluid
   b. Direct pressure of contracting fundus on the fetus
   C. Contraction of maternal diaphragm and abdominal muscles in second stage
2. Degree of descent is gauged by station of presenting part.
3. This continues throughout labor; all other mechanisms are superimposed on it.

Flexion (descending head meets resistance from cervix, pelvic wall, or pelvic floor; chin is brought closer to fetal chest).
1. Fetal head brought to smaller suboccipitobregmatic diameter.
2. This is accomplished by pressure.

Internal Rotation (long axis of fetal head must fit into long axis of maternal pelvis)
1. Head, which entered pelvis in transverse diameter, must rotate to anteroposterior diameter.
2. This is accomplished when contact with pelvic floor (levator ani) causes rotation 45 degrees to right (LDA → OA).

Extension (fetal head reaches perineum and is deflected anteriorly by perineum)
1. Occiput acts as fulcrum and passes through outlet slowly under lower border of symphysis pubis.
2. Nape of neck pivots in subpubic angle.
3. Head is born by extension.

Restitution and External Rotation (once head is born it rotates briefly to position it occupied when engaged in inlet-restitution)
1. External rotation occurs as shoulders engage and descend similar to head
2. Anterior shoulder is born first.

Expulsion (after delivery of shoulders, remaining fetal body is delivered by movement of lateral flexion in direction of symphysis pubis)
1. End of second stage of labor

Table 3-5 *Stages of Labor*

Stage	Duration Nullipara	Duration Multipara	Description	Source of Pain
First State				
Latent phase	20 hrs	14 hrs	More progress in effacement of cervix, little increase in descent	Hypoxia of uterine muscle cells Stretching of lower uterine segment Cervical dilation at height of contraction—no O_2 exchanged
Active phase	½ cm/hr	1.5 cm/hr	More rapid dilation of the cervix and descent of presenting part	Pressure on pelvic viscera Pain felt in lower abdominal wall and back, with greater intensity at lower back, area just above symphysis, and area over iliac crest
Second Stage	2 hrs	1.5 hrs	From full dilation of cervix to delivery of neonate	Hypoxia due to contracting uterine muscle Distension of vagina and perineum Pressure on adjacent structures as fetus descends
Third Stage	5 to 60 minutes		From delivery of neonate to delivery of placenta Placental separation begins with contraction that delivers baby's trunk and is completed with first contraction after birth of baby	Uterine contractions Cervical dilation as placenta is expressed
Fourth Stage	Approximately 2 hrs after delivery of placenta		Period of immediate recovery Homeostasis reestablished by "living ligature" of uterine myometrium	Contraction of uterine muscle

PHARMACOLOGIC CONTROL OF DISCOMFORT

Nursing management of obstetric analgesia and anesthesia combines the nurse's expertise in maternity care with a knowledge and understanding of anatomy and physiology, and of medications and their desired and undesired side effects and methods of administration.

Anesthesia encompasses analgesia, amnesia, relaxation, and reflex activity. It is the abolition of pain perception by interrupting the nerve impulses going to the brain. Analgesia is a component of anesthesia. The term *analgesia* is best reserved to describe only the alleviation of the sensation of pain or the raising of one's threshold for pain perception. An *agonist* is an agent that does something; an *antagonist* is an agent that blocks something from happening.

Table 3-6   *Comparison of Modalities for Obstetric Analgesia*

Therapeutic Modality/Drug	Usual Parenteral Dose	Time of Administration	Advantages for Parturient	Disadvantages for Neonate	Nursing Concerns
Psychoprophylaxis		Late pregnancy Labor stages 1-3	No drugs Training in self-reliance	None	Pain controlled but not eliminated
Hypnosis		Late pregnancy Labor stages 1-3	No drugs In rare women, pain free	None	Suggestion reinforcement essential
Medications *Sedatives*					
Secobarbital sodium (Seconal)	50-100 mg IM	Early stage 1, midstage 1, or postdelivery	Disinhibition or somnolence (no pain relief in usual doses)	Hypoactive "sleepy" neonate	Either subdued or excited; may become dehydrated
Pentobarbital (Nembutal) sodium	50-100 mg IM				
Narcotic Analgesics					
Morphine	8-15 mg IM or IV	Midstage 1	Analgesia excellent	Moderate to marked CNS depression if delivery <2 hr after administration	Emesis common
Meperidine	50-100 mg IM or IV	Midstage 1	Analgesia good	Slight CNS depression	Routine care
Narcotic Agonist-Antagonist Compounds					
Butorphanol tartrate (Stadol)	1-3 mg IM; 0.5-2 mg IV	Midstage 1	Analgesia without respiratory depression	None anticipated; monitor for CNS depression	If woman is dependent on narcotics, reversal of narcotic effect results in withdrawal symptoms
Nalbuphine (Nubain)	0.2 mg/kg SC/IM; 0.1-0.2 mg/kg IV				
Narcotic Antagonist					
Naloxone (Narcan)	Adult—0.4 mg IM or IV; Neonate—0.01 mg/kg body weight, IV or SC	Stage 2 or to neonate	Reverses narcotic side effects (nausea, vomiting, tachycardia, hypertension, pruritus, respiratory depression)	None	Abrupt reversal of narcotic effect; withdrawal symptoms in narcotic addicts
Analgesic-Potentiating Drugs (Ataractics, Tranquilizers)					
Promethazine (Phenergan)	25-50 mg IM	Early stage 1, midstage 1, and postdelivery	Apprehension, anxiety, depression relieved; narcotic effects potentiated; antiemetic	Drug enhances narcotic effect (CNS depression)	Closer supervision may be necessary because of mild pseudohypnotic state
Hydroxyzine pamoate (Vistaril)	25-50 mg IM or SC				
Promazine (Sparine)	50 mg IM				

Summary of Nursing Actions—cont'd

PHARMACOLOGIC CONTROL OF DISCOMFORT

I. Goals
  A. For the mother: to achieve adequate pain relief without adding to maternal risk.
  B. For the unborn and newborn: to maintain well-being and adjustment to extrauterine life.
  C. For the family: to know of their needs and rights in relation to use of analgesia or anesthesia.
II. Priorities
  A. Differentiate between the woman's need for pharmacologic control and her need for physiologic control of discomfort.
  B. Select the most effective techniques for each woman.
  C. Prepare the medication and administer it correctly.
  D. Monitor the effects of pharmacologic control on maternal, fetal, and newborn well-being and on maternal pain relief.
III. Assessment
  A. Interview
    1. Health history: allergies or unusual reactions to medications
    2. Psychosocial: level of understanding of analgesia or anesthesia; preferences; assessed need for pharmacologic relief; fatigue
    3. Review of systems: present respiratory problem (cold); amount, type, time of last food taken
  B. Physical examination
    1. Vital signs, blood pressure, fetal heart rate (FHR); uterine contractions, station, effacement and dilatation; degree of hydration
  C. Laboratory tests: none specific
  D. Informed consent, obtained before woman is sedated
  E. Physician's orders
  F. Before administration of analgesia or anesthesia:
    1. Labor: contractions, cervical effacement and dilatation, station; FHR; maternal response and desire for medication
    2. Degree of hydration: input and output; moisture of mucous membranes, skin turgor, temperature
    3. Bladder distension
    4. Client understanding of the analgesia or anesthesia to be administered
  G. During administration of analgesia/anesthesia
    1. Maternal or fetal response
  H. Following administration of analgesia/anesthesia
    1. Safety precautions: side rails; use of restraints on stirrups
    2. Labor: maternal or fetal response (as just given)
    3. Bladder distension
IV. Potential nursing diagnoses
  A. Ineffective breathing pattern
  B. Altered health maintenance
  C. Potential for injury
  D. Anxiety
  E. Fear
  F. Knowledge deficit
  G. Powerlessness

H. Potential for trauma
I. Impaired physical mobility
J. Personal identity disturbance
K. Self esteem disturbance: situational low self esteem
L. Body image disturbance
M. Ineffective individual coping
N. Pain
O. Alteration in tissue perfusion (fetal): cerebral, cardiopulmonary, renal, gastrointestinal, peripheral
P. Potential fluid volume deficit
Q. Spiritual distress
R. Sensory/perceptual alterations (specify)
S. Altered patterns of urinary elimination
T. Sleep pattern disturbance
U. Altered nutrition: less than body requirements
V. Fatigue
W. Activity intolerance
V. Plan/implementation
  A. Support person
    1. Provides explanation of procedure and what will be asked of the woman (e.g., to maintain flexed position during insertion of epidural).
    2. Coaches woman regarding sensations she can expect.
  B. Teacher/counselor/advocate
    1. Reviews or validates woman's choices for relief from discomfort.
    2. Clarifies mother's information, as necessary
    3. Describes how medication is to be given, degree of discomfort to expect from administration of medication, skin preparation, time requirement for administration, interval before medication "takes hold"
    4. Explains need for keeping bladder empty
  C. Technician
    1. Monitors labor: contractions, cervical effacement and dilatation, descent, status of membranes.
    2. Monitors maternal and fetal response to labor: vital signs, blood pressure, and fetal heart rate.
    3. Monitors maternal perception of, response to, and coping with discomfort.
    4. Assists mother to keep bladder empty.
    5. Assists mother with position changes, hygiene needs, fluids and calories, as needed.
    6. Initiates and maintains intravenous infusions.
    7. Administers medications as needed.
    8. During administration of anesthesia:
      a. *Ensures safety* by selecting wrapped supplies that are sterile and are not outdated; prepares mother's skin (nurse [and physician] practices *good handwashing techniques*).
      b. Aids woman in assuming proper position and assists her in maintaining it.
      c. Assists physician, as appropriate, if needed; opens sterile trays and packages; adds medications.

Continued.

Summary of Nursing Actions—cont'd

9. After the procedure the nurse does the following:
   a. Repeats all nursing actions implemented when preparing the woman for the procedure.
      (1) Answers questions.
      (2) Keeps woman's bladder empty.
      (3) Monitors vital signs, blood pressure, contractions, and FHR.
   b. Monitors and records woman's response to medication:
      (1) Level of pain relief.
      (2) Return of sensations and perception of pain.
      (3) Allergic or untoward reactions (e.g., hypotension).
   c. Raises side rails; places call bell in easy reach; monitors medicated woman closely. Avoids prolonged pressure on an anesthetized part (e.g., lying on one side with weight on one leg; tight bed clothes on feet). If stirrups are used, pads stirrups; adjusts stirrups at same level and angle; places both legs into stirrups simultaneously and avoids pressure to popliteal angle; applies restraints without restricting circulation.
10. Maintains records.

VI. Evaluation
   A. Before administration of analgesia/anesthesia:

1. Woman decides on the type of medication she wants.
2. Woman states she understands the medication selected.
3. Woman signs the Informed Consent form.
   B. During administration of analgesia/anesthesia:
   1. Injury does not occur from needle if woman moves during injection.
   2. Woman receives the correct medication and dose by the appropriate method.
   3. Aseptic technique is used.
   C. After administration of analgesia/anesthesia:
   1. Injury does not occur from falls or from prolonged pressure on anesthetized tissues.
   2. Physician is informed when
      a. Pain sensation returns.
      b. Maternal vital signs change.
      c. Uterine contractions change (decrease in intensity, frequency, duration).
      d. FHR pattern changes.
   3. Hydration is maintained with solutions such as lactated Ringer's.
   4. Nurse maintains records.
      a. Evidence of need for medication.
      b. Medication: type, amount, dose, time, route of administration.
      c. Effects of woman ("discomfort lessened") or effects on fetus ("FHR 140").

FETAL MONITORING

Fetal monitoring is one of the newest technologic advances in maternal child health and is surrounded by controversy and uncertainty. The nurse must be competent in this skill to care for the mother and fetus safely. Competence is based on an understanding of the stress that labor places on the fetus and recognition of both normal and abnormal fetal responses to uterine contractions.

Since labor represents a period of stress for the fetus, continuous monitoring of fetal health is instituted as part of the nursing care during labor. The fetal oxygen supply must be maintained during labor to prevent severe debilitating conditions after birth. Fetal stress can result in death in utero or shortly after birth. The fetal oxygen supply can be reduced in a number of ways:

1. Reduction of blood flow through the maternal vessels as a result of maternal hypertension or hypotension (systolic blood pressure of 100 mm Hg in brachial artery is necessary for placental perfusion)
2. Reduction of the oxygen content of the maternal blood as a result of hemorrhage or severe anemia
3. Alterations in fetal circulation, occurring with compression of the cord, placental separation, or head compression (Head compression causes increased intracranial pressure and vagal nerve stimulation with slowing of the heart rate.)

Fetal well-being during labor is measured by the *response of the FHR to uterine contractions*. In general, normal, active labor is characterized by:

1. An FHR between 120 and 160 beats/min with normal baseline variability and no ominous periodic changes.
2. Uterine contractions with the following characteristics (Tucker, 1978):
   a. Frequency of every 3 to 5 minutes
   b. Duration of 30 to 60 seconds
   c. Intensity resulting in a rise in intrauterine pressure to 50 to 70 mm Hg at the peak of a contraction
   d. An average resting intrauterine pressure of between 8 and 15 mm Hg

Fetal Blood Sampling. The blood sample is obtained from the fetal scalp transcervically after rupture of membranes. The scalp is swabbed with a disinfecting solution before the puncture is made. Fetal acidosis follows fetal hypoxia, and some perinatologists insist that true fetal distress can be diagnosed only when serious FHR changes can be correlated with fetal blood acidosis (pH $\leq$ 7.20).

Most infants who have low Apgar scores have scalp blood readings of pH 7.15 or less. If there are consecutive blood samples with a pH below 7.20, prompt delivery of the infant is imperative.

The normal values are:

pH: 7.25 to 7.35
O_2 saturation: 30% to 50%
Po_2: 18 to 22 torr.
Pco_2: 40 to 50 torr.
Base excess: 0 to -10 mEq/L.

Meconium-Stained Amniotic Fluid. The passage of meconium from the fetal bowel before birth may indicate fetal distress. Peristalsis of the bowel increases during hypoxia, and the contents are likely to be expelled. Although the presence of meconium-stained amniotic fluid is not always an indication of fetal difficulty, its presence requires immediate notification of the physician.

Electronic Fetal Monitoring

Electronic fetal monitoring has become a virtually routine aspect in the care of women in labor. The nurse should become familiar with the various modes used in fetal monitoring and must adhere to nursing standards set by NAACOG regarding this nursing function. This section concludes with a summary of nursing actions to help the nurse to provide competent, comprehensive care.

Table 3-7 *External and Internal Modes of Monitoring*

External Mode	Internal Mode
Fetal Heart Rate (FHR) *Ultrasound transducer:* High-frequency sound waves reflect mechanical action of the fetal heart. Used during the antepartum and intrapartum period. *Phonotransducer:* Microphone amplifies sound, reflects excessive noise when woman is in labor. Used infrequently for antepartum monitoring. *Abdominal electrodes:* Fetal ECG is obtained when electrodes are properly positioned. Used infrequently for antepartum monitoring because of ease and reliability of ultrasound transducer.	*Spiral electrode:* Electrode converts fetal ECG as obtained from the presenting part to FHR via a cardiotachometer. This method can only be used when membranes are ruptured and cervix is sufficiently dilated during the intrapartum period. Electrode penetrates fetal presenting part 1.5 mm and must be on securely to ensure a good signal.
Uterine Activity *Tocotransducer:* This instrument monitors frequency and duration of contractions by means of pressure-sensing device applied to the maternal abdomen. Used during both the antepartum and intrapartum periods.	*Intrauterine catheter:* This instrument monitors frequency, duration, and *intensity of contractions.* Catheter filled with sterile water is compressed during contractions, placing pressure on a strain gauge converting the pressure into millimeters of mercury on the uterine activity panel of the strip chart. It can be used when membranes are ruptured and cervix is sufficiently dilated during the intrapartum period.

Table 3-8 *Nursing Standards: Electronic Fetal Monitoring**

Fetal Heart Rate Patterns	Characteristics	Clinical Significance	Nursing Interventions
Baseline changes 1. Tachycardia	Normal 120-160 bpm	Smooth or flat baseline—(no variability: 0-2 bpm): warning sign of fetal problems	Count baseline rate between contractions.
a. Moderate	160-180 bpm		None
b. Marked	Above 180 bpm	May be ominous when associated with late or variable decelerations and absence of variability	Collaborate with physician in alleviating primary cause. Monitor maternal vital signs closely, change maternal position (left lateral preferred). Check hydration status and increase rate of maintenance intravenous fluid until specific order can be obtained from physician. Administer oxygen at 5 L/min.† Observe for presence of meconium-stained fluid.
2. Bradycardia			
a. Moderate	100-120 bpm, transitory		Check maternal pulse.
b. Marked	Below 100 bpm	Ominous sign when associated with loss of variability or when preceded by or associated with late or variable decelerations	Check maternal pulse. Change maternal position (left lateral preferred). Increase rate of maintenance intravenous until specific order can be obtained from physician. Discontinue Pitocin drip, if infusing. Administer oxygen at 5 L/min. Observe for presence of meconium-stained fluid. Notify physician.
3. Variability	Normal fluctuations of fetal baseline. Refers to the intervals between beats.	Represents fetal reserve	
a. Marked			None
b. Average			None
c. Minimal		May be ominous if associated with changing baseline or decelerations	Observe closely for signs of decelerations and absence of variability. Optimize fetal blood flow by changing maternal position. Notify physician.
d. Absent		Ominous sign of fetal distress when preceded by a period of acute insult	Change maternal position (left lateral preferred). Increase rate of maintenance intravenous until specific order can be obtained from physician. Administer oxygen at 5 L/min. Observe for presence of meconium-stained fluid. Notify physician.

From Blank JJ: Electronic fetal monitoring: nursing management defined, JOGN Nurs **14**:463, Nov/Dec, 1985.

*As part of fetal assessment and in keeping with NAACOG standards, the intrapartum nurse has the responsibility of observing, assessing, evaluating information received from the fetal monitor, and intervening appropriately. The ability to recognize and interpret FHR patterns and uterine activity is inherent in the nurse's role in EFM.

†Some hospital protocols specify 10-12 L/min.

Table 3-8, cont'd   *Nursing Standards: Electronic Fetal Monitoring*

Fetal Heart Rate Patterns	Characteristics	Clinical Significance	Nursing Interventions
4. Sinusoidal	Predominant pattern of rhythmic long-term variability with absence of beat-to-beat changes	When persistent, this pattern may be ominous.	Collaborate with physician in determining the significance and treatment of this pattern.
Decelerations 1. Early	Uniform shape, onset, and recovery correspond with contraction Repetitive Degree of deceleration usually not exceeding 110 bpm	Indicates head compression	None
2. Late	Uniform shape with late onset (usually 20 sec after beginning of contraction) Depth of deceleration proportional to amplitude of contraction Repetitive	May be ominous sign, especially when associated with change in baseline and absence of variability	Change maternal position, (left lateral preferred). Increase rate of maintenance intravenous until specific order can be obtained from physician. Discontinue Pitocin if infusing. Administer oxygen at 5 L/min. Observe for presence of meconium-stained fluid. Notify physician. Anticipate fetal scalp sampling.
3. Variable deceleration a. Mild	Variable shape with sudden drop not to go below 80, lasting less than 30 s Onset can be anytime. Recovery occurs rapidly. Baseline rate and variability remain unchanged.		Try alternate positions to minimize effects of cord compression. Notify physician.
b. Deep	Variable shape with sudden drop below 80 lasting longer than 30 s Onset can be any time. Recovery slow, may be accompanied by overshoot of baseline. Associated with rising or falling baseline or decrease in variability	May be ominous pattern when associated with changing baseline and loss of variability	Try alternate position to minimize effects of cord compression. Increase rate of maintenance intravenous fluid until order can be obtained from physician. Discontinue Pitocin if infusing. Administer oxygen at 5 L/min. Notify physician.
4. Prolonged deceleration	Drop in fetal heart rate at least 30 bpm, lasting 2½ min or more. Not necessarily in relation to contraction pattern.		Collaborate with physician in eliminating primary cause such as hyperstimulation. Alternate maternal position (left lateral preferred). Increase rate of maintenance intravenous until order can be obtained from physician. Discontinue Pitocin if infusing. Check maternal BP and pulse. Administer oxygen at 5 L/min. Observe for presence of meconium-stained fluid. Notify physician.

Summary of Nursing Actions

FETAL HEART MONITORING

I. Goal
  A. To maintain fetal well-being during labor and delivery.
II. Priorities
  A. To maintain adequate fetal oxygenation
  B. To identify and treat fetal distress
III. Assessment
  A. The interview, physical examination, and laboratory tests reveal normal findings.
  B. Woman does not report any changes in fetal movement.
IV. Potential nursing diagnoses
  A. Altered health maintenance
  B. Knowledge deficit
  C. Potential for injury
  D. Fear
  E. Anxiety
V. Plan/implementation
  A. Support person
    1. To allay anxiety, the nurse:
      a. Explains the basic functions of the monitor.
      b. Describes briefly the type of information printed on the upper and lower panels of the chart paper.
      c. Explains that the information regarding fetal status can be assessed continuously, even during contractions.
      d. Explains that although the digital display cannot print out every heart beat, it provides a sampling of FHR.
      e. Explains that the flucuations and variability in the heart rate result in numbers such as 88 and 156 when the baseline rate is actually 120 beats/min.
    2. To reassure and encourage some women, set the volume to an audible beep.
  B. Teacher/advocate/counselor
    1. To help gravida and family to adapt learning from prepared childbirth classes:
      a. Teaches them to effleurage upper thighs instead of abdomen.
      b. Teaches them to look at monitor to identify onset of the contraction to coach her to start the desired breathing sequence before she senses the contraction. The coach can note the peak of the contraction and relay this information to the woman so that she knows the contraction is half over and that the intensity will diminish.

    2. To assist couples who are adamantly opposed to the fetal monitor:
      a. Notes that the physician has obtained a signed informed consent.
      b. Answers questions as necessary.
      c. Monitors FHR intermittently per hospital protocol.
  C. Technician
    1. To ensure the woman's comfort and proper functioning of the monitor:
      a. Cleans the ultrasound transducer and reapplies transmission gel every 2 hours as needed.
      b. Repositions the belts and tocotransducer every 1 to 2 hours; massages any reddened areas; provides a light dusting of powder under the belts often.
      c. Repositions the leg plate strap when ECG paste is reapplied.
      d. Uses a checklist to trouble-shoot the monitor.
        (1) Avoids dropping the transducers.
        (2) Avoids tight rolling of the cords (damages the wires and leads to an unsatisfactory signal).
    2. If an abnormal tracing appears, to ensure fetal wellbeing, the nurse immediately effects the following measures.
      a. Changes the woman's position from supine to side or from one side to another.
      b. Administers oxygen by mask (10 to 12 L/min).
      c. Stops oxytocin administration; changes to bottle of Ringer's lactate solution or 5% dextrose in water and increases drip rate to deliver 80 to 125 ml/h or more.
      d. Notifies the physician of the tracing and the effect of repositioning and oxygen administration.
      e. Completes preparation for cesarean delivery if the pattern persists.
VI. Evaluation
  A. FHR and pH remain within normal limits; no meconium-stained amniotic fluid is seen.
  B. Gravida receives nursing care specific to the mode of monitoring used.
  C. Gravida and family understand functions of the monitor.
  D. Gravida is able to use learning derived from prepared childbirth classes.
  E. The monitor functions accurately.

FIRST STAGE OF LABOR

Nursing care of the woman during the first stage of labor is directed toward safe delivery of a live, healthy baby and a happy and fulfilling childbirth experience. The first stage of labor begins with the onset of regular uterine contractions and culminates when the cervix has reached full dilation. Care of the woman in labor begins with the woman's report of the following:

1. Onset of progressive, regular uterine contractions that increase in strength and frequency
2. Rupture of the membranes
3. Bloody vaginal discharge (bloody show)

When the woman arrives in labor, the nurse must make a thorough assessment of her status, including the signs and symptoms she exhibits. It is helpful to have her prenatal records available for review; most hospitals keep them handy. Important information for her care can be made part of her labor chart.

Table 3-9   *Minimum Assessment of Progress of First Stage of Labor*

	Cervical Dilation		
	0-5 cm	6-7 cm	8-10 cm
Vital signs*	Every 4 hr	Every 4 hr	Every 4 hr
Blood pressure	Every 60 min	Every 30 min	Every 30 min
Contractions	Every 30 min to 1 hr	Every 15 min	Every 5-10 min
Fetal heart rate (FHR)	Every 15 min†	Every 15 min†	Every 15 min†
Show	Every 60 min	Every 30 min	Every 10-15 min
Behavior, appearance, energy level	Every 30 min	Every 15 min	Every 5 min
Vaginal examination‡	To be done only for following reasons:		

1. To confirm diagnosis when symptoms indicate change (e.g., strength, duration, or frequency of contractions; increase in amount of bloody show; membranes rupture; or woman feels pressure on her rectum)
2. To determine whether dilation and descent are sufficient for administration of anesthetic
3. To reassess progress if labor takes longer than expected
4. To determine station of presenting part

*If membranes have ruptured, check temperature every 2 hours.
†For a period of 30 seconds immediately after a uterine contraction (Zuspan and Quilligan, 1982).
‡In presence of vaginal bleeding, physician performs vaginal examination, usually under double setup.

Table 3-10   *Maternal Progress in First Stage of Labor Within Normal Limits*

	Phases Marked by Cervical Dilation*		
Criterion	0-3 cm	4-7 cm	8-10 cm Transition
Duration	About 8-10 hr	About 3 hr	About 1-2 hr
Contractions			
Magnitude (strength)	Mild	Moderate	Strong to expulsive
Rhythm	Irregular	More regular	Regular
Frequency	5-30 min apart	3-5 min apart	2-3 min apart
Duration	10-30 sec	30-45 sec	45-60 (few to 90) sec
Descent			
Station of presenting part	Nulliparous: 0	About +1 to +2 cm	+2 to +3 cm
	Multiparous: 0 to −2 cm	About +1 to +2 cm	+2 to +3 cm

*The pace of progress in cervical dilation (according to Friedman and Sachtleben, 1965) varies as follows: from 0 to 2 cm (**latent phase**), progress is slow; from 2 to 4 cm (**phase of acceleration**), pace quickens; from 4 to 9 cm (**phase of maximal acceleration**), pace is most rapid; and from 9 to 10 cm (**phase of deceleration**), pace slows again.
In the nullipara, effacement is often complete before dilation begins; in the multipara, it occurs simultaneously with dilation.

Continued.

Table 3-10, cont'd. *Minimum Maternal Progress in First Stage of Labor Within Normal Limits*

	Phases Marked by Cervical Dilation*		
Criterion	0-3 cm	4-7 cm	8-10 cm Transition
Show			
Color	Brownish discharge, mucous plug or pale, pink mucus	Pink to bloody mucus	Bloody mucus
Amount	Scant	Scant to moderate	Copious
Behavior and appearance	Excited; thoughts center on self, labor, and baby; may be talkative or mute, calm or tense; some apprehension; pain controlled fairly well; alert, follows directions readily; open to instructions	Becoming more serious, doubtful of control of pain, more apprehensive; desires companionship and encouragement; attention more inner directed; fatigue evidenced; malar flush; has some difficulty following directions	Pain described as severe; backache common; feelings of frustration, fear of loss of control, and irritability surface; vague in communications; amnesia between contractions; writhing with contractions; nausea and vomiting, especially if hyperventilating; hyperesthesia; circumoral pallor, perspiration on forehead and upper lips; shaking tremor of thighs; feeling of need to defecate, pressure on anus

Procedures

Certain procedures are performed in the labor and delivery room, and the practitioner must be prepared to perform them (or assist) skillfully and efficiently. The following pages present nursing actions and rationales for the most commonly performed procedures.

Procedure 3-1

PERFORMING OR ASSISTING WITH A VAGINAL EXAMINATION

DEFINITION

The periodic assessment of the condition of the cervix, membranes, and fetus before and during labor.

PURPOSE

To assess the cervix: degree of softness (readiness for labor), effacement, and dilation.
To assess fetal presentation and position.
To assess degree of fetal descent or station.
To assess degree of molding of the fetal head, if presenting.
To assess the membranes: intact, bulging, or ruptured.
To assess how well the presenting part is applied to the cervix.
To assess the presence and amount of stool in the maternal rectum.
To apply internal fetal monitor (scalp clip).
To insert intrauterine pressure catheter for internal monitoring of uterine contractions.

EQUIPMENT

Sterile gloves.
Antiseptic solution, sterile water, or water-soluble gel.
Drapes.
Light source.
Nitrazine (Litmus) paper.
Intrauterine pressure catheter (optional).
Scalp clip (optional).

Procedure 3-1—cont'd

NURSING ACTIONS	RATIONALE
Assess for vaginal bleeding, one indication of placenta previa, a cause of life-threatening hemorrhage.	To prevent hemorrhage should a placenta previa exist.
If no bleeding is present, ask woman to empty her bladder.	To increase maternal comfort and facilitate accurate assessment.
Drape appropriately.	To respect woman's modesty and to protect privacy.
Position light source.	To permit visualization of vulva.
Assist woman to a supine position with one pillow under her head and her knees flexed and separated.	To facilitate examination. To relax abdominal musculature and increase comfort.
Place small rolled towel under woman's right hip.	To displace uterus to the left, off major blood vessels to prevent supine hypotension syndrome.
Wash hands, apply gloves, or help examiner put on gloves.	To maintain asepsis for the mother and the examiner.
Lubricate examining fingers with sterile water, antiseptic solution or water-soluble gel.	To facilitate examination; maintain asepsis; prevent interference with reading of Nitrazine (Litmus) paper when water is used.
Separate labia with one gloved hand, introduce middle and index finger of examining hand into vagina with palmar surface downward. Maintain downward pressure toward less sensitive posterior vaginal wall.	To prevent rolling of labia into vagina as fingers of examining hand enter vagina and to aid in preventing infection. To lessen discomfort by directing pressure toward less sensitive posterior vaginal wall.
Curl last two fingers.	To lessen chance of contamination or infection from anal area.
Place other hand on uterine fundus and exert a gentle downward pressure.	To facilitate assessment by steadying the fetus and applying the presenting part to the cervix.
Rotate fingers as necessary to complete assessment of fetus, station, cervix, status of amniotic membrances, and rectal fullness.	To perform assessment. To assess need for enema, if physician deems necessary.
Coach woman with breathing and focusing.	To assist with perineal relaxation.
Remind woman to keep her eyes open and her hands relaxed.	To assist woman to relax perineum and "stay in control."
If woman shows signs of supine hypotension or vasovagal syncope (i.e., she becomes pale, breathless, and faint, with clammy skin), turn her on her left side.	To relieve the signs and symptoms.
After completing the examination, clean the woman's vulva and place a clean pad on bed under her; Dispose of soiled articles per hospital protocol, remove and discard gloves, and wash hands, reposition bed covers according to woman's preference.	To increase comfort, both physical and emotional. To implement universal precautions when handling body fluids To maintain cleanliness and decrease possibility of infection. To respect woman's dignity.
Answer any questions about the findings.	To help decrease anxiety and increase woman's (couple's) sense of control over the situation.
Enter initial findings on admission form:	To establish data base to compare future findings.

Cervix		To provide data base for next steps in the nursing process.
Dilation	0 to 10 cm	
Effacement	0 to 100%	
Consistency	Thick/firm to soft ("ripe")	
Position	Anterior/posterior	To promote collaboration with other members of the health care team.
Fetus		
Presentation and position	Vertex, left occipito-anterior	
Station	Floating to 0 to +4	

Procedure 3-2

ABDOMINAL PALPATION: LEOPOLD'S MANEUVERS

DEFINITION

Four maneuvers for assessing fetal position by external palpation of the mother's abdomen.

PURPOSE

To identify number of fetuses.

To identify fetal presentation, lie, presenting part, degree of descent, and fetal attitude.

To identify point of maximum intensity (PMI) of FHR in relation to the woman's abdomen.

To monitor the descent and internal rotation of the fetus.

EQUIPMENT

Fetal monitoring device.

NURSING ACTIONS	RATIONALE
Wash hands	To prevent nosocomial infection.
Ask woman to empty bladder.	To increase maternal comfort during examination.
	To facilitate accurate assessment.
Position woman supine with one pillow under her head and with her knees slightly flexed.	To ensure comfort.
	To relieve tension of abdominal musculature.
Place small rolled towel under woman's right hip.	To displace uterus to left off of major blood vessels. (Avoids supine hypotensive syndrome).
If right-handed, stand at woman's right, facing her:	To facilitate examination by using dominant hand.
1. Identify fetal part that occupies the fundus. The head feels round, firm, freely movable, and palpable by ballottement; the breech feels less regular and softer.	To identify fetal lie (vertical or horizontal) and presentation (vertex or breech).
2. Using palmar surface of one hand, locate and palpate the smooth convex contour of the fetal back and the irregularities that identify the small parts (feet, hands, elbows).	To assist in identifying fetal presentation.
3. With the right hand, determine which fetal part is presenting over the inlet to the true pelvis. Gently grasp the lower pole of the uterus between the thumb and fingers, pressing in slightly. If the head is presenting and not engaged, determine the attitude of the head.	Confirms presenting part. Helps identify degree of descent. If the presenting part is not engaged, it can be rocked from side to side; if engaged, it cannot be rocked.
4. Turn to face gravida's feet. Using two hands, outline the fetal head.	When presenting part has descended deeply, only a small portion of it may be outlined.
	Palpation of cephalic prominence assists in identifying attitude of head.
	If the cephalic prominence is found on the same side as the small parts, the head must be flexed, and the vertex is presenting. If the cephalic prominence is on the same side as the back, the presenting head is extended.
Determination of PMI of FHR	
Wash hands	To prevent nosocomial infection.
Perform Leopold's maneuvers.	To locate fetal back, presentation, and position.
Auscultate FHR.	To assist in estimating PMI.
Apply monitor prn.	To assist in assessing fetal well-being.
Wash hands.	To implement universal precautions when handling body fluids.
Chart fetal presentation, position, and lie; whether presenting part is flexed or extended, engaged or free floating.	To provide data base for future findings.
	To provide data base for next steps in the nursing process.
Use hospital's protocol for charting (e.g., "Vtx, LOA, floating")	To promote collaboration with other members of the health care team.
Chart PMI of FHR using a two-line figure to indicate the four quadrants of the maternal abdomen, right upper quadrant (RUQ), left upper quadrant (LUQ), left lower quadrant (LLQ), and right lower quadrant (RLQ):	To provide data base for future comparison.
	To provide data base for nursing process.

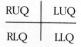

RUQ	LUQ
RLQ	LLQ

Procedure 3-2—cont'd

NURSING ACTIONS	RATIONALE
The umbilicus is the point where the lines cross. The PMI for the fetus in vertex presentation, in general flexion with the back on the mother's right side, is commonly found in the mother's right lower quadrant, and is recorded with an "x" or with the FHR as follows:	To assist other examiners.

```
      |                          |
 —————+—————      or      ——————+——————
      |                          |
  x   |                  140     |
```

Procedure 3-3

ASSISTING WITH PLACEMENT OF AN INTRAUTERINE PRESSURE CATHETER (IUPC)

DEFINITION

The use of an internal pressure catheter and transducer to monitor labor contractions.

PURPOSE

To assess contractions more accurately.
To monitor dysfunctional labor patterns.
To titrate oxytocin more accurately.

EQUIPMENT

Sterile IUPC kit.
Sterile water for injection.
10-ml syringe.
19-gauge needle.
Strain gauge apparatus, transducer, and sterile dome.

NURSING ACTIONS	RATIONALE
Wash hands before and after touching woman or equipment.	To prevent nosocomial infection and implement universal precautions.
Explain procedure to woman/couple.	To decrease anxiety and gain cooperation.
Assist woman into dorsal lithotomy position with sterile drapes under buttocks.	To assist in passage of catheter and provide a clean environment.
Using aseptic technique, open sterile kit. Attach dome to transducer and fill with sterile water; keep air bubbles out of dome.	To avoid contamination of equipment. To prepare equipment for use.
While physician is placing catheter, provide support to the woman.	To ensure accurate measurement. To help facilitate catheter insertion.
Stand by and observe while physician calibrates machine.	To ensure correct interpretation of monitor strip.
Flush catheter every hour with sterile water while monitoring.	To remove vernix or air bubbles that may enter the catheter and cause a false reading.
Ask woman to cough or apply fundal pressure periodically while observing graph.	To check functioning of catheter.
Chart insertion and functioning of catheter.	To aid in collaboration of health care team.
Apply gentle traction to remove catheter before delivery.	To allow delivery of baby without obstruction.

Procedure 3-4

TESTS FOR RUPTURE OF MEMBRANES

DEFINITION

Affirmation of rupture of membranes or leakage of amniotic fluid by using definitive diagnostic measures.

PURPOSE

To determine if membranes have ruptured. To determine if fluid leakage is urine or amniotic fluid.

EQUIPMENT

Nitrazine paper.
Sterile glove, water, swab.
Microscope, clean glass slide.
Nile blue stain.

NURSING ACTIONS	RATIONALE
Nitrazine Test for pH	
Explain procedure to woman (couple).	To diminish anxiety and assist her (them) to maintain sense of control.
Procedure	
Use Nitrazine paper, a dye 1-1 impregnated test paper for pH.	To differentiate amniotic fluid, which is slightly alkaline, from urine and purulent material (pus), which are acidic.
Wearing a sterile glove lubricated with water, place a piece of test paper at the cervical os.	To maintain asepsis.
	To avoid affecting pH.
OR	To ensure testing for amniotic fluid.
Use a sterile, cotton-tipped applicator to dip deep into vagina to pick up fluid; touch applicator to test paper.	To maintain asepsis.
	To ensure testing for amniotic fluid.
Read results:	To complete the test.
Membranes probably intact:	To identify vaginal and most body fluids that are acidic.
Yellow pH 5.0	
Olive yellow pH 5.5	
Olive green pH 6.0	
Membranes probably ruptured:	To identify amniotic fluid that is alkaline.
Blue-green pH 6.5	
Blue-gray pH 7.0	
Deep blue pH 7.5	
Realize that false tests are possible because of presence of bloody show or insufficient amniotic fluid.	To minimize misdiagnosis.
Remove gloves and wash hands.	To implement universal precautions while handling body fluids.
Chart results: positive or negative.	To provide data base.
Test for Ferning or Fern Pattern (usually performed by physician)	
Explain procedure to client/couple	To reduce anxiety.
Wash hands, apply gloves, obtain specimen of fluid.	To minimize nosocomial infection.
Spread a drop of fluid from vagina on a clean glass slide with a sterile, cotton-tipped applicator.	To prepare specimen for assessment.
	To maintain asepsis.
Allow fluid to dry.	To prepare specimen.
Assess slide under microscope: observe for appearance of ferning (a frondlike crystalline pattern) (do not confuse with cervical mucus test, when high levels of estrogen are responsible for the ferning).	To support finding of ruptured membranes.
Observe for absence of ferning.	To alert staff to possibility that specimen was inadequate or that specimen was urine, vaginal discharge, or blood.
Remove gloves and wash hands.	To implement universal precautions when handling body fluids.
Chart results, either a positive or negative fern test.	To provide a data base.
Test for Lanugo Hairs or Fetal Squamous Cells (usually performed by physician)	
Explain procedure to client/couple.	To reduce anxiety.
Wash hands and apply gloves.	To prevent nosocomial infection.

Procedure 3-4—cont'd

NURSING ACTIONS	RATIONALE
Aspirate fluid from posterior vaginal vault with sterile aspiration syringe.	To obtain specimen.
	To maintain asepsis.
Place on clean glass slide.	To prepare specimen for assessment.
Observe under microscope for presence of fetal lanugo hairs or fetal squamous cells.	To support finding of ruptured membranes.
Stain with Nile blue stain to identify fetal cells because some squamous cells that contain lipids stain yellow; other squamous cells and hairs stain blue.	To support finding of ruptured membranes.
Assess findings.	To provide data for analysis.
Remove gloves and wash hands.	To implement universal precautions when handling body fluids.
Chart results: Nile blue stain shows some squamous cells and some blue squamous cells and hair.	To provide data base.

Procedure 3-5

PREPARATION OF THE VULVA AND THE MINI-PREP

DEFINITION

The act of cutting and or shaving the pubic and perineal hairs before delivery of the baby.

PURPOSE

To cleanse the vulva.
To facilitate cutting and repairing of episiotomy.
To curtail infection.

EQUIPMENT

Soap.
Warm water.
Bedpan prn.
Underpads.
Razor (sterile, disposable) or scissors or Prep Kit.
Examination gloves.
Drape.

NURSING ACTIONS	RATIONALE
Check physician's orders.	To confirm physician's orders.
Explain procedure to woman.	To reduce anxiety.
Explain to woman that she may experience itching as the hair grows back.	To prepare woman.
Put on gloves.	To prevent nosocomial infection and to implement universal precautions while handling body fluids.
Cleanse vulvar area with soap solution or nonirritating detergent preparation: on admission, after elimination, after vaginal examination, and for vaginal discharge.	To maintain cleanliness.
	To curtail infection.
	To promote comfort.
If voided urine specimen is indicated, obtain after cleansing vulva.	To minimize potential for contamination with vaginal discharge.
Proceed with mini-prep after checking hospital protocol. A mini-prep varies with the institution and physician. It is the clipping of vulvar hair with scissors or shaving of a small area between the vagina and the anus, the site used for episiotomies.	
Use extreme care in shaving because even in expert hands the razor leaves nicks and scrapes that serve as portals of entry for infection.	To minimize danger of opening portals for infection and of inadvertently cutting off small warts or moles.
Accomplish prep quickly between contractions.	To promote comfort and minimize danger of nicking.
Following the prep, pat the area dry with a dry towel. Change to a dry underpad.	To promote comfort.

General Nursing Care

Nursing care during the first stage of labor includes physiologic, sociocultural, and emotional aspects. The nurse needs to recognize and respond to emergencies such as prolapse of the cord and inadequate uterine relaxation. This section ends with a sample care plan and a summary of nursing actions for the first stage of labor.

Table 3-11   *Fluid Intake, Voiding, Bowel Elimination, and General Hygiene: Nursing Actions and Rationales*

Need	Nursing Actions	Rationale
Fluid Intake		
Oral	Per physician's orders: Offer clear fluids, which are fluids you can see through; tea with honey and lemon, homemade broth (not salt-loaded bouillon), apple juice, and lollipops are sources of clear fluids.	Meets standard of care; provides hydration; provides calories; warm teas are used by many cultural groups to counteract the effects of heat loss during labor and delivery; absorb quickly and are less likely to be vomited; provides positive emotional experience.
	Offer small amounts of ice chips, if ordered.	Deters vomiting and its potential sequelae, aspiration, and tracheal irritation.
IV	Establish and maintain IV	IV medications can be administered quickly if needed.
Nothing by mouth (NPO)	Inform family of NPO and rationale.	A precautionary measure if anesthesia is a possibility; deters vomiting and its possible sequelae.
	Provide mouth care.	Promotes comfort.
Voiding	Encourage voiding at least every 2 hours.	A full bladder may impede descent of presenting part; overdistension may cause bladder atony and injury and difficulty in voiding postnatally.
Ambulatory	Ambulate to bathroom per physician's orders, *if*: The presenting part is engaged, or The membranes are not ruptured, and The woman is not medicated.	Reinforces normal process of labor. Precautionary measure against prolapse of umbilical cord. Precautionary measure against injury.
Bedrest	Offer bedpan.	Prevents hazards of bladder distension and ambulation.
	Turn on the tap water to run; pour warm water over the vulva; and give positive suggestion.	Encourages voiding.
	Provide privacy.	Shows respect for gravida.
	Put up side rails on bed.	Prevents injury from fall.
	Place call bell within reach.	
	Offer washcloth for hands.	Maintains cleanliness and comfort.
	Wash vulvar area.	Maintains standard of care.
Catheterization	Catheterize per physician's order per hospital protocols.	Prevents hazards of bladder distension.
	Insert catheter between contractions.	Minimizes discomfort.
	Avoid force if obstacle to insertion is noted.	"Obstacle" may be caused by compression of urethra by presenting part.
	If presenting part is low, introduce 2 fingers of free hand into introitus to apply upward pressure on presenting part while other hand inserts the catheter.	Minimizes potential for injury and subsequent infection to urethra.
Bowel elimination	After careful assessment *experienced* nurse ambulates woman to bathroom or offers bedpan.	Women often misinterpret rectal pressure from the presenting part as the need to defecate.

Table 3-11, cont'd. *Fluid Intake, Voiding, Bowel Elimination, and General Hygiene: Nursing Actions and Rationales*

Need	Nursing Actions	Rationale
General hygiene		Improves woman's morale and comfort. Maintains cleanliness.
Showers/bed baths	Assess for progress in labor.	Determines appropriateness for the activity.
	Supervise showers closely if gravida is in true labor.	Prevents injury from fall; labor may accelerate.
	Suggest allowing warm water to strike lower back.	Aids relaxation; increases comfort.
Vulva	See Procedure 3-5.	
Oral hygiene	Offer toothbrush, mouthwash, or wash the teeth with an ice-cold wet washcloth every hour.	Refreshes mouth; improves morale; helps counteract dry, thirsty feeling.
Hair	Comb, braid per gravida's wishes	Improves morale; helps maintain a "nonsick" attitude.
Hand-washing	Offer washcloths before and after voiding and prn.	Maintains cleanliness; improves morale and comfort.
Gowns/linens	Change prn; fluff pillows.	

Table 3-12 *Sociocultural Basis of Pain Experience*

	Woman in Labor	Nurse
Perception of meaning	Origin: cultural concept of and personal experience with pain; for example: Pain in childbirth is inevitable, something to be borne Pain in childbirth can be avoided completely Pain in childbirth is punishment for sin Pain in childbirth can be controlled	Origin: Cultural concept of and personal experience with pain; in addition, nurse becomes accustomed to working with certain "expected" pain trajectories. For example, in obstetrics, pain is expected to increase as labor progresses, be intermittent in character, and have end point; relief can be derived from drugs once labor is well established and fetus or newborn can cope with amount and elimination of drug; relief can also come from woman's knowledge and attitude and support from family or friends
Coping mechanisms	Woman may do the following: Be traditionally vocal or nonvocal; crying out or groaning or both may be part of her response to pain Use counterstimulation to minimize pain; for example, rubbing, applying heat, or counterpressure Have learned to use relaxation, distraction, autosuggestion as pain-countering techniques Resist any use of "needles" as modes of administering pain relief	Nurse may do the following: Have learned to use self effectively; for example, tone of voice, closeness in space, touch, as media for message of interest and caring Use avoidance, belittling, or other distancing actions as protective device for self Use pharmacologic resources at hand judiciously Be skilled in use of comfort measures Assume accountability for control and management of pain
Expectations of others	Nurse may be seen as someone who will accept woman's statement of pain and act as her advocate Medical personnel may be expected to relieve woman of all pain sensations Nurse may be expected to be interested, gentle, kindly, and accepting of behavior exhibited	Nurse may accept only certain verbal or nonverbal behaviors as responses to pain Nurse may expect couple who are prepared for childbirth to refuse medication and to wish to "do everything on their own" Nurse may find it difficult to accept woman's definition of pain; that is, woman may wish to experience and participate in controlling pain or might not be able to accept any pain as reasonable

Table 3-13   *Summary of Woman's Expected Responses and Support Person's Actions by Phase of Cervical Dilation*

	Woman	Support Person
Dilation of Cervix 0-3 cm		

Contractions 10-30 sec long, 5-30 min apart, mild to moderate
 	
Mood: alert, happy, excited, mild anxiety
	Settles into labor room; selects focal point
	Rests or sleeps if possible
	Uses breathing techniques: begin contraction with deep breath in through nose and out through pursed lips; slow chest breathing, 6-9/min through contraction; end contraction with deep breath in and out
	Uses effleurage; focusing and relaxation techniques
		Provides encouragement, feedback for relaxation, companionship
		Assists with contractions
		  Alerts woman to the following: beginning of contraction; time called out at 15 sec, 30, etc.; ending of contraction
		  Uses focusing techniques: concentration on fixed point in room; "Listen to me and follow my breathing"; "Watch my face"
		  Concentration on breathing technique
		Uses comfort measures
		  Position most comfortable for woman
		  Keeps woman aware of progress, explains procedures and routines
		  Gives praise
		  Offers ataractics as ordered

Dilation of Cervix 4-7 cm		

Contractions 30-40 sec long, 3-5 min apart, moderate to strong
 	
Mood: seriously labor oriented, concentration and energy needed for contractions, alert, more demanding
	Continues relaxation, focusing techniques
	Uses breathing techniques
	Begin contraction with deep breath in and out, then slow chest breathing until contraction intensifies, then shallow, effortless breathing, moderate pace, high in chest through peaking of contraction; slow chest breathing as contraction subsides
	OR
	Use abdominal breathing to raise abdominal wall away from uterus; end contraction with deep breathing in and out
		Acts as buffer, limits assessment techniques to between contractions
		Assists with contractions
		  May need to encourage woman to help her maintain breathing techniques
		  Uses same instructions
		  Uses same focusing devices as in early phase
		Uses comfort measures
		  Positions woman on side to minimize pressure of uterus on vena cava and aorta
		  Encourages voluntary relaxation of muscles of back, buttocks, thighs, and perineum; effleurage
		  Uses counterpressure to sacrococcygeal area
		  Encourages and praises
		  Keeps woman aware of progress
		  Offers analgesics and anesthetics as ordered
		  Checks bladder, encourages to void
		  Gives mouth care, ice chips

Dilation of Cervix 8-10 cm (transition)		

Contractions 45-60-90 sec long, 2-3 min apart, strong
 	
Mood: irritable, intense concentration, symptoms of transition
	Continues relaxation, needs greater concentration to do this
	Breathing techniques
	Uses 4:1 pattern if possible
	Uses panting to overcome response to urge to push
		Stays with woman, provides constant support
		Assists with contractions
		  Probably will need to remind, reassure, and encourage to reestablish breathing pattern and concentration
		  If sedated or drowsy, woman needs warning to begin breathing pattern before contraction becomes too intense
		  If woman begins to push, institutes panting respirations
		Uses comfort measures
		  Accepts woman's inability to comply with instructions
		  Accepts irritable response to helping, such as counterpressure
		  Supports woman who has nausea and vomiting, gives mouth care as needed, gives reassurance regarding symptomatology of end point of first stage
		  Uses countertension techniques (effleurage and voluntary relaxation)
		  Keeps woman aware of progress, tells woman when time to push

Emergency Procedure

PROLAPSE OF CORD

DEFINITION

Protrusion of the umbilical cord in advance of the presenting part.

PURPOSE

To stop compression of the umbilical cord.
To stop umbilical cord from drying out.
To facilitate a delivery that will be the least harmful to mother and fetus.

EQUIPMENT

Fetoscope or doppler; sterile gloves; towels; oxygen equipment; IV fluid and equipment; sterile, normal saline.

NURSING ACTIONS	RATIONALE
Preprocedure	
Explain what is happening to woman (couple). Explain procedure.	To reduce anxiety and elicit cooperation of woman (couple).
Procedure	
Glove the examining hand quickly and insert two fingers into the vagina to the cervix. With one finger on either side of the cord or both fingers to one side, exert upward pressure against the presenting part to relieve compression of the cord. Apply a rolled towel under the woman's right hip.	To maintain asepsis. To reinsert cord without compressing it. To stop compression from the presenting part. To stop supine hypotensive syndrome.
Place woman into extreme Trendelenburg's, modified Sims', or knee-chest position.	To allow gravity to pull presenting part down and relieve compression of the cord.
Notify physician immediately.	Delivery must be done at once.
If cord is protruding from vagina, wrap loosely in a sterile towel wet with sterile normal saline.	To stop cord from drying out and becoming nonfunctioning.
Administer oxygen by mask 10 to 12 L/min to the woman until delivery is accomplished.	To increase oxygen to fetus. To increase placental perfusion.
Start IV fluids or increase existing drip rate.	To increase circulating fluid volume to fetus. To maintain maternal blood pressure and hydration.
Deliver fetus immediately. If cervix is completely dilated, vaginal delivery is possible.	To allow for a favorable outcome and good prognosis for mother and baby.
If cervical dilation is incomplete, cesarean delivery is the method of choice.	To decrease trauma to mother and baby.
Postprocedure	
Vaginal delivery: assess mother and baby for trauma or untoward effects. Pediatrician should examine infant in nursery. Assess mother for emotional stress and trauma.	Stressful situation may have physical or emotional sequela following. Be alert for any problems. Any high-risk delivery should have a pediatrician or neonatologist in attendance to care for the infant.
Cesarean delivery: same as above, add postoperative assessment and observation of postanesthesia problems.	
Chart incident and results of treatment.	To provide data base for future comparison. To provide information for implementation of nursing process. To promote collaboration between members of health care team.

Prolapsed Cord

1. Premature rupture of membranes
2. Presenting part not engaged
3. Fetal distress or abnormal fetal heart rate pattern
4. Protruding cord from vagina

Emergency Procedure

INADEQUATE UTERINE RELAXATION

DEFINITION

Inadequate resting tone between uterine contractions. May cause fetal distress caused by poor delivery of oxygen to the placenta and fetus.

EQUIPMENT

Oxygen mask or cannula; mechanical oxygen source; IV fluid without oxytocin added.

PURPOSE

To increase uterine muscle relaxation. To increase placental perfusion.

NURSING ACTIONS	RATIONALE
Preparation	
Assess problem by monitoring labor and its effects on the fetus.	Uterine contractions are monitored continuously during labor. FHR observed for unusual patterns.
Explain procedure to client.	Elicits cooperation through understanding.
Procedure	
Change maternal position. Turn woman to her left side, if that is ineffectual, put woman in modified Sim's position.	Increases placental perfusion and increases oxygen delivered to the fetus.
Stop oxytocin infusion (if there is one running) and replace it with a plain IV.	Stops stimulation of the uterine muscle. Allows muscle to relax.
Notify physician.	Allows collaboration in decision-making and informs him/her of possible problems.
Administer oxygen by face mask or nasal cannula at 10 to 12 L per min until physician arrives and decides course of action.	Increases amounts of oxygen available to the muscle and the fetus.
Record problems observed and actions taken by medical/nursing personnel.	Provides information for future care and collaboration.

Sample Nursing Care Plan

FIRST STAGE OF LABOR

ASSESSMENT	NURSING DIAGNOSES (ND)/ PLAN (P)/GOAL (G)	RATIONALE/ IMPLEMENTATION	EVALUATION
Term pregnancy. Admission to labor unit in labor. Latent phase of labor. Assess level of knowledge.	ND: Anxiety, mild, related to excitement of onset of labor and fear of unknown. ND: Knowledge deficit related to latent phase of first stage of labor. P: Reduce anxiety by providing adequate and relevant teaching and relaxation techniques. G: Woman (and her family) verbally and nonverbally communicates less anxiety, more comfort, and ability to collaborate with her care.	*To provide reassurance and help woman relax, the nurse will:* Support woman's knowledge of labor. Explain all procedures. Answer all questions and provide information as needed. Orient women and support person to environment. Support woman's preference for breathing and relaxation techniques to be used at this time. Provide comfort measures. Monitor vital signs, FHR, and progress of labor. Provide privacy.	Woman remains calm and retains psychologic and physiologic control.
Diminished oral intake. Monitor intake and output; vital signs, FHR, blood pressure, and respirations, and amount of diaphoresis.	ND: Fluid volume deficit related to decreased intake and increased loss of fluid with the work of labor. P: Provide and maintain adequate fluid intake. G: Woman remains appropriately hydrated.	*To maintain adequate hydration the nurse will:* Explain to woman and support person why oral fluids are restricted or stopped at this time. Start and maintain an IV infusion. Provide ice chips or sips of clear fluids if allowed. Provide mouth care as needed.	Woman's temperature, skin turgor, and moisture of mucous membranes remain normal. Specific gravity of urine remains within normal limits. Woman verbalizes understanding of procedures and information given. Woman does not suffer the fatigue associated with dehydration.
Rupture of membranes: baseline data of maternal vital signs and FHR; fetal lie, station, presentation, and position; status of membranes (bulging?); character of vaginal discharge.	ND: Potential for injury, maternal and fetal, related to contamination, infection, prolapsed cord, abnormal fetal position. P: Decrease or prevent potential complications related to rupture of membranes. G: Woman and fetus are not compromised as a result of rupture of membranes.	*To prevent potential problems the nurse will:* Maintain asepsis during vaginal examinations. Change dirty linen or underpads frequently. Continue to monitor: maternal vital signs (especially temperature and pulse); FHR for tachycardia; vaginal secretions; fetal lie and position, using Leopold's maneuvers. Observe for physical signs of umbilical cord prolapse, and implement emergency procedure, prn.	Woman verbalizes understanding of procedures and information. Woman reports subjective symptoms as necessary. Woman and infant are not compromised as a result of rupture of membranes. FHR indicates continued fetal well-being. Fetal scalp pH indicates continued fetal well-being. Cesarean delivery is accomplished in a timely fashion; mother and infant are in good condition.

Continued.

Sample Nursing Care Plan—cont'd

ASSESSMENT	NURSING DIAGNOSES (ND)/ PLAN (P)/GOAL (G)	RATIONALE/ IMPLEMENTATION	EVALUATION
First stage of labor. Woman in active phase. Baseline data: maternal vital signs; FHR; labor pattern. Degree of perceived discomfort.	ND: Pain, related to increasing frequency and intensity of uterine contractions. P: Decrease maternal discomfort without compromising mother or fetus. G: Mother perceives decreased discomfort; FHR remains within normal limits.	*To provide pain relief the nurse will:* Assess woman's verbal and nonverbal communication. Promote the use of psychoprophylactic breathing techniques. Provide comfort measures. Assess vital signs, including blood pressure, FHR, frequency, and intensity of uterine contractions. Administer analgesics as ordered.	Woman verbalizes understanding of information presented. Woman participates in her care as much as possible and within her personal preferences. Baseline data remains within normal limits.
Bladder fullness.	ND: Altered patterns of urinary elimination related to discomfort, effects of analgesia, or fetal position. P: Monitor degree of bladder fullness and ensure bladder emptying. G: Bladder will be emptied periodically.	Offer bedpan frequently to avoid bladder distension; catheterize prn. Assess vaginal discharge. Assess for side effects from analgesics or anesthetics. Administer oxygen as needed. Monitor IV or po fluids.	Bladder fullness is prevented.
Woman in stressful and threatening situation.	ND: Ineffective individual coping related to anxiety, fear, and decreased problem-solving capability. P: Support woman's (family's) coping and self-esteem. G: Woman's self-esteem is maintained or increased as her perception of her behavior during labor matches her self-expectations.	*To help woman cope with increasing pain and anxiety of active labor the nurse will:* Assess anxiety level. Assess behavior of support person and its effect on the woman. Provide information. Provide comfort measures. Assist woman and support person in focusing on breathing and relaxation techniques to maintain control. Give quiet reassurance. Support woman's decisions for pain medications.	Woman remains calm and in control. Support person providing necessary help and reassurance to woman. Woman and support person express satisfaction with their behavior during labor and with the management of their labor.

Summary of Nursing Actions

NURSING CARE DURING THE FIRST STAGE OF LABOR

I. Goals
  A. For the mother: a safe and satisfying first stage of labor
  B. For the unborn: an uncompromised adjustment to the labor process
  C. For the family: an experience that fulfills their expectations for the first stage of labor
II. Priorities
  A. Validate onset of true labor.
  B. Determine maternal and fetal status.
  C. Identify and initiate immediate therapy for deviations from normal labor processes.
  D. Facilitate family's achievement of personal goals.
III. Assessment
  A. Before admission to unit
    1. Review prenatal record, if possible.
  B. Interview
    1. Health history: family history, medical history, sexual history, obstetric history, present pregnancy.
    2. Psychosocial history: identifying data such as age
    3. Review of systems
  C. Physical examination
    1. Findings during this pregnancy, such as pattern and amount of weight gain, blood pressure, symptomatology experienced, height, nutritional status
  D. Laboratory tests
    1. Hemoglobin, hematocrit, blood type, Rh, CBC, antibody titers; urinalysis; amniocentesis and ultrasound, if done; other
  E. Following admission to unit
    1. Assess general appearance and behavior.
    2. Check vital signs and blood pressure.
    3. Assess fetal status:
      a. FHR
      b. Leopold's maneuvers: fetal presentation, lie, position, engagement
      c. Fetal activity
    4. Assess for onset of true labor
    5. Assess progression of labor
      a. Contractions: time begun, intensity, frequency, regularity
      b. Vaginal discharge, bloody show
      c. Effacement and dilatation of cervix
      d. Station of presenting part
      e. Degree of molding of fetal head (if head is presenting)
    6. Assess status of amniotic membranes
      a. Bulging
      b. Ruptured: time, color, character, amount, odor
    7. Assess bladder distension; presence and amount of stool in rectum
    8. Assess for complications
      a. Inquire regarding symptoms of infection.
      b. Recheck for allergies.
      c. Check for edema.

    d. Otain specimen of urine for routine analysis and presence of albumin, glucose, and acetone.
    e. Check woman's dietary intake for last 4 hours.
    9. Assess psychologic status and support
      a. Assess psychologic status and support:
        (1) Preparation for childbirth
        (2) Expectations of woman and family
        (3) Response to first stage
IV. Potential nursing diagnoses
  A. Potential for injury
  B. Alteration in health maintenance
  C. Ineffective individual coping
  D. Ineffective family coping: compromised
  E. Impaired verbal communication
  F. Spiritual distress
  G. Altered sexuality patterns
  H. Knowledge deficit
  I. Altered nutrition: less or more than body requirements
  J. Pain
  K. Anxiety
  L. Fear
  M. Powerlessness
  N. Body image disturbance
  O. Personal identity disturbance
  P. Self esteem disturbance: situational low self esteem
  Q. Altered role performance
  R. Potential for infection
  S. Ineffective airway clearance
  T. Sensory/perceptual alteration (specify)
  U. Sleep pattern disturbance
V. Plan/implementation
  A. Admit to unit per hospital protocol; ascertain that necessary permits are signed and identification bracelet is accurate and secure.
  B. Welcome and greet by name, orient to personnel and unit, and to procedures, as necessary.
  C. Measure vital signs and blood pressure, record findings, and report any deviations from normal limits per hospital protocol and physician directives.
  D. Assist physician or midwife with general and obstetric examinations to:
    1. Determine general health of body systems.
    2. Determine diagnosis of true labor.
    3. Determine progress of labor.
    4. Determine maternal and fetal health status.
    5. Follow medical directives for preparation of vulva, administration of enema.
    6. Monitor contractions by uterine palpation or by electronic monitor; record findings; report deviations from normal limits.
    7. Share findings and their significance with gravida and family, if appropriate.
    8. Record findings and report deviations from normal limits.
    9. Complete vaginal examination using aseptic technique.

Continued.

Summary of Nursing Actions—cont'd

10. Advise gravida that ambulation and bedrest are directed by fetal station and status of amniotic membranes.
11. Following rupture of membranes, institute appropriate assessments, reporting and recording; if cord prolapses, institute emergency care.

E. Record on partogram; assess and report deviations from expected pattern for nullipara or multipara.

F. Limit dietary intake to clear fluids (ice chips) as ordered by physician.

G. Monitor intravenous fluids (may be ordered to counteract dehydration and to meet energy needs). If permitted, offer ice chips, tea with lemon and sugar, and hard sour candy suckers.

H. Encourage woman to void frequently; catheterize as necessary.

I. Provide comfort measures
1. Maintain supportive attitude: calm manner, gentleness in carrying out necessary procedures, and acceptance of gravida's definition of pain and desires for alleviation of discomfort; willingly repeat instructions and stay with gravida having unavoidable pain; orient partner to unit and inform where fluids or meals may be obtained.
2. Work through a number of contractions with gravida and husband, noting effectiveness of their method of relaxation, breathing, and other supportive techniques. If none are used, introduce techniques and coach husband in their use (for example, counterpressure against sacrum during contractions, effleurage, assuming position of comfort, breathing techniques).
3. Provide for general hygiene: showers or bed baths, if allowed; frequent washing of vulva; mouthwash and mouth care.
4. Although most women feel very warm as result of labor, a number complain of feeling cold—promote comfort by placing warm blanket over her and wrapping another around her feet; if available, apply bedsocks.
5. Maintain comfortable, quiet environment and control temperature, light, and ventilation in room.
6. Administer analgesia as ordered.
7. Assist with anesthesia as necessary.
8. Orient to unit.
9. Provide information as requested and if appropriate
10. Treat with respect (refer to them by name, offer coffee).

11. Support them if husband needs a break and if they and couple wish.
12. Involve siblings per hospital protocol.
13. Orient the babysitter to place where siblings can wait if not involved in the labor or birth or when distraction is needed.
14. Provide acceptance of behaviors.
15. Explain behavior to family.
16. Provide continual support, comfort measures, and explanations.
17. Help partner with or provide coaching.

VI. Evaluation
A. Admission routines are completed.
B. Woman, family, and personnel establish therapeutic relationship.
C. Parturient
1. Vital signs and blood pressure remain within normal limits.
2. Progress in labor is within normal limits.
3. Fluid and nutrient needs are met.
4. Elimination needs are met.
D. Stress in labor
1. Maternal and paternal stress is minimized.
2. Support person(s) participates in supporting relaxation and in providing comfort measures; partner meets self and parturient's expectations.
3. Parturient and family express satisfaction with labor experience.
4. Granparental stress is minimized or eliminated.
5. Sibling stress is minimized or eliminated.
6. Maternal behavior follows the expected course: from excited (usually) and alert to introspective (concentrating on self and and what is happening inside her); to perhaps irritable, vague in communication, amnesic between contractions: to appearance of circumoral pallor, perspiration on forehead and upper lip, shaking, belching, and feeling need to defecate.
E. Fetus
1. Perfusion of uterus is maintained as evidenced by FHR.
2. Fetal response throughout first stage indicates continued well-being, as follows:
    a. Rate: between 120-160 beats per minute
    b. Normal baseline variability
    c. No abnormal variability
    d. No periodic changes
3. Preparation for delivery is completed.
4. Records are completed concurrently with care given; all care given is documented thoroughly.

SECOND AND THIRD STAGES OF LABOR

The second stage of labor is the stage of expulsion of the fetus. It extends from full cervical dilation (10 cm) through the birth of the baby. The three phases of the second stage are latency/resting, descent, and final transition. A woman normally responds to this stage by changing body positions, pushing in response to the urge, and vocalizing as she bears down. It is extremely advantageous for the woman to have some preparation in breathing techniques that can help her maintain control of her body and the birth process. A support person can keep the laboring woman focused on the task of delivering the baby.

The third stage of labor is on the stage of separation and expulsion of the placenta. The nurse's primary responsibility at this time is to care for the newborn and to perform a minimal examination immediately following birth. A more extensive examination and assessment is performed later.

TRANSFER TO DELIVERY ROOM

Parity	Stage	Characteristic
Nulliparas	Second	When the presenting part begins to distend the perineum
Multiparas	First	When the cervix is dilated to 8 to 9 cm

Table 3-14 *Maternal Progress in Second Stage of Labor*

Criterion	Latent/Resting (10-20 min)	Descent	Final/Transition

Contractions
  Magnitude (intensity)
  Frequency
  Duration
	Period of physiologic lull for all criteria
	Period of peace and rest (Carr, 1983; Mahan and McKay, 1984)
		Significant increase
		
		2½ min
		90 sec
			Overwhelmingly strong
			Expulsive
			2½ min
			90 sec

Descent		Increases and **Ferguson's reflex*** activated	Rapid
Show: color and amount		Significant increase in dark red bloody show	Fetal head visible at introitus; bloody show accompanies birth of head
Spontaneous bearing-down efforts	Slight to absent except with peaks of strongest contractions (Carr, 1983)	Increased urgency to bear down	Greatly increased
Vocalization		Grunting sounds or expiratory vocalization (Carr, 1983; Mahan and McKay, 1984)	Grunting sounds and expiratory vocalizations continue
Maternal behavior (Carr, 1983)	Experiences sense of relief that transition to second stage is finished Feels fatigued and sleepy Feels a sense of accomplishment and optimism, since the "worst is over" Feels in control	Senses increased urgency Alters respiratory pattern: has short 4 to 5 sec breath-holds with regular breaths in between, 5-7 times per contraction Makes grunting sounds or expiratory vocalizations	Expresses sense of extreme pain Expresses feelings of powerlessness Shows decreased ability to listen or concentrate on anything but giving birth Describes the **"ring of fire"**† Often shows excitement immediately following delivery of head

*Ferguson's reflex. Pressure of presenting part on stretch receptors of pelvic floor stimulates release of oxytocin from posterior pituitary, resulting in more intense uterine contractions.

†Ring of fire. Burning sensation of acute pain as vagina stretches and fetal head crowns.

Table 3-15 *Summary of Woman's Expected Responses and Support Person's Actions by Phase of Second Stage of Labor*

Phase	Woman	Nurse/Support Person
Latent/resting	Experiences a short period (10-20 min) of peace and rest	Encourages woman to listen to her body (Carr, 1983) Continues support measures If descent phase does not begin after 20 min, suggests upright position to encourage progression of descent
Descent	Senses increased urgency to bear down as Ferguson's reflex is elicted Notes increase in intensity of uterine contractions Demonstrates change in respiratory pattern, e.g., 5-second breath-holds, 5 to 7 per contraction Makes grunting sounds or expiratory vocalizations	Endorses respiratory pattern (short breath-holds with glottis closed) Stresses normalcy and benefits of grunting sounds and expiratory vocalizations Encourages pushing *with* urge to push Encourages/suggests maternal movement and position changes (upright, if descent is not occurring) If descent is occurring, encourages woman to listen to her body regarding movement and position change Discourages long breath holding If transfer to a delivery room (DR) cannot be avoided, nurse transfers her early to avoid rushing or offers her option of walking to DR if permitted If descent is too fast, places woman in lateral recumbent position to slow descent (Carr, 1983)
Final/transitional	Behaves in manner similar to transition during first stage (8-10 cm) Experiences a sense of severe pain and powerlessness (Carr, 1983) Shows decreased ability to listen Concentrates on delivery of baby until head is born Experiences contractions as overwhelming in intensity Reports "ring of fire" as head crowns Maintains respiratory pattern of 3 to 5, 5-second breath-holds per contraction followed by forced expiration Eases head out with short expirations Responds with excitement and relief after head is born	Encourages slow, gentle pushing (Carr, 1983) Explains that "blowing away the contraction" facilitates a slower birth of the head Provides mirror or guides woman to see/touch emerging fetal head (best to extend over 2 to 3 contractions) to help her understand the perineal sensations Coaches relaxation of mouth, throat, and neck to relax pelvic floor Applies warm compresses to perineum to aid relaxation

Emergency Childbirth: When the Nurse Assists the Mother to Give Birth

Even under the best of circumstances there will probably come a time when the maternity nurse will be required to deliver an infant without medical assistance. Consider the precipitous multipara who arrives at the community hospital fully dilated in the middle of the night. As it is impossible to prevent an impending delivery, the maternity nurse needs to be able to function independently and to be skilled in safely delivering a vertex fetus.

Emergency Birth of Fetus in Vertex Presentation. The following measures are necessary for the emergency birth of a fetus in the vertex position:

1. The woman will usually assume the position most suitable for her. If she is in a bed and there is time, elevate the head of the bed about 45 degrees. This position, in addition to facilitating perfusion of the uterus, allows you to maintain eye-to-eye contact with the woman. Occasionally the woman will assume the crawling position, on hands and knees. Some women will stand and lean either over a bed or over their support person's shoulder. Others will assume a side-lying position.

2. Reassure the woman verbally with eye-to-eye contact and a calm, relaxed manner. If there is someone else available (e.g., the father), that person could help support her in position, assist with coaching, and compliment her on her efforts.

3. Wash your hands with soap and water or wash-and-dry pledgets if possible.

4. Place under woman's buttocks whatever clean material or clean newspapers are available.

5. Avoid touching the vaginal area to decrease the possibility of infection. (If there is time, scrub your hands and fingernails for 5 minutes before touching the parturient.) If hands are clean or sterile gloves are available, massage or support perineum as needed.

6. The perineum thins and distends. As the head begins to crown, the birth attendant should do the following:
   a. Tear the amniotic membrane (caul) if it is still intact.
   b. Instruct the woman to pant or pant-blow, thus avoiding the urge to push.
   c. Place the flat side of the hand on the exposed fetal

head and apply *gentle* pressure toward the vagina to prevent the head from "popping out". The mother may participate by placing her hand under yours on the emerging head.

NOTE: Rapid delivery of the fetal head must be prevented because (1) it is followed by a rapid change of pressure within the molded fetal skull, which may result in dural or subdural tears, and (2) it may cause vaginal or perineal lacerations.

7. Instruct the mother to pant or pant-blow as you check for an umbilical cord. If the cord is around the neck, try to slip it up over the baby's head or pull *gently* to get some slack and slip it down over the shoulders.

8. Support the fetal head as restitution (external rotation) occurs. After restitution, with one hand on each side of the baby's head, exert *gentle* pressure downward so that the anterior shoulder emerges under the symphysis pubis and acts as a fulcrum; then as *gentle* pressure is exerted in the opposite direction, the posterior shoulder, which has passed over the sacrum and coccyx, is delivered.

9. Be alert! Hold the baby securely because the rest of the body may deliver quickly. The baby will be slippery!

10. Cradle the baby's head and back in one hand and the buttocks in the other, keeping the head down to drain away the mucus. Use a bulb syringe to remove mucus if one is available.

NOTE: Do not hold the baby upside down by the ankles because to do so (1) hyperextends the spine, which has been flexed since conception; (2) increases intracranial pressure and the danger of capillary rupture; (3) may cause direct tissue trauma to the ankles; and (4) increases the possibility of dropping a wet, slippery baby.

11. Dry the baby rapidly (to prevent rapid heat loss), keeping the baby at the same level as the mother's uterus.

NOTE: Keep the baby at the same level to prevent gravity flow of baby's blood to or from the placenta and the resultant hypovolemia or hypervolemia. Also, do not "milk" the cord: hypervolemia can cause respiratory distress initially or hyperbilirubinemia subsequently; and if isoimmunization has occurred, the baby may receive an additional inoculation of harmful antibodies (e.g., anti-Rh positive or anti-A or anti-B antibodies).

12. As soon as the infant is crying, place the baby on mother's abdomen, cover baby (remember to keep head warm too) with her clothing, and have her cuddle baby. Compliment her (them) on a job well done and on the baby if appropriate. (If something appears to be the matter with the baby, do not lie!) She may wish to expose the part of the baby that will be touching her skin for skin-to-skin contact.

NOTE: Soon after the Wharton's jelly in the cord is exposed to cool air and shrinks and the infant cries, the umbilical vessels stop pulsating and the blood flow ceases. The baby's presence on the mother's abdomen stimulates the release of oxytocin from the posterior pituitary and thus stimulates uterine contractions, which aid in placental separation.

13. *Wait* for placenta to separate; *do not* tug on the cord.

NOTE: Injudicious traction may tear the cord, separate the placenta, or invert the uterus. Signs of placental separation include (1) a slight gush of dark blood from the introitus, (2) lengthening of the cord, and (3) change in uterine contour from discoid to globular.

14. Instruct the mother to push to deliver the separated placenta. Gently ease out the placental membranes, using an up-and-down motion until membranes are removed. To minimize complications do not cut the cord without proper clamps or ties and a sterile cutting tool and inspect the placenta for intactness. Place the baby on the placenta and wrap the two together for additional warmth.

NOTE: There is no hurry to cut the cord. The infant will not lose blood through the placenta because the cord circulation ceases (clots) within minutes of birth.

15. Check the firmness of the uterus. Gently massage the uterus and demonstrate to the mother how she can massage her own uterus properly.

16. Clean the area under the mother's buttocks.

17. Prevent or minimize hemorrhage.

    a. Hemorrhage from uterine atony.

       (1) *Gently* massage fundus to stimulate uterine musculature to contract.

          NOTE: Overstimulation may fatigue the myometrium and cause atony.

       (2) Put the baby to the breast as soon as possible. Sucking or nuzzling and licking the breast stimulate the release of oxytocin from the posterior pituitary.

          NOTE: If the baby does not nurse, manually stimulate the mother's breasts.

       (3) If medical assistance is delayed, do not allow the mother's bladder to become distended.

       (4) Expel any clots from her uterus.

          NOTE: The fundus should be firm to prevent accidental inversion during this procedure. While holding the bottom of the uterus just above the symphysis pubis, apply gentle pressure on the firm fundus downward toward the vagina.

    b. Hemorrhage from perineal lacerations.

       (1) Apply a clean pad to the perineum.

       (2) Instruct the mother to press her thighs together.

18. Comfort or reassure the mother and her family or friends. Keep her and the baby warm. Give her fluids if available and tolerated.

19. In a multiple birth, identify infants in order of birth.

20. Make notations on the birth.

    a. Fetal presentation and position.

    b. Presence of cord around neck or other parts and number of times cord encircles part.

    c. Color, character, and amount of amniotic fluid.

    d. Time of delivery.

    e. Estimated time of Apgar score, resuscitation, and ultimate condition of baby.

    f. Sex of baby.

    g. Approximate time of placental expulsion, its appearance, and completeness.

    h. Maternal condition: affect, amount of bleeding, and status of uterine contractions.

    i. Any unusual occurrences during the delivery.

Table 3-16 *Nursing Care of the Neonate: Implementation and Rationales*

Implementation	Rationale
Airway	
Hold baby with head lowered (10 to 15 degrees).	Uses gravity to help remove fluids.
Suction oral pharynx with a small bulb syringe as soon as head is born.	Expedites drainage and prevents aspiration of amniotic fluid, mucus, and blood (maternal).
Suction nares next.	Prevents inspiration following stimulation of nares before mouth is clear.
Avoid deep suctioning with a catheter, if possible.	May cause bradycardia or laryngospasm or both.
Avoid suspending neonate by the ankles.	Results in hyperextension of baby whose entire development occurred in the flexed position (may be detrimental or painful).
Cord Clamping	
Immediately following birth, neonate is kept at about the same level as the uterus, until cord clamp is applied or until cord has stopped pulsating. Cord pulsations usually cease within seconds after respiration is initiated.	If neonate is held above level of uterus, allows gravity to drain blood to the placenta. If neonate is held below level of uterus, allows gravity to drain blood from placenta to neonate.
Without "stripping" ("milking") it, the cord is clamped close to the umbilicus approximately 30 seconds after birth if neonate appears normal and mature.	Some parents want the baby to receive an extra supply of blood and advocate "stripping" the cord toward the baby. Ordinarily it is unwise to strip the cord before clamping and cutting because postdelivery red blood cell destruction, which normally occurs neonatally, will be increased and hyperbilirubinemia may ensue. In addition, polycythemia (increased number of red blood cells) increases blood viscosity, leading to cardiopulmonary problems in the neonate.
The cord is clamped 8 to 10 cm from the umbilicus if there is a possibility for exchange transfusion.	Permits access to umbilical vessels.
Assess cord for two arteries and one vein.	Alerts physician for need of further assessment if there is only one artery.
Attachment and Warmth	
If neonate is full term, of adequate weight for gestational age, and in good condition, dry quickly and place her or him on mother's abdomen and cover both of them with a warm blanket. Or wrap neonate in warm blanket first.	Facilitates attachment, especially if there is skin-to-skin contact. Assures and relaxes mother. Prevents cold stress to neonate.
Caution parents to keep neonate's head covered.	Prevents cold stress to neonate.
Apgar Score	
Appraise neonate at 1 minute and again at 5 minutes. Use the Apgar scoring method.	Permits a rapid and semiquantitative assessment based on five signs indicative of the physiologic state of the neonate; heart rate, based on auscultation with stethoscope; respiration, based on observed movement of chest wall; muscle tone, based on degree of flexion and movement of the extremities; reflex ability, based on response to gentle slaps on the soles of the feet; and color (pallid, cyanotic, or pink). The 5-minute score correlates with neonatal mortality and morbidity.
Eye Prophylaxis	
Instill medication in conjunctival sacs.	Meets the legal requirement for all newborns to have treatment to prevent conjunctival infections: gonococcal, pneumococcal, or chlamydial. Such infections, known as ophthalmia neonatorum, can lead to varying degrees of blindness.
OR	
If family objects to eye prophylaxis, physician requests parent(s) to sign an informed consent. Note parents' refusal in neonate's record.	
May delay instillation safely until the fourth stage (about 2 hours after birth).	
Newborn Weight and Length	
Weigh and measure the neonate. This may be delayed until the fourth stage.	Pleases parents who are anxious to know and who want to spread the word to relatives and friends.
Identification	
Identify the neonate by one of a number of techniques *before mother or baby leaves the delivery area.*	Although rare, an occasional mix-up in the identity of newborns occurs. Identification and care to check both mother's and baby's ID numbers prevent unnecessary anxiety and legal complications.

Summary of Nursing Actions

NURSING CARE DURING THE SECOND AND THIRD STAGES OF LABOR

I. Goals
   A. For the mother: a safe and satisfying second and third stage of labor
   B. For the unborn child: a continuing state of well-being
   C. For the newborn: a satisfactory adjustment to extrauterine existence
   D. For the family: a satisfying experience in the second stage of labor and in the first meeting with the newborn

II. Priorities
   A. Early identification and immediate therapy for any deviations from normal processes
   B. Cheerful, comfortable, and supportive environment
   C. Encouragement to facilitate the natural rhythm of the second stage
   D. Safe transition into extrauterine life for the neonate
   E. Environment to facilitate individual and family coping and growth

III. Assessment
   A. Second stage
      1. Monitor the following continuously:
         a. FHR
         b. Contractions
         c. Show, excessive bleeding
         d. Amniotic fluid
         e. Maternal response to labor: energy level, ability to relax between contractions, ability to push
      2. Monitor per hospital protocol:
         a. Descent of presenting part and readiness for delivery
         b. Respirations and blood pressure (between contractions)
      3. Assess family's response
      4. Assess physician's or midwife's need for equipment and supplies
      5. Assess woman for comfort and safety needs
   B. Third stage: mother and family
      1. Assess mother's level of anxiety, excitement, or restlessness
      2. Assess for signs of placental separation and note time of delivery of placenta
      3. Observe physician or midwife in case other supplies or equipment is needed while:
         a. Cervix, vagina, perineum, placenta, and membranes are checked
         b. Uterine fundus is checked for degree of firmness and position
         c. Episiotomy or laceration is repaired
      4. After physician or midwife completes care, assess:
         a. Uterine fundus
         b. Lochia
         c. Perineum
         d. Comfort level
         e. Maternal response to baby and family

           f. Family's response to baby (taking into consideration the family's culture and ethnicity)
           g. Mother's mobility of lower limbs (postanesthesia effects)
           h. Check labor and delivery records
   C. Third stage: newborn
      1. Assess respirations
      2. Estimate infant's health status using Apgar rating at 1 and 5 minutes of age
      3. Examine cord and count vessels
      4. Complete the physical examination
      5. Confirm time of birth, sex, and presentation and position (e.g., LOA) for medical records
      6. Collect cord blood for analysis (Rh factor, blood group, and hematocrit)
      7. Assess for safety and comfort

IV. Potential nursing diagnoses
   A. Potential for injury
   B. Altered health maintenance
   C. Knowledge deficit
   D. Powerlessness
   E. Ineffective family coping: compromised
   F. Pain
   G. Anxiety
   H. Altered parenting
   I. Activity intolerance
   J. Ineffective individual coping
   K. Spiritual distress
   L. Impaired physical mobility
   M. Self-esteem disturbance: situational low self esteem
   N. Potential ineffective airway clearance
   O. Potential for aspiration
   P. Alteration in nutrition: less than body requirements
   Q. Potential fluid volume deficit
   R. Potential impaired gas exchange
   S. Potential for infection
   T. Altered role performance
   U. Potential toileting self care deficit
   V. Body image disturbance
   W. Potential for trauma
   X. Altered patterns of urinary elimination
   Y. Impaired tissue integrity
   Z. Impaired skin integrity
   AA. Potential altered tissue perfusion (renal, cerebral, cardiopulmonary, gastrointestinal, peripheral)
   BB. Decreased cardiac output
   CC. Potential ineffective thermoregulation

V. Plan/implementation
   A. Monitor respirations, blood pressure, and maternal progress in labor per hospital protocol; record findings; and report deviations from normal limits.
   B. Assist woman to use her expulsive powers to expedite descent and birth of infant.
      1. Encourage woman to push with urge to bear down until vertex crowns.
      2. When presenting part crowns, instruct woman to control urge to push by panting to permit

Continued.

Summary of Nursing Actions—cont'd

slow delivery of head and eventually of entire infant.

3. Give woman simple, clear directions.
4. If necessary, transfer woman to delivery area at appropriate time for nullipara and rate of progress of labor.
5. If stirrups are used, use care to pad stirrups and to position and restrain woman's legs properly.

C. Provide care for delivery.

D. Record time of birth, sex, and other items required on the delivery record.

E. Report any findings that deviate from normal limits.

F. Monitor flow rate. Adjust arm position and protect IV site during woman's movements or transfer from bed to table.

G. Moisten lips and teeth with cold, wet washcloths, but usually prohibit oral fluids.

H. Encourage voiding, or catheterize bladder if fullness is seen as interfering with descent or if bladder is in danger of trauma.

I. Monitor maternal behavior.

J. Coach as necessary; use simple, clear instructions. NOTE: only one person should coach at a time; all other conversation is avoided.

K. Monitor FHR continuously electronically or manually after each contraction; report any deviations immediately; implement emergency action for ominous FHR decelerations immediately; when appropriate, record event, therapy given, and results.

L. Assist physician or midwife as needed.

M. Administer oxytocin as ordered.

N. Check respirations and blood pressure before transferring from delivery area.

O. Provide opportunities for parents to verbalize reactions to newborn and to the experience.

P. Share in excitement and joy over birth.

Q. Facilitate mother-father-sibling-newborn attachment.

R. Accept any expressions of disappointment from parents and reassure them that such feelings are expected.

S. Reassure mother that her behavior during labor was acceptable if she appears worried about this.

T. Assist with breast feeding if desired.

U. Remove legs from stirrups; put perineal pad in place.

V. Cover with warm blanket and change gown.

W. Help woman to move from delivery table to bed or stretcher (if epidural or spinal anesthetic has been used, with help, lift or roll her into position on her bed).

X. Transfer woman to recovery area.

Y. Ensure clear airway.

Z. Ensure warm environment; prevent cold stress.

AA. Protect from injury and infection.

BB. Report findings that deviate from normal limits.

CC. Complete and record Apgar score at 1 and 5 min.

DD. Initiate resuscitation as necessary.

EE. Identify the newborn per hospital protocol (bands, footprints).

FF. Assist with breast feeding if mother wishes.

VI. Evaluation

A. Second stage: parturient-mother

1. Vital signs and blood pressure remain within normal limits.
   a. Respirations: altered by pushing, hyperventilation prevented
   b. Blood pressure: altered by pushing or anesthesia; hypertension or hypotension prevented
   c. Temperature: assessed when indicated

2. Maternal progress through second stage: within normal limits
   a. Cervix: completely effaced and dilated; lacerations do not occur during birth
   b. Show: copius amounts of mixed blood and mucus with no evidence of excessive bleeding
   c. Contractions: magnitude is expulsively powerful (50-75 mm Hg); frequency, 2-3 min; duration, 60 s; rhythm, regular
   d. Descent: constant
      (1) For *nulliparas,* it takes ½-1 h for descent from station +1 to station +4 cm; from station +4 cm to birth of infant, approximately 20 contractions needed
      (2) For *multiparas,* it takes 10-30 min for descent from station 0 to station +4 cm; from station +4 cm to birth of infant, approximately 10 contractions needed
   e. Duration of labor: within normal limits for nullipara or multipara

3. Birth: no lacerations of vagina or perineum

4. Fluids/nutrients: intravenous flow rate maintained

5. Elimination: bladder and urethra not traumatized by labor or delivery

6. Maternal behavior and appearance: pain sensations decrease in early phases of second stage; urge to push controlled by panting; woman eager to cooperate and give birth to infant and fretful and irritable if progress is not deemed fast enough; needs coaching to work with contractions and will experience amnesia between contractions; fatigue becomes apparent, especially in nulliparas; woman can follow simple, clear directions; will often comment with surprise at sensation of birth

B. Second stage: fetus

1. Well-being continues
   a. Fetal heart rate: within normal pattern
   b. No evidence of meconium staining of amniotic fluid (in vertex presentations)

C. Third stage: parturient/mother

1. Maternal progress through third stage of labor: within normal limits

Summary of Nursing Actions—cont'd

  a. Placenta: delivered intact, with membranes, within 30 min (usually 3-5 min)

  b. Uterine muscles: contract sufficiently to limit loss of blood from placental site

  c. Bleeding from cervical tears: within normal limits or controlled by ligation of torn vessels

  d. After delivery, uterus remains firm, positioned in midline

  e. At birth: 2 cm below or at the umbilicus

2. Vital signs and blood pressure: remain within her normal range

3. Immediate maternal response to infant within normal limits (e.g., open expression of concern for infant's health, joy or disappointment tempered by her physical state and amount of pain or fatigue experienced); reactions vary from euphoria to sleepy exhaustion, with lack of awareness of surroundings

4. Opportunity for parent(s) to begin attachment to (or acquaintance with) newborn

D. Third stage: newborn

1. Infant is in good health: Apgar rating of 7-10 (at birth); respirations present; color dusky to pink; muscle tone good; if neonate is crying, crying is strong; reflexes present; no obvious malformations

2. Apgar score: 7-10 at 5 min

3. Respirations: established within 30-60 s

4. Cord clamped and cut after pulsations cease and respirations are established; no obvious malformations noted

5. Gestational age characteristics are appropriate for estimated date of confinement

6. Infant identified

7. Findings from minimal physical examination are within normal limits

8. Cold stress is avoided

FOURTH STAGE OF LABOR

The fourth stage of labor, the stage of recovery, is a critical period for the mother and newborn, who not only are recovering from the physical process of birth but are also initiating new relationships.

During the 2 hours after the birth, the maternal organism makes its initial readjustment to the nonpregnant state, and body systems begin to stabilize. The newborn continues with the transition from intrauterine to extrauterine existence. This is a period of readjustment for the woman, her infant, and her family. The nurse must be aware of these adjustments to recognize problems and danger signs. These definitions must be understood for optimum care:

puerperium: Variable period, usually 6 to 8 weeks, that begins with the delivery of the placenta and ends either with the resumption of ovulatory menstrual periods or when involuntary changes that result in the nonparous state are complete (e.g., after postdelivery hysterectomy); the postpartum period; the postnatal period; the postdelivery period.

involution: Process that results in the healing of the birth canal and the return of the uterus and all systems to or almost to the prepregnant state. Generally, changes reflect reversals of the anatomic and physiologic adaptations to pregnancy.

atonic uterus: A lack of tone in the uterine muscle caused by interference with the ability of the muscle to contract and retract.

Nursing responsibilities during this stage include assessment of the mother, reporting of information to the postpartum nurse, recognizing and treating dangerous problems, and administering medications as ordered. Client teaching regarding both physical and emotional factors is very important at this stage.

Table 3-17 *Physical Assessment of the Mother During Fourth Stage of Labor*

Factors	Minimum Assessment	Findings and Comments
Blood pressure	Every 15 min for 1 hr or until stable, then every 30 min times 2	Slightly elevated from excitement and effort of delivery; returns to normal within 1 hr
Pulse	Every 15 min for 1 hr or until stable; then every 30 min times 2	Normal rate for individual within 1 hr; slight bradycardia may occur (50-70 bpm)
Temperature	Once, at 1 hr; then as per hospital protocol	May be elevated if dehydrated or fatigued
Fundus	Every 15 min for 1 hr or until stable; then every 30 min times 2	Firm: midline, 2 cm below or at umbilicus Soft: massage until firm and express clots until contracted to midlevel Right of midline: check bladder for distension
Bladder	Every time fundus is assessed	Fills quickly because of postdelivery diuresis and intravenous fluids.
Lochia	Every 15 min (in conjunction with assessment of fundus)	Moderate flow: normal; if flow comes in spurts, suspect cervical tear Heavy flow: recheck in 3-5 min and report
Perineum	Check in conjunction with assessment of lochia	Condition of episiotomy and perineum: clean, edematous, discolored, stitches intact

Table 3-18 *Recovery Nurse's Report to Postpartum Nurse*

Item	Example
Type of labor and delivery; unusual observations, if any, of the placenta	Spontaneous or assisted (forceps) vaginal delivery; vertex presentation
Gravidity and parity, age	GI, PI, 22 years old
Anesthesia and analgesia used	None; epidural, low spinal, local
Condition of perineum	Episiotomy; repair of lacerations
Events since delivery	Vital signs, blood pressure, fundus, lochia, intake and output, medications (dosage, time of administration, and results), response to newborn, observation of family interactions, including siblings, if present
Condition and sex of newborn; other information	Apgar at 1 and 5 min; time of birth; eye prophylaxis given; weight; whether breast- or bottle-feeding; if breast-feeding, whether newborn was at breast; name of pediatrician
Relevant information from prenatal record	Need for rubella vaccination
Miscellaneous information	
Intravenous drip	If IV drip is infusing, rate of infusion, medications added (e.g., Pitocin), whether to keep open or discontinue after completion of bag that is hung
Social factors	If woman is giving baby up for adoption, whether she wants to see baby, breast-feed, allow visitors, or other preferences she may have

Table 3-19 *Recovery Nurse's Report on Newborn*

Item	Example
Type of labor and delivery; unusual events (e.g., cord around neck)	Spontaneous or assisted (forceps, vacuum extractor) vaginal birth in vertex presentation
Gravidity and parity, age of mother	GI, PI, 22 years old
Analgesia and anesthesia	None; epidural, low spinal, or local
Condition at birth	Apgar scores at 1 and 5 min
Sex and weight	Male; 3400 g (7 lb, 8 oz)
Events since birth	Nursed at breast; took nipple well Voided ×1; meconium ×1 Eye prophylaxis Vitamin K injection Held by siblings who are happy (or have other response) to newborn
Relevant information from prenatal record	Unremarkable pregnancy

DANGER SIGNS

Hypovolemic Shock

1. Persistent significant bleeding—perineal pad soaked within 15 minutes; *may not be accompanied by a change in vital signs or maternal color or behavior*
2. Mother states she feels light-headed, "funny," "sick to my stomach," or sees "stars"
3. Mother begins to act anxious, or exhibits air hunger
4. Woman's color turns ashen or grayish
5. Temperature of skin feels cool and clammy
6. Increasing pulse rate
7. Falling blood pressure

Emergency Procedure

HYPOVOLEMIC SHOCK

DEFINITION

State of physical collapse and prostration caused by massive blood loss, circulatory malfunction, and inadequate tissue perfusion.

PURPOSE

To identify and control bleeding.
Prompt replacement of blood and fluid volumes.
Prevention of total collapse and death.

EQUIPMENT

IV fluid; IV tubing, needles, angiocaths; aromatic spirits of ammonia; oxytoxic medication; oxygen with nasal prongs or mask.

NURSING ACTIONS	RATIONALE
Preprocedure	
Observe mother for persistent heavy bleeding: the soaking of a second perineal pad in 15 minutes, may or may not be accompanied by a change in vital signs, skin color, or behavior.	Fast diagnosis leads to quick action and a favorable prognosis.
	Blood volume still sufficient for body to compensate for loss.
Assess mother for signs of shock (i.e., feels light-headed, sick feeling in stomach, sees "stars," starts to act anxious, ashen or grayish color appears, skin feels cool and clammy, exhibits air hunger). Pulse rate increases as blood pressure falls.	Compensatory mechanisms becoming ineffective.
	Sympathetic nervous system stimulated.
	Hypoxia of brain cells.
	Hypoxia of tissue cells.
	β-adrenergic receptor stimulation. Attempt made to compensate for tissue hypoxia and metabolic acidosis.
Procedure	
Call for help immediately or bring help *to* you.	*Do not leave* the woman.
Tilt woman onto her side and raise her legs *high*. Increase flow of IV drip.	To increase circulating blood volume; prevent supine hypotension.
If uterus is atonic, massage gently and expel clots to allow uterus to contract; compress uterus manually, as needed, using two hands. Add oxytocic to IV drip, as ordered.	To prevent further loss of blood by stimulating uterine contractions.
	To stimulate uterine contractions.
Break ampule of aromatic amonia, a respiratory stimulant; give oxygen by face mask or nasal prongs at 8 to 10 L/min.	To facilitate oxygen by stimulating respirations and increasing available oxygen.
Postprocedure	
Chart incident and medical and nursing interventions employed. Chart results of treatments.	To provide data base for future comparison.
	To provide information for implementation of nursing process.
Reassure woman (couple).	To decrease anxiety.

MEDICATIONS FOR THE FOURTH STAGE OF LABOR

Oxytocin (prescription)

Brand names: Pitocin, Syntocinon
Dosage forms: injection (IM/IV)
Use: for both stage 3 and 4 of labor.
    Stage 3: to stimulate uterine contractions
    Stage 4: to control postpartum hemorrhage
Side effects: Cardiac arrhythmia, postpartum hemorrhage, fetal bradycardia (stage 3), nausea, vomiting, pelvic hematoma, uterine hypertonicity, spasms, tetanic contractions, uterine rupture
Drug interactions: with vasopressors can produce severe hypertension
Client education: Explain rationale for use to patient and family. Explain recurrence of contractions and relation techniques and comfort measures.

Methylergonovine, Ergonovine maleate (prescription)

Brand names: Methergine, Ergotrate
Dosage forms-IM, IV, pO
Use: treatment of hemorrhage associated with postpartum
Side effects: headache, dizziness, nausea, vomiting, chest pain, palpitations, hypertension, tinnitus, sweating, rash, abdominal cramps
Drug interactions: none known
Client education: Explain menstrual-like cramps. Report increased blood loss, foul-smelling lochia.

Guidelines For Client Teaching

PHYSICAL FACTORS DURING THE FOURTH STAGE OF LABOR

ASSESSMENT

1. Woman has given birth within the last 2 hours.
2. Physical parameters must be observed to prevent harm to postpartum woman.
3. Uterus must remain firm to prevent hemorrhage.
4. Urinary bladder must be emptied periodically to prevent distension and boggy, or atonic, uterus.
5. Interest in breast-feeding established.
6. Breast-feeding may begin in recovery room if all parameters are normal.
7. Watch for verbal and nonverbal cues of pain and discomfort.
8. Woman complains of fatigue.
9. Woman has elevated temperature.
10. Woman's fluid intake (oral and intravenous) is limited.
11. Woman states she is hungry.
12. Effects of analgesia or anesthesia given for later part of labor and the delivery are wearing off.

NURSING DIAGNOSES

Pain, related to episiotomy, hemorrhoids, involution of the uterus, full bladder
Knowledge deficit related to the fourth stage of labor.
Potential fluid volume deficit related to decreased oral fluid intake and IV administration.
Altered nutrition: potential for less than body requirements, related to having nothing by mouth during labor and delivery.
Impaired skin integrity related to lacerations of the perineum or episiotomy.
Sleep pattern disturbance related to labor and delivery.
Activity intolerance related to fatigue.
Potential for infection related to alteration in skin integrity.

GOALS

Short-term

Woman will get rest and sleep.
Woman's hunger and thirst will be satisfied.
Woman's bladder will be emptied periodically.
Woman's pain and discomfort will be diminished.
Anesthesia from delivery will wear off.

Intermediate

Woman's perineal swelling will start to subside and healing will begin.
Woman's fundus will remain firm and lochia rubra will remain within normal limits.
Woman will begin to breast-feed.
Woman will ambulate with assistance to the bathroom to void.

Long-term

Woman will ambulate to bathroom by herself to void.
Woman will begin self-care activities.
Woman will continue to breast-feed.
Uterus will begin to involute.

REFERENCES AND TEACHING AIDS

Prelabor and delivery counseling using pamphlets and booklets explaining the physiologic changes that take place during the fourth stage of labor.

CONTENT/RATIONALE	TEACHING ACTIONS
To **prevent hemorrhage** *through direct care and through teaching woman self-care, the nurse shares the following:* Uterus must remain firm to become the *living ligature.* When uterus becomes boggy, or atonic, living ligature is no longer working to stop excessive bleeding. If gentle massage does not work, further assessment must be performed. When lochia is heavy, reassessment of source of bleeding, uterine tone, and bladder distension must be made. Clots should be expelled. Note size and amount.	Identify for woman the location and size of the uterus. Show mother how to massage uterus gently to firm up uterine fundus. Explain what the term *involution* means. Discuss lochia and clot formation. Give rationale for assessing, discuss meaning of terms. Teach woman about expected regression (color and amount) during involution. Explain that atony and subsequent hemorrhage can be the result of a distended bladder. Bleeding may be from another source. Clots prevent the living ligature from working.
To prevent hemorrhage by averting bladder problems: Assess woman's intake of fluids, oral and intravenous. Assess rate of diuresis as evidenced by bladder filling. Assess woman's ability to void. Share information related to diuresis and postdelivery bladder function	Discuss rationale for keeping bladder empty: prevent uterine atony and trauma to bladder. Provide privacy, sound of running water, fluids to drink. If available, expose urinary meatus to vapors from spirits of peppermint. Offer analgesia to assist woman to relax urinary meatus. Suggest she void while in sitz bath or while using surgigator. Discuss possible catheterization if trauma and edema to tissues or anesthesia impairs normal urination pattern.
To prevent hemorrhage through stimulation of endogenous oxytocin and help woman meet her goal to breast-feed: Review the benefits to the newborn (who is healthy and ready to nurse) and to her. *To foster* **comfort:** Reassure woman that discomfort is "normal." Episiotomy: positioning, icepacks, medication (local or systemic). Afterpains: warm blanket, empty bladder, medication. *To maintain* **hydration,** *the nurse is aware that:* Drinking small amounts of fluids slowly prevents nausea and vomiting. There is a relationship between fluid deficit and temperature rise and fatigue. *To maintain* **nutrition,** *the nurse is aware that:* Giving birth consumes considerable energy. There is a relationship between food deficit and fatigue and rate of recovery. *To prevent dysfunction in* **bladder elimination,** *the nurse is aware that:* Overdistension can lead to bladder atony and delayed recovery. Urine retention can predispose to bladder infection. *To maintain* **safety,** *the nurse is aware that:* Postdelivery splanchnic engorgement predisposes the woman to orthostatic hypotension. Recovery from effects of analgesia/anesthesia varies: Some analgesics affect the woman's balance. Spinal anesthesia requires a period of bed rest with only a small flat pillow under the woman's head Childbirth increases the woman's vulnerability to infection for a variety of reasons, including fluid and calorie deficit and tissue trauma.	Show woman how to put the infant to breast and explain that nipple stimulation results in the release of oxytocin, which causes the uterus to contract and assists involution. Validate that woman's discomfort is expected and interventions are available to help. Implement care (icepacks, medications); show rationale and expected outcomes. Provide explanations. Maintain intravenous fluids or provide oral fluids, as ordered. Caution against drinking large amounts at one time or rapidly. Provide rationale. Provide foods as ordered. Begin postpartum nutrition counseling. Provide rationale for need to prevent bladder distension. Encourage woman to void. Catheterize as needed, per physician's order. Request that woman ask for assistance to ambulate. Put side rails up and call bell within reach, and provide rationale. Help woman maintain flat position for specified time after spinal anesthesia, and provide rationale. Explain rationale to promote comfort and healing, and prevent infection. Demonstrate perineal care. Teach woman signs and symptoms to report after discharge home.

EVALUATION The nurse can be reasonably assured that teaching and care were effective when all goals for care have been achieved. The uterus retains tone. Mother locates and massages uterus. The lochia is moderate or less with a few small clots. The mother voids completely so that uterus is firm, in midline, and below umbilicus; is emptied without additional trauma and by using strict aseptic technique. Mother understands cause of possible severity of afterpains during breast-feeding. Woman's nonverbal and verbal responses validate that she is comfortable and able to rest comfortably. Woman is well hydrated (elevated temperature and fatigue take time to resolve). Her hunger is satisfied. She takes oral fluids and foods without difficulty. Before ambulating, woman requests assistance, ambulates without difficulty, and incurs no injury. Woman understands rationale for all care provided her.

Guidelines For Client Teaching

EMOTIONAL FACTORS DURING THE FOURTH STAGE OF LABOR

ASSESSMENT

1. Woman has completed labor and given birth within previous 2 hours.
2. Woman gives verbal cues that suggest failure, loss of self-esteem (e.g., "I was such a baby").
3. Woman embarrassed about behavior during labor and delivery (e.g., "I'm sorry for screaming").
4. Woman indicates desire to hold newborn; other family members desire to hold newborn.
5. Woman indicates desire to breast-feed.
6. Woman (couple) talks about met and unmet expectations.
7. Woman (couple) reacts to newborn.

NURSING DIAGNOSES

Situational low self-esteem related to labor and delivery experience.

Potential altered parenting related to care of newborn.

Potential short-term memory deficit related to events of labor and delivery and body's potential for natural amnesia.

Knowledge deficit related to care of newborn, breast-feeding, and process of integration of the birth experience.

Potential altered thought processes related to sensory overload during labor and delivery.

GOALS

Short-term

Woman (couple) will relive and replay birth experience.

Woman will begin to feel comfortable with her behavior.

Woman will begin to breast-feed.

Woman will begin to bond with her newborn.

Intermediate

Woman (couple) will resolve feelings of birth experience and begin to feel satisfaction from the process.

Woman will gain satisfaction from breast-feeding.

Woman (couple) and family will become attached to newborn.

Long-term

Woman (couple) will have joyous memories of the birth experience.

Woman will continue to derive satisfaction from breast-feeding.

Woman (couple) will cherish her new infant and provide love and care for her/him.

REFERENCES AND TEACHING AIDS

Printed material explaining normal reactions to labor and delivery processes.

Breast-feeding information.

Pamphlets and booklets describing newborn care.

CONTENT/RATIONALE	TEACHING ACTIONS
To foster self-esteem and facilitate integration of experience, the nurse is aware that: Women approach labor with certain self-expectations. "Normal" behavior during labor includes behaviors that are unacceptable to many people, such as loss of control, moaning, belching, grunting. Normal amnesia, medications, and labor preclude a clear recall of events; gaps in recall or misinterpretations prevent positive coping and self-esteem.	Implement communication techniques. Listen to mother's replay of her experience. Phrase questions and answers in manner that indicates that her responses during all stages of labor were within expected range.
To foster parent-child attachment, the nurse is aware that: Attachment to newborn is a continuous process. Fatigue of either mother or baby may delay but will not adversely influence attachment response.	Assess woman's readiness (absence of sedation or fatigue) and newborn's condition. Wrap baby warmly. Position baby in woman's arms for maximum safety. Ensure woman's comfort. Point out newborn's individual characteristics. Help the mother put baby to breast if she wishes to.

To foster individual and family satisfaction, the nurse is aware that:
 Each ethnic and cultural group and individual couple have developed workable ways for family interactions. There is no one "right" way.
	Meet family's ethnic and cultural and couple's expectations for care:
	    Accept degree of involvement of individuals regarding overt expression of joy or love.
	    Accept family's desires regarding neonate (e.g., some may want newborn to be cared for in nursery).

EVALUATION Woman gives nonverbal cues that she is beginning to accept her behavior and the experience. Woman (couple) begins attachment process. Family indicates satisfaction with the experience.

Summary of Nursing Actions

NURSING CARE DURING THE FOURTH STAGE OF LABOR

I. Goals
  A. For the mother: an uncomplicated immediate recovery from the birth process and an adequate beginning for integration of the birth experience
  B. For the newborn: a continuation of a healthy extrauterine existence
  C. For the family: a continuation of a positive process of attachment to the newborn and an adequate beginning for integration of the birth experience

II. Priorities
  A. Identification of the potential risks for hemorrhage and initiation of preventive measures if needed
  B. Implementation of immediate interventions if hemorrhage does occur
  C. Promotion of recovery through the use of supportive and comfort measures (e.g., nourishment, fluids, safety precautions, and medications)
  D. Promotion of attachment of family members to newborn
  E. Promotion of opportunities for family to begin to integrate the experience

III. Assessment
  A. Mother
    1. Obtain information from delivery room personnel (or check record) regarding significant findings from prenatal and intrapartum periods.
    2. Complete assessment for physical findings every 15 min:
      a. Fundus
      b. Lochia
      c. Perineum
      d. Blood pressure
      e. Pulse
      f. Bladder distension
    3. Assess temperature before transfer to postpartum unit.
    4. Assess comfort; locate discomfort.
    5. Assess energy level.
    6. Assess recovery from analgesia and anesthesia
      a. Regional anesthesia—return of sensation
      b. General—awake and alert
      c. Nerve block—return of sensation, proper position and body alignment
    7. Assess emotional response to birth and to the newborn, taking into consideration cultural and ethnic variations.
    8. Assess fluids and nutrients.
    9. Assess mother's (family's) educational needs:
      a. Postpartum care and recovery
      b. Breast- or bottle-feeding
      c. Newborn characteristics
      d. Newborn care
    10. Assess and summarize findings, charting some, before transfer to postpartum unit.
  B. Newborn
    1. Evaluate maternal history, including labor, to identify potential problems for newborn.
    2. Assess respirations and newborn's ability to keep airway clear.
    3. Assess for meconium staining of fingernails, vernix, or cord.
    4. Assess temperature and color.
    5. Assess weight, length (may be delayed until temperature is stabilized).
    6. Reassess for gestational age and possible complications, including structural malformations.
    7. Note passage of meconium or urine.

IV. Potential nursing diagnoses
  A. Potential for injury
  B. Potential fluid volume deficit
  C. Altered health maintenance
  D. Ineffective individual coping
  E. Knowledge deficit
  F. Pain
  G. Potential for infection
  H. Sleep pattern disturbance
  I. Potential activity intolerance
  J. Impaired physical mobility
  K. Sleep pattern disturbance
  L. Ineffective individual coping
  M. Ineffective family coping: compromised
  N. Potential altered parenting
  O. Altered family process
  P. Body image disturbance
  Q. Self esteem disturbance: situational low self esteem
  R. Altered role performance
  S. Alteration in nutrition: less than body requirements
  T. Potential altered body temperature
  U. Potential ineffective airway clearance
  V. Potential for aspiration
  W. Potential for trauma
  X. Impaired skin integrity
  Y. Potential altered patterns of urinary elimination
  Z. Potential impaired breast-feeding

V. Plan/implementation
  A. Recovery room
    1. Massage gently as necessary to maintain firmness; expel clots if present. Teach mother how and why this is done.
    2. Encourage to void completely. If distension occurs and woman is unable to void, catheterize and record amount, character, and type. Send specimen to laboratory if indicated.
    3. Caution her to drink fluids slowly and in small amounts to prevent nausea or vomiting.
    4. Explain return of sensation to legs after spinal or epidural anesthestics.
    5. Monitor vital signs and blood pressure.
    6. Check record for completeness and prepare record for transfer to postdelivery area. Collect woman's possessions; raise side rails on bed; check intravenous bottle, lines, and pole to ensure safe transfer.
    7. Give report to admitting nurse.
  B. On postpartum floor
    1. Assist nurse to help woman into bed.
    2. Introduce her to postpartum nurse and to other women sharing her room.

Continued.

Summary of Nursing Actions—cont'd

3. Check record to see that consent form has been signed.
4. Administer the medication per physician's order.
5. If woman is to receive bromocriptine mesylate (Parlodel), delay administration until the vital signs have been stabilized and administer no sooner than 4 hours after delivery.
6. Settle the mother comfortably in bed; explain routine care.
7. Change perineal pads as necessary; wash vulva with soap and water as needed.
8. Teach mother about lochia—amount and color to expect and time periods for change in character and amount.
9. Apply ice pack to perineum per physician's order.
10. If blood pressure is too low: turn her on her side, give oxygen by face mask is she is breathless, give intravenous fluids; massage uterus until firm; place in Trendelenburg's position; call physician if blood pressure does not return to normal quickly.
11. If blood pressure elevated: assess deep tendon reflexes (DTR) and for other signs of pregnancy-induced hypertension (PIH); record and report to physician.
12. Provide fluids, oral or intravenous, per hospital and physician protocol.
13. If infection is diagnosed, treat per physician order.
14. Teach regarding "afterpains," lochia, reasons for checking fundus and expressing clots, return of sensation to legs after regional anesthesia, and need to keep bladder empty.
15. Give medications for pain if other comfort measures do not work, if woman desires medication, and if appropriate.
16. Provide general hygiene.
17. Help her into positions of comfort.
18. Make environment conducive to rest (e.g., temperature, ventilation, quiet).
19. Provide emotional support as needed (e.g., answer questions).
20. Provide fluids and nourishment per hospital and physician's protocol.
21. Record amounts and types.
22. Assist to ambulate for the first time to prevent injury in case of fall secondary to splanchnic engorgement.
23. Keep side rails up and call bell within easy reach until woman is fully recovered.
24. Provide assurance by answering questions simply and directly; encourage questions regarding labor and recovery experience.
25. Share in excitement and joy over birth.
26. Facilitate mother-family-child attachment: provide a warm, quiet, darkened environment (newborn is more apt to open eyes), encouraging parents to hold newborn en face within

2.5 to 20 cm (1 to 8 in, the distance at which most newborns can focus).
27. Accept any expressions of disappointment from parents and reassure them that such feelings are common.
28. Reassure mother and family that her behavior during labor was acceptable if she or they appear worried about it.
29. Assist with breastfeeding as necessary.
30. Inquire of mother and family what they expect in terms of care during the recovery from childbirth. Accommodate them as much as possible. Use services of interpretor if indicated.

C. Newborn
1. Ensure clear airway.
2. Maintain warmth by mother's body heat, warm blankets, a stockinette cap for head, overhead heating panel, or a warmed bassinet, following hospital protocol.
3. Share data with parents, if appropriate.
4. Meet parents' needs for knowledge regarding eye prophylaxis; provide eye prophylaxis.
5. Facilitate mother-father-child attachment.
6. Suggest breast feeding and assist with process if mother indicated she planned to breast feed.
7. Keep newborn with parents during recovery phase if new-born remains in good condition. Check record for transfer to postdelivery area.
8. Accomplish transfer per hospital protocol, e.g., father may carry newborn to nursery and place in heated crib; mother may carry baby in bed with her; nurse may carry newborn.
9. Give report to admitting nurse.
10. Give postpartum nurse information regarding mother's (family's) knowledge as well as noting this on her record.

VI. Evaluation
A. Mother
1. Physical findings are assessed every 15 min × 4 (at least) until stable within normal limits:
   a. Uterus remains firm, in midline, at or slightly above umbilicus for, first 2 hours.
   b. Lochia is moderate.
   c. Perineum is intact; or repair of episiotomy or laceration is intact; perineal edema is minimal.
   d. Blood pressure remains within her normal limits.
   e. Pulse may be slow, often between 50 and 70 beats/min.
   f. Bladder distension is prevented.
   g. Temperature is within normal limits.
2. Woman states she feels comfortable and rested.
3. Desire to rest if not hampered because of discomfort from pain, thirst, hunger, or emotional upset.
4. Mother's fluids and nutrients are met.
5. Mother takes fluids and food without nausea and vomiting.
6. Mother recovers from analgesics or anesthetics.

Summary of Nursing Actions—cont'd

7. Mother's and family's questions are answered.
8. Initial mother-family-child interactions are enough to satisfy the need to touch, hold, and examine the newborn; to reassure as to the normalcy of the newborn's appearance and behavior; to provide eye contact with the newborn (if possible); and to initiate breast feeding of the newborn (if desired).
9. Maternal behavior and appearance are within normal limits.
10. Initial excitement replaced with drowsy satisfaction.
11. Mother and family indicate that care given is within their religious, cultural, and ethnic prescriptions and proscriptions.
12. Transfer to postdelivery area is accomplished when mother's condition is stabilized within normal limits, fundus is remaining contracted, bladder is empty, and record is complete.
13. If woman does not want to breast feed, administer antilactogenic medications. If antilactogenic hormones are used, in some hospitals the woman is asked to sign an informed consent (before delivery) before receiving these hormones.

B. Newborn

1. Physical health is satisfactory as measured by the following:
   a. Temperature is 37° C (98.6° F).
   b. Heart rate, rhythm, regularity are within normal limits.
   c. Color and respiration are within normal limits.
2. Data base established through physical examination and assessment for gestational age; by end of 2 hours after birth, newborn is weighed, length and suboccipital bregmatic diameter are measured, and eye prophylaxis is completed.
3. Newborn is alert with eyes open during first 30-60 min, followed by sleep; during alert period when sucking reflex is present, newborn is put to the breast.
4. Transfer of newborn is accomplished per parent's choice and hospital protocol, e.g., to transitional nursery where constant surveillance, external heat sources, and emergency care are available until newborn is stabilized; then to normal newborn unit or rooming-in unit; or, from delivery area directly to rooming-in unit where nursing personnel, mother, or family member share responsibility for continuous surveillance and care needed by newborn.

References

Blank JJ: Electronic fetal monitoring, JOGN Nurs 14:463, Nov/Dec 1985.
Carr KG: Management of the second stage of labor, NAACOG update series, lesson 9, vol 1, 1983.
Friedman FA and Sachtleben MR: Station of the presenting part, Am J Obstet Gynecol 93:522, 1965.
Mahan CS and McKay S: Are we overmanaging second stage labor? Contemp OB/GYN 24:37, Dec 1984.
Tucker SM: Pocket guide to fetal monitoring, St. Louis, 1988, The CV Mosby Co.
Zuspan FF and Quilligan EJ, editors: Practical manual of obstetric care, St. Louis, 1982, The CV Mosby Co.

Bibliography

American College of Obstetricians and Gynecologists: Standard for obstetric-gynecologic services, ed 6, Washington, DC, ACOG, 1985.
Fields LM, Haire MF, and Troiano NH: Current concepts in fetal monitoring (data media), Sharon, Mass, 1985, PPG Biomedical Systems, Inc.
Friedman FA: Labor: clinical evaluation and management, ed 2, New York, 1978, Appleton-Century-Crofts.
Pritchard JA, MacDonald PC, and Gant NF, editors: Williams' obstetrics, ed 17, Norwalk, Conn, 1985, Appleton-Century-Crofts.

UNIT

4

The Normal Newborn

The newborn baby, a miracle of life and growth, usually astounds the woman and her family. Very often the nurse will find the mother sitting with the unclothed infant, counting fingers and toes. The nurse's assessment and care of the newborn is a bit more comprehensive. Newborns face a critical period of adjustment to extrauterine life. Their successful adjustment is determined by their biologic and behavioral readiness and the care provided them by families and health care professionals.

The nurse's responsibilities during this period focus on complete and extensive assessment of the newborn and on provision of the care needed for a smooth transition to extrauterine life. This care should include teaching the mother and family how to care for the infant. Teaching is especially important regarding the nutritional needs of the newborn, which must be met for optimum growth and development.

CHARACTERISTICS OF THE NEWBORN

By term the infant's various anatomic and physiologic systems have reached a level of development and functioning that permits a physical existence apart from the mother and a readiness for social interaction. The newborn and adult learn about each other and about themselves—a feeling of mutuality, of identification with the "other" is accom-

plished. The nurse uses knowledge of the biologic and behavioral characteristics of the newborn as a basis for the infant care and parental teaching and counseling.

Biologic Characteristics

A thorough physical assessment of the newborn provides the data needed to plan nursing care and client-teaching activities. The nurse must be knowledgeable about normal parameters to be able to identify indications of problems requiring nursing or medical intervention. Some of the most significant changes that occur in the newborn during the transfer to extrauterine life involve the cardiovascular system. This section begins with information regarding these changes and goes on to provide extensive information regarding the complete physical examination, including average findings, normal variations, and deviations from the normal range. Assessment of the newborn's early reflexes provides important information about the infant's nervous system and the state of neurologic maturation. The nurse should assess for these reflexes as early as possible because abnormal signs that appear in the early neonatal period may disappear, only to reappear months or years later as abnormal functions. This section concludes with techniques for eliciting significant reflexes and the characteristic responses.

Table 4-1 *Cardiovascular Changes at Birth (See Box, Schematic of Fetal Circulation, below)*

Prenatal Status	Postdelivery Status	Associated Factors
Primary Changes		
Pulmonary circulation: high pulmonary vascular resistance; increased pressure in right ventricle and pulmonary arteries	Low pulmonary vascular resistance; decreased pressure in right atrium, ventricle, and pulmonary arteries	Expansion of collapsed fetal lung with air
Systemic circulation: low pressures in left atrium, ventricle, and aorta	High systemic vascular resistance; increased pressure in left atrium, ventricle, and aorta	Loss of placental blood flow
Secondary Changes		
Umbilical arteries: patent; carry blood from hypogastric arteries to placenta	Functionally closed at birth; obliteration by fibrous proliferation may take 2-3 months; distal portions become lateral vesicoumbilical ligaments; proximal portions remain open as superior vesicle arteries	Closure precedes that of umbilical vein; probably accomplished by smooth muscle contraction in response to thermal and mechanical stimuli and alteration in oxygen tension; mechanically severed with cord at birth
Umbilical vein: patent; carries blood from placenta to ductus venosus and liver	Closed; after obliteration it becomes *ligamentum teres hepatis*	Closure shortly after umbilical arteries; hence blood from placenta may enter neonate for short period after birth; mechanically severed with cord at birth
Ductus venosus: patent; connects umbilical vein to inferior vena cava	Closed; after obliteration it becomes *ligamentum venosum*	Loss of blood flow from umbilical vein
Ductus arteriosus: patent; shunts blood from pulmonary artery to descending aorta	Functionally closed almost immediately after birth; anatomic obliteration of lumen by fibrous proliferation requires 1-3 months; becomes *ligamentum arteriosum*	High systemic resistance increases aortic pressure; low pulmonary resistance reduces pulmonary arterial pressure Increased oxygen content of blood in ductus arteriosus creates vasospasm of its muscular wall
Foramen ovale: forms a valve opening that allows blood to flow directly to left atrium	Functionally closes at birth; constant apposition gradually leads to fusion and permanent closure within a few months or years in majority of infants	Increased pressures in left atrium together with decreased pressure in right atrium cause closure of valve over foramen

From Whaley LF and Wong DL: Nursing care of infants and children, ed 3, St Louis, 1987, The CV Mosby Co.

SCHEMATIC OF FETAL CIRCULATION

Total

Placenta → umbilical vein → ductus venosis → inferior vena cava → right atrium → foramen ovale → left atrium → left ventricle → ascending aorta (supplies coronary arteries cerebral arteries, arteries of upper extremities → head and upper extremities → superior vena cava → right atrium → tricuspid valve → right ventricle → pulmonary artery → ductus arteriosus → descending aorta → inferior vena cava → viscera of abdomen and pelvis, lower extremities → hypogastric arteries → umbilical arteries → placenta.

Simplified

Placenta → umbilical vein → ductus venosis → inferior vena cava → right atrium → foramen ovale → left atrium → ductus arteriosis → descending aorta → umbilical arteries → placenta.

Table 4-2 *Physical Assessment of Newborn*

Area Assessed and Appraisal Procedure	Normal Findings		Deviations from Normal Range (Possible Causes)
	Average Findings	Normal Variations	
Posture			
Inspect newborn before disturbing for assessment	Vertex: arms, legs in moderate flexion; fists are clenched	Frank breech: more straight and stiff, so that newborn will assume intrauterine position in repose for a few days	Lack of muscle tone, relaxed posture while awake: prematurity or hypoxia in utero
Refer to maternal chart for fetal presentation, position, and type of birth (vaginal, surgical), since newborn readily assumes prenatal position	Newborn resists having extremities extended for examination or measurement and will cry when this is attempted	Prenatal pressure of limb or shoulder may cause temporary facial asymmetry or resistance to extension of extremities	Hypertonia: drug dependence, CNS disorder
	Crying ceases when allowed to reassume curled-up fetal position		Opisthotonos: CNS disturbance
	Normal spontaneous movement is bilaterally asynchronous (legs move in bicycle fashion) but equally extensive in all extremities		Limitation of motion in any of extremities: see Extremities, below
Vital Signs			
Blood pressure (BP)	75/42 (approximately)	Varies with change in activity level: awake, crying, sleeping	Difference between upper and lower extremity pressures may provide early clue to coarctation of aorta
Electronic monitor	At birth		
BP cuff: BP cuff width affects readings; use cuff 2.5 cm (1 in) wide and palpate radial pulse	Systolic: 60-80 mm Hg		Hypotension
	Diastolic: 40-50 mm Hg		Hypertension: coarctation of aorta
	At 10 days		
	Systolic: 95-100 mm Hg		
	Diastolic: slight increase		
Heart rate and pulses	Pulsations visible in left midclavicular line; fifth intercostal space	100 (sleeping) to 160 (crying); may be irregular for brief periods, especially after crying	Tachycardia (persistent; ≥170): RDS
Thorax	Apical pulse; fourth intercostal space 120-140/min	Murmurs, especially over base or at left sternal border in interspace 3 or 4 (foramen ovale anatomically closes at about 1 yr)	Bradycardia (persistent; ≤120): congenital heart block
Inspection	Quality: *first sound* (closure of mitral valves) and *second sound* (closure of aortic and pulmonic valves) should be sharp and clear	Average pulses (slightly faster for girls)	Murmurs: may be functional
Palpation		2 yr: 105	Arrhythmias: irregular rate
Auscultation		6 yr: 100	Sounds
Apex: mitral valve		8-12 yr: 85-90	Distant: pneumomediastinum
Second interspace, left of sternum: pulmonic valve		16 yr: 80	Poor quality
Second interspace, right of sternum: aortic valve		18 yr: 70	Extra
Junction of xiphoid process and sternum: tricuspid valve			Heard on right side of chest: dextrocardia (often accompanied by reversal of intestines)
Femoral pulse palpation: flex thighs on hips; place fingers along inguinal ligament about midway between symphysis pubis and iliac crest; feel bilaterally at same time	Femoral pulses should be equal and strong		Weak or absent femoral pulses
			Hip dysplasia
			Coarctation of aorta
			Thrombophlebitis
Temperature	Axillary: 36.5°-37° C (97.6°-98.6° F)	36.4° to 37.2° C (97.5° to 99° F)	Subnormal—may reflect the following: Prematurity, infection, low environmental temperature, inadequate clothing, and dehydration
Axillary: method of choice until 6 yr of age; hold in axillary fold for 5 min	Rectal: may be misleading—even in cold stress may remain unchanged until metabolic activity can no longer maintain core temperature	Heat loss: 200 kcal/kg/min from evaporation, conduction, convection, radiation	Increased (pyrexia)—may reflect the following: Infec-
Rectal: before passage of meconium check			

Table 4-2, cont'd. *Physical Assessment of Newborn*

Area Assessed and Appraisal Procedure	Normal Findings		Deviations from Normal Range (Possible Causes)
	Average Findings	Normal Variations	
Vital Signs—cont'd			
for patent anus; insert thermometer with great caution no further than 1 to 2 cm (¼ to ½ in) into rectum, gently; hold in place for 5 min, keeping legs immobilized to prevent thermometer from being dislodged or broken (there is a risk of traumatizing or perforating rectal mucosa) Electronic: thermistor probe (avoid taping over bony area)	Temperature stabilization by 8-10 hr of age Shivering mechanism undeveloped		tion, high environmental temperature, excessive clothing, proximity to heating unit or in direct sunshine, drug addiction (following increased activity level of infant), and diarrhea and dehydration Temperature not stabilized by 10 hr after birth If mother received magnesium sulfate, newborn is less able to conserve heat by vasoconstriction; maternal analgesics may reduce thermal stability in newborn
Respiratory rate and effort	Infants are obligatory nose breathers		Reflex to open mouth to maintain airway not present for about 3 weeks
Observe respirations when infant is at rest Count respirations for full minute Apnea monitor Listen for sounds audible without stethoscope Observe respiratory effort	40/min Tend to be shallow, and when infant is awake, irregular in rate, rhythm, and depth No sounds should be audible on inspiration or expiration Breath sounds: bronchial; loud, clear, near	30-60/min May appear to be Cheyne-Stokes with short periods of apnea and with no evidence of respiratory distress First period (reactivity): 50-60/ min Second period: 50-70/min Stabilization (1-2 days): 30-40/ min	Apneic episodes: ≥15/sec Preterm or premature infant: "periodic breathing" Rapid warming or cooling of infant Bradypnea: ≤25/min Maternal narcosis from analgesics or anesthetics Birth trauma Tachypnea: ≥60/min RDS Aspiration syndrome Diaphragmatic hernia Sounds Rales, rhonchi, wheezes Expiratory grunt Distress: Nasal flaring, retractions, chin tug, labored breathing
Weight*			
Put protective liner in place and adjust scale to 0 Take weight at same time each day Protect newborn from heat loss	3400 g (7 lb 8 oz) Regains birth weight within first 2 weeks	2500-4000 g (5 lb 8 oz to 8 lb 13 oz) Acceptable weight loss: 10% or less	Weight ≤2500 g Prematurity Small for gestational age Rubella syndrome Weight ≥4000 g Large for gestational age (LGA): maternal diabetes Hereditary: normal for these parents Weight loss over 10%: dehydration?

*NOTE: Weight, length, and head circumference should all be close to same percentile for any child.

Continued.

Table 4-2, cont'd. *Physical Assessment of Newborn*

Area Assessed and Appraisal Procedure	Normal Findings		Deviations from Normal Range (Possible Causes)
	Average Findings	Normal Variations	
Head Circumference			
Measure head at greatest diameter: occipitofrontal circumference	33-35.5 cm (13-14 in) Circumferences of head and chest may be about the same for first 1 or 2 days after birth	32-37 cm (12½-14½ in)	Microcephaly (under 32 cm) Rubella Toxoplasmosis Cytomegalic inclusion disease (CMV) Hydrocephaly (≥4 cm more than chest) Increased intracranial pressure Hemorrhage Space-occupying lesion
May need to remeasure on second or third day after resolution of molding and caput succedaneum			
Chest Circumference			
Measure at nipple line	2 cm (¾ in) less than head circumference; averages between 30-33 cm (12-13 in)		Prematurity: ≤30 cm Postmaturity: some SGA and some LGA
Abdominal Circumference			
Measure below umbilicus	Abdomen enlarges after feeding because of lax abdominal muscles		Enlarging abdomen between feedings may indicate abdominal mass or blockage in intestinal tract
Length			
Measure recumbent length from top of head to heel; difficult to measure in full-term infant because of presence of molding, incomplete extension of knees	50 cm (20 in)	45-55 cm (18-22 in)	Chromosomal aberration Heredity: normal for these parents
Integument			
Color Inspection and palpation Inspect naked newborn in well-lit, warm area without drafts; natural daylight provides best lighting Inspect newborn when quiet and when active	Varies with ethnic origin; skin pigmentation begins to deepen right after birth in basal layer of epidermis Generally pink Acrocyanosis, especially if chilled	Mottling Harlequin sign Plethora Telangiectases ("stork bites" or capillary hemangiomas) Erythema toxicum neonatorum ("newborn rash")	Dark red: prematurity Pallor Cardiovascular problem CNS damage Blood dyscrasia; blood loss; twin transfusion Nosocomial problem (e.g., infection) Cyanosis Hypothermia Infection Hypoglycemia Cardiopulmonary diseases Malformations: cardiac, neurologic, or respiratory
Check for jaundice			Jaundice Gray: hypotension, poor perfusion
		Petechiae over presenting part	Petechiae over any other area

Table 4-2, cont'd. *Physical Assessment of Newborn*

Area Assessed and Appraisal Procedure	Normal Findings		Deviations from Normal Range (Possible Causes)
	Average Findings	Normal Variations	
Integument—cont'd			
			may be caused by the following: Clotting factor deficiency Infection
		Ecchymoses from forceps in vertex births or over buttocks and legs in breech births	Ecchymoses in any other area: hemorrhagic disease
Birthmarks Inspect and palpate for location, size, distribution, characteristics, color	Transient hyperpigmentation Areolae Genitals Linea nigra	Mongolian spotting Infants of black, Oriental, and American Indian origin; 70% Infants of white origin: 9%	Hemangiomas (vascular tumors) Nevus flammeus (port-wine stain) Strawberry mark Cavernous hemangiomas
Condition Inspect and palpate for intactness, smoothness, texture, edema	No skin edema Texture: thick; superficial or deep cracking Opacity: few large blood vessels seen indistinctly over abdomen	Slightly thick; superficial cracking, peeling, especially of hands, feet No blood vessels seen; a few large vessels clearly seen over abdomen Some fingernail scratches	Prematurity Edema on hands, feet; pitting over tibia Texture thin, smooth, or of medium thickness; rash or superficial peeling seen Numerous vessels easily seen over abdomen Postmaturity Texture thick, parchmentlike Skin tags; webbing Papules, pustules, vesicles, ulcers, maceration: impetigo, candidiasis, herpesvirus Diaper rash
Hydration and consistency Weigh infant routinely Inspection and palpation Gently pinch skin between thumb and forefinger over abdomen and inner thigh to check for turgor Check subcutaneous fat deposits (adipose pads) over cheeks, buttocks	Dehydration: best indicator is loss of weight After pinch is released, skin returns to original state immediately	Normal weight loss after birth is up to 10% of birth weight May feel puffy Amount of subcutaneous fat varies	Loose, wrinkled skin Prematurity Postmaturity Dehydration: fold of skin persists after release of pinch Tense, tight, shiny skin: edema, extreme cold, shock, infection Lack of subcutaneous fat (e.g., clavicle or ribs prominent): prematurity, malnutrition
Check voiding	Voids 6-10 times per day		
Vernix caseosa Observe amount		Amount varies; usually more is found in creases, folds	Absent or minimal: postmaturity Excessive: prematurity
Observe its color and odor before bath or wiping If not readily apparent	Whitish, cheesy, odorless		Yellow color Possible fetal anoxia 36 hours or more before birth

Continued.

Table 4-2, cont'd.   *Physical Assessment of Newborn*

Area Assessed and Appraisal Procedure	Normal Findings		Deviations from Normal Range (Possible Causes)
	Average Findings	Normal Variations	
Integument—cont'd			
over total body, check in folds of axilla and groin			Rh or ABO incompatibility Green color: possible in utero release of meconium because of fetal anoxia less than 36 hr before birth or presence of bilirubin Odor; possible intrauterine infection (e.g., amnionitis)
Lanugo Inspect for this fine, downy hair: amount, distribution	Over shoulders, pinnae of ears, forehead	Amount varies	Absent: postmaturity Excessive: prematurity, especially if lanugo is abundant and long and thick over back
Head			
Palpate skin		Caput succedaneum; may show some ecchymosis	Cephalohematoma

Palpate, inspect, measure fontanels	Anterior fontanel 5 cm diamond; increases as molding resolves
	Posterior fontanel triangle; smaller than anterior
		Fontanel size varies with degree of molding
		Fontanels may be difficult to feel because of molding
			Fontanels
			  Full, bulging: possible intracranial lesion (e.g., tumor, hemorrhage, infection)
			  Large, flat, soft: malnutrition, hydrocephaly, retarded bone age (hypothyroidism)
			  Depressed: dehydration
			  Large mastoid and sphenoid fontanels: hydrocephaly

Palpate sutures	Sutures palpable and not joined	Sutures may overlap with molding	Sutures
			  Widely spaced: hydrocephaly
			  Premature synostosis (closure)

Inspect pattern, distribution, amount of hair; feel texture	Silky, single strands, lies flat; growth pattern is toward face and neck	Amount varies	Fine, wooly: prematurity Unusual swirls, patterns, hairline or coarse, brittle: endocrine or genetic disorder

Inspect shape and size	Makes up one fourth of body length
	Molding
		Slight asymmetry from intrauterine position	Molding
			  Severe molding may result from birth trauma
			  Lack of molding: prematurity, breech presentation, cesarean birth
			  Circumference ≥4 cm larger than chest circumference: hydrocephaly; ≤32 cm: prematurity, microcephaly

Eyes			
Placement on face Symmetry in size, shape	Symmetric in size, shape		

Table 4-2, cont'd. *Physical Assessment of Newborn*

Area Assessed and Appraisal Procedure	Normal Findings		Deviations from Normal Range (Possible Causes)
	Average Findings	Normal Variations	
Eyes—cont'd			
Eyelids: size, movement, blink	Blink reflex Epicanthal folds: normal racial characteristic	Edema from instilling silver nitrate	Epicanthal folds, when present with other signs, may be caused by chromosomal disorders (e.g., Down's syndrome, cri-du-chat syndrome)
Discharge	None	Some discharge from silver nitrate	
Eyeballs: presence, size, shape	No tears Both present and of equal size; both round, firm	Occasionally has some tears Subconjunctival hemorrhage	Agenesis or absence of one or both eyeballs Small eyeball size: rubella syndrome Lens opacity or absence of red reflex: congenital cataracts, possibly from rubella Lesions: coloboma (absence of part of iris) Pink color of iris: albinism Jaundiced sclera Discharge: purulent Pupils: unequal, constricted, dilated, fixed
Eyeball movement	Random, jerky, uneven, can focus momentarily, can follow to midline	Transient strabismus or nystagmus until third or fourth month	Persistent strabismus
Eyebrows: amount, pattern	Distinct		
Nose			
Observe shape, placement, patency, configuration of bridge of nose	Midline Apparent lack of bridge, flat, broad Some mucus but no drainage Obligatory nose breathers Sneezes to clear nose	Slight deformity from passage through birth canal	Copious drainage, with or without regular periods of cyanosis at rest and return of pink color with crying: choanal atresia, congenital syphilis Malformed: congenital syphilis, chromosomal disorder Flaring of nares
Ears			
Observe size, placement on head, amount of cartilage, open auditory canal Hearing	Correct placement: line drawn through inner and outer canthi of eye should come to top notch of ear (at junction with scalp) Well-formed, firm cartilage	Size: small, large, floppy Darwin's tubercle (nodule on posterior helix)	Agenesis Lack of cartilage: possible prematurity Low placement: possible chromosomal disorder, mental retardation, kidney disorder Preauricular tags Size: may have overly prominent or protruding ears
Facies			
Observe overall appearance of face	Infant looks "normal"; features are well placed, proportionate to face	"Positional" deformities	Infant looks "odd" or "funny" Usually accompanied by other features (low-set ears, other structural disorders)

Continued.

Table 4-2, cont'd. *Physical Assessment of Newborn*

Area Assessed and Appraisal Procedure	Normal Findings		Deviations from Normal Range (Possible Causes)
	Average Findings	Normal Variations	
Mouth			
Inspection and palpation	Pink gums	Transient circumoral cyanosis	Gross anomalies
Placement on face	Symmetry of lip movement	Short frenulum	Placement, size, shape
Lips: color, configuration, movement, rooting reflex, sucking	Tongue does not protrude, is freely movable; symmetric in shape, movement		Cleft lip and/or palate, gums
			Cyanosis; circumoral pallor
Gums			Asymmetry in movement of lips: seventh cranial nerve paralysis
Tongue: attachment, mobility, movement, size			
Cheeks	Sucking pads inside cheeks		Macroglossia
Palate (soft, hard)		Anatomic groove in palate to accommodate nipple; disappears by 3-4 yr of age	Prematurity
Arch	Soft and hard palates intact		Chromosomal disorder
Uvula	Uvula in midline		Excessive saliva
Saliva: amount, character	Reflexes present	Epstein's pearls (Bohn's nodules): whitish, hard nodules on gums	Esophageal atresia
Chin			Tracheoesophageal fistula
Reflexes		Reflex response dependent on state of wakefulness and hunger	Micrognathia: Pierre Robin or other syndrome
			Teeth: predeciduous or deciduous
			Thrush: white plaques on cheeks or tongue that bleed if touched
Neck			
Inspection and palpation	Short, thick, surrounded by skinfolds; no webbing	Transient positional deformity apparent when neonate is at rest: head can be moved passively	Webbing
Length			Restricted movement; head held at angle; torticollis (wryneck), opisthotonos
Movement of head	Head held in midline, i.e., sternocleidomastoid muscles are equal; no masses		
Sternocleidomastoid muscles; position of head			Masses: enlarged thyroid
Trachea: position; thyroid gland	Freedom of movement from side to side and flexion and extension; cannot move chin past shoulder		Distended veins: cardiopulmonary disorder
Reflex response	Thyroid not palpable		Skin tags
			Positive owl's sign: prematurity
			Absence of head control: prematurity; Down's syndrome
Chest			
Inspection and palpation	Almost circular; barrel shaped	Occasional retractions, especially when crying	Bulging of chest
Shape	Symmetric chest movements; chest and abdominal movements synchronized during respirations		Pneumothorax
Clavicles			Pneumomediastinum
Ribs			Malformation: funnel chest (pectus excavatum)
Nipples: size, placement, number	Breast nodule: approximately 6 mm	Breast nodule: 3-10 mm	Fracture of clavicle
Breast tissue		Secretion of witch's milk	Nipples
Respiratory movements	Nipples prominent, well formed; symmetrically placed		Supernumerary, along nipple line
Amount of cartilage in rib cage			Malpositioned or widely spaced
Auscultation			Lack of breast tissue: possible prematurity
Heart tones and rate and breath sounds (see Vital signs, above)			Poor development of rib cage and musculature: possible prematurity
			Sounds: bowel sounds (see Abdomen, below)
			Retractions with or without respiratory distress

Table 4-2, cont'd. *Physical Assessment of Newborn*

Area Assessed and Appraisal Procedure	Normal Findings		Deviations from Normal Range (Possible Causes)
	Average Findings	Normal Variations	
Abdomen			
Inspect, palpate, and smell umbilical cord	Two arteries, one vein (AVA) Whitish gray Definite demarcation between cord and skin; no intestinal structures within cord Dry around base; drying Odorless	Reducible umbilical herniation	One artery: internal anomalies Bleeding or oozing around cord: hemorrhagic disease Redness or drainage around cord: infection, possible persistence of urachus Hernia: herniation of abdominal contents into area of cord (e.g., omphalocele); defect covered with thin, friable membrane, may be extensive Gastroschisis: congenital fissure of abdominal cavity Meconium stained: intrauterine distress
Inspect size of abdomen and palpate contour Auscultate for bowel sounds	Rounded, prominent, dome shaped because abdominal musculature is not fully developed No distension Bowel sounds heard 1 hr after birth	Some diastasis of abdominal musculature	Distension At birth Ruptured viscus Genitourinary masses or malformations: hydronephrosis; teratomas Abdominal tumors Mild Aerophagia Overfeeding High gastrointestinal tract obstruction Marked Lower gastrointestinal tract obstruction Imperforate anus Intermittent or transient Aerophagia Overfeeding Partial intestinal obstruction from stenosis of bowel Annular pancreas Malrotation of bowel or adhesions Sepsis
Auscultate for bowel sounds and note number, amount, and character of stools, and behavior—crying, fussiness—before and during elimination Color	Sounds present within 1-2 hr after birth Meconium stool passes within 24-48 hr after birth	Linea nigra may be apparent; possibly caused by hormone influence during pregnancy	Scaphoid, with bowel sounds in chest and respiratory distress: diaphragmatic hernia
Movement with respiration	Respirations primarily diaphragmatic; abdominal and chest movements synchronous		Decreased abdominal breathing Intrathoracic disease Diaphragmatic hernia

Continued.

Table 4-2, cont'd. *Physical Assessment of Newborn*

Area Assessed and Appraisal Procedure	Normal Findings		Deviations from Normal Range (Possible Causes)
	Average Findings	Normal Variations	
Genitals			
Girl			
Inspection and palpation			
General appearance	Female genitals	Increased pigmentation caused by pregnancy hormones	Ambiguous genitals—enlarged clitoris with urinary meatus on tip; fused labia: chromosomal disorder; maternal drug ingestions
Clitoris	Usually edematous		
Labia majora	Usually edematous; cover labia minora in term neonates	Edema and ecchymosis following breech birth	
Labia minora	May protrude over labia majora	Vaginal tag	Stenosed meatus
Discharge	Smegma	Blood-tinged discharge from pseudomenstruation caused by pregnancy hormones	Labia majora widely separated and labia minora prominent: prematurity
Vagina	Orifice open		
	Mucoid discharge	Some vernix caseosa may be between labia	Absence of vaginal orifice or imperforate hymen
			Fecal discharge: fistula
Urinary meatus	Beneath clitoris; hard to see—watch for voiding	Rust-stained urine (uric acid crystals) (To determine whether rust color is caused by uric acid or blood, wash under running warm tap water. Uric acid washes out, blood does not)	
Boy			
Inspection and palpation			
General appearance	Male genitals	Increased size and pigmentation caused by pregnancy hormones	Ambiguous genitals
Penis	Meatus at tip of penis		Urinary meatus not on tip of glans penis
Urinary meatus seen as slit			
Prepuce	Prepuce (foreskin) covers glans penis and is not easily retractable	Prepuce removed at circumsion	Hypospadias ⎱ May be associated with other anomalies
		Size of genitals varies widely	Epispadias ⎰
Scrotum	Large, edematous, pendulous; covered with rugae	Scrotal edema and ecchymosis if breech birth	
Rugae (wrinkles)		Hydrocele, small, noncommunicating	Adherent or tight prepuce: phimosis
			Scrotum smooth and testes undescended: prematurity, cryptorchidism
			Hydrocele
			Inguinal hernia
			Round meatal opening
Testes	Palpable on each side	Bulge palpable in inguinal canal	If not palpable may be in abdomen
Urination	Voiding before 24-48 hr, stream adequate, amount adequate	Rust-stained urine (uric acid crystals)	
Reflexes			
Erection	Erection may occur when genitals are touched		
Cremasteric	Testes are retracted, especially when neonate is chilled		
Extremities			
Clavicles	Intact		Fracture
General			

Table 4-2, cont'd. *Physical Assessment of Newborn*

Area Assessed and Appraisal Procedure	Normal Findings		Deviations from Normal Range (Possible Causes)
	Average Findings	Normal Variations	
Extremities—cont'd			
Inspection and palpation	Assumes position maintained in utero	Transient (positional) deformities	Limited motion: malformations
Degree of flexion	Attitude of general flexion		Poor muscle tone
Range of motion	Full range of motion, spontaneous movements		Positive scarf design
Symmetry of motion			
Muscle tone			
Arms			
Inspection and palpation	Longer than legs in newborn period	Slight tremors may be seen at times	Asymmetry of movement
Color	Contours and movement are symmetric	Some acrocyanosis, especially when chilled	Fracture
Intactness			Brachial nerve trauma
Appropriate placement	Should be intact		Malformations
Number of fingers	Fist often clenched with thumb under fingers		Asymmetry of contour
Palpate humerus			Malformations
Joints	Full range of motion; symmetric contour		Fracture
Shoulder			Amelia or phocomelia
Elbow			Webbing of fingers: syndactyly
Wrist			Absence or excess of fingers
Fingers			Palmar creases
Reflex: grasp			Simian line (commonly seen in Down's syndrome) seen with short, incurved little fingers
			Strong, rigid flexion; persistent fists; fists held in front of mouth constantly: CNS disorder
			Increased tonicity, clonicity, prolonged tremors (especially if whole body is involved): CNS disorder
Legs			
Inspection and palpation	Appear bowed since lateral muscles more developed than medial muscles	Feet appear to turn in but can be easily rotated externally, also positional defects tend to correct while infant is crying	Amelia, phocomelia
Intactness			Chromosomal defect
Length—in relation to arms and body and to each other	Major gluteal folds even		Teratogenic effect
	Femur should be intact	Acrocyanosis	Webbing, syndactyly: chromosomal defect
Major gluteal folds	No click should be heard; femoral head should not override acetabulum		Absence or excess of digits
Number of toes			Chromosomal defect
Femur	Feet flat; soles well lined (or wrinkled) over two-thirds		Familial trait
Head of femur as legs are flexed on hips and abducted; placement in acetabulum; femoral pulses	Plantar fat pad gives flat-footed effect		Femoral fracture: after difficult breech delivery
	Inspection and palpation		Congenital hip dysplasia
	Joints		Absent femoral pulses
	Hip		Soles of feet
Color	Knee		Poorly lined: prematurity
	Ankle		Covered with lines: postmaturity
	Toes		Simian line: Down's syndrome
	Reflexes		Congenital clubfoot
			Hypermobility of joints: Down's syndrome
			Yellowed nail beds
			Temperature of one leg differs from that of the other

Continued.

Table 4-2, cont'd. *Physical Assessment of Newborn*

Area Assessed and Appraisal Procedure	Normal Findings		Deviations from Normal Range (Possible Causes)
	Average Findings	Normal Variations	
Back			
Anatomy			
Inspection and palpation	Spine straight and easily flexed	Temporary minor positional deformities, which can be corrected with passive manipulation	Limitation of movement: fusion of deformity of vertebrae
Spine	Infant can raise and support head momentarily when prone		Pigmented nevus with tuft of hair when located anywhere along the spine is often associated with spina bifida occulta
Shoulders	Shoulders, scapulae, and iliac crests should line up in same plane		
Scapulae			
Iliac crests			Spina bifida cystica
Base of spine—pilonidal area			Meningocele
			Myelomeningocele
Reflexes (spinal related)			
Test reflexes			
Anus			
Inspection and palpation	One anus with good sphincter tone	Passage of meconium within 48 hr after birth	Low obstruction: anal membrane (thermometer cannot be inserted)
Placement	Passage of meconium within 24 hr after birth		High obstruction: anal or rectal atresia (thermometer may be inserted, but there is no passage of meconium)
Number	Good "wink" reflex of anal sphincter		
Patency			
Test for patency and sphincter response (active "wink" reflex)			
Observe for following:			Drainage of fecal material from vagina in female or urinary meatus in male: possible rectal fistula
Abdominal distension			
Passage of meconium			
Passage of fecal drainage from surrounding orifices			
Stools	Meconium transitional	First stool within 24 hours, appears on third to fourth day	Meconium may be passed in utero due to hypoxia
	Typical milk stool		Breast-fed infants' stools are different in color (yellow to golden) and consistancy and have an odor similar to that of sour milk

Table 4-3 *Assessment of Newborn's Reflexes*

Reflex	Eliciting the Reflex	Characteristic Response	Comments

Sucking and root-ing	Touch infant's lip, cheek, or cor-ner of mouth with nipple	Infant turns head toward stimulus, opens mouth, takes hold, and sucks	Difficult if not impossible to elicit after infant has been fed; if weak or absent, consider prematurity or neurologic defect
			Parental guidance
			    Avoid trying to turn head toward breast or nipple; allow infant to root.
			    Disappears after 3-4 months but may persist up to 1 year*

Swallowing	Swallowing usually follows suck-ing and obtaining fluids; suck and swallow are often uncoordi-nated in early-born infant and may also occur during first few hours of term (normal) infant's life	Swallowing is usually coordinated with sucking and usually occurs without gagging, coughing, or vomiting	If weak or absent, may indicate pre-maturity or neurologic defect
Extrusion	Touch or depress tongue	Newborn forces tongue outward	Disappears at about fourth month
Glabellar (Myer-son's)	Tap over forehead, bridge of nose, or maxilla of neonate whose eyes are open	Newborn blinks for first 4 or 5 taps	Continued blinking with repeated taps is consistent with extrapyra-midal disorder
Tonic neck or "fencing"	With infant falling asleep or sleep-ing, turn head quickly to one side	With infant facing left side, arm and leg on that side extend; op-posite arm and leg flex (turn head to right, and extremities assume opposite postures)	Responses in legs more consistent Complete response disappears by 3-4 months; incomplete response may be seen until third or fourth year After 6 weeks persistent response is sign of possible cerebral palsy

Grasp
    Palmar
    Plantar
	Place finger in palm of hand
	Place finger at base of toes
		Infant's fingers curl around exam-iner's fingers; toes curl down-ward	Palmar response lessens by 3-4 months; parents enjoy this con-tact with infant; plantar response lessens by 8 months

Moro's	Hold infant in semisitting position; allow head and trunk to fall backward to an angle of at least 30 degrees Place infant on flat surface; strike surface to startle infant	Symmetric abduction and exten-sion of arms; fingers fan out and form a **C** with thumb and forefinger; slight tremor may be noted; arms are adducted in embracing motion and return to relaxed flexion and move-ment Legs may follow similar pattern of response Premature infant does not com-plete "embrace," instead, arms fall backward because of weak-ness	Present at birth; complete response may be seen until 8 weeks* of age; body jerk only, between 8-18 weeks; absent by 6 month if neu-rologic maturation is not delayed; may be incomplete if infant is deeply asleep; give parental guid-ance about normal response Asymmetric response; possible in-jury to brachial plexus, clavicle, or humerus Persistent response after 6 months: possible brain damage
Startle	Loud noise of sharp hand clap elicits response; best elicited if newborn is 24-36 hours old or older	Arms abduct with flexion of el-bows; hands stay clenched	Should disappear by 4 months Elicited more readily in premature newborn (inform parents of this characteristic)
Pull-to-sit (traction)	Pull infant up by wrists from su-pine position	Head will lag until infant is in up-right position; then head will be held in same plane with chest and shoulder momentar-ily before falling forward; head will right itself spontaneously for a few moments	Depends on general muscle tone, maturity, and condition of infant

*All durations for persistence of reflexes are based on time elapsed since 40 weeks' gestation, that is, if this newborn was born at 36 weeks' gestation, add 1 month to all time limits given.

Continued.

Table 4-3, cont'd. *Assessment of Newborn's Reflexes*

Reflex	Eliciting the Reflex	Characteristic Response	Comments
Trunk incurvation (Galant)	Infant should be prone on flat surface; run finger down back about 4-5 cm (1½-2 in) lateral to spine, first on one side, and then down other	Trunk is flexed and pelvis is swung toward stimulated side	Response disappears by fourth week
Magnet	Infant should be supine; partially flex both lower extremities and apply pressure to soles of feet	Both lower limbs should extend against examiner's pressure	
Crossed extension	Infant should be supine; extend one leg, press knee downward, stimulate bottom of foot; observe opposite leg	Opposite leg flexes, adducts, and then extends	
Babinski's sign (plantar)	On sole of foot, beginning at heel, stroke upward along lateral aspect of sole, then move finger across ball of foot	All toes hyperextend, with dorsiflexion of big toe	Absence requires neurologic evaluation; should disappear after 1 year of age
Stepping or "walking"	Hold infant vertically, allowing one foot to touch table surface	Infant will simulate walking, alternating flexion and extension of feet; term infants walk on soles of their feet, and premature infants walk on their toes	Normally present for 3-4 weeks
Neck righting	Place newborn in supine position and turn head to one side	Shoulder and trunk and then pelvis will turn to be in alignment with head	Disappears at 10 months of age; absence: implications same as for absent tonic neck reflex
Otolith righting	Hold newborn erect and tilt body	Head returns to erect, upright position	Absence: implications same as for absent tonic neck reflex
Crawling	Place newborn on abdomen	Newborn makes crawling movements with arms and legs	Should disappear about sixth week of age
Deep tendon	Use finger instead of percussion hammer to elicit patellar, or knee jerk, reflex; newborn must be relaxed	Reflex jerk is present; even with newborn relaxed, nonselective overall reaction may occur	
Landau	Over a crib or a table, using two hands, suspend infant in prone position	Infant attempts to hold spine in horizontal plane	Absence suggests need for neurologic examination
Yawn, stretch, burp, hiccup, sneeze	Spontaneous behaviors	May be slightly depressed temporarily because of maternal analgesia or anesthesia, fetal hypoxia, or infection	Parental guidance Most of these behaviors are pleasurable to parents Parents need to be assured that behaviors are normal Sneeze is response to lint, etc., in nose and (usually) not an indicator of a cold
Sweat	Usually not present in term newborn	Sweat response usually not present in term infant; may be seen in infants with cardiac response	Parental guidance Amount of clothing for infant: indoors, outside Room temperature
Shiver	Usually not present in term newborn	Shiver response usually not present in term infant; if seen, check infant for postmaturity	See above
Kernig's sign	Flex thigh on hip and extend leg at knee	Procedure should be accomplished easily and without inflicting pain	Pain and resistance to extension of knee suggest meningeal irritability
Brudzinski's sign	Place infant in supine position; flex neck and observe knees	Infant does not move legs when neck is flexed	Spontaneous flexion of knees suggests meningeal irritability
Paradoxic irritability	Ascertain that infant is not hungry; hold and cuddle infant	Infant usually responds by quieting down	Infant cries when touched and held; response suggests meningeal irritability

Behavioral Characteristics

The behavioral characteristics of the newborn include purposeful (not only reflex) action, organization, and direction. Behavioral characteristics provide the basis of the social capabilities of the infant. To plan holistic care, the nurse should be knowledgeable about the newborn's behavioral characteristics and the parents' responses to them.

Table 4-4 *Behavioral States and State Behavior*

State	Characteristics of State				
	Body Activity	Eye Movements	Facial Movements	Breathing Pattern	Level of Response
Sleep States					
Deep sleep	Nearly still, except for occasional startle or twitch	None	Without facial movements, except for occasional sucking movement at regular intervals	Smooth and regular	Threshold to stimuli is very high so that only very intense and disturbing stimuli will arouse infants
Light sleep	Some body movements	Rapid eye movements (REMS), fluttering of eyes beneath closed eyelids	May smile and make brief fussy or crying sounds	Irregular	More responsive to internal and external stimuli; when these stimuli occur, infants may remain in light sleep, return to deep sleep, or arouse to drowsy
Awake States					
Drowsy	Activity level variable, with mild startles interspersed from time to time; movements usually smooth	Eyes open and close occasionally, are heavy-lidded with dull, glazed appearance	May have some facial movements; often there are none, and face appears still	Irregular	Infants react to sensory stimuli although responses are delayed; state change after stimulation commonly noted
Quiet alert	Minimum	Brightening and widening of eyes	Faces have bright, shining, sparkling looks	Regular	Infants attend most to environment, focusing attention on any stimuli that are present; optimum state of arousal
Active alert	Much body activity; may have periods of fussiness	Eyes open with less brightening	Much facial movement; faces not as bright as quiet alert state	Irregular	Increasingly sensitive to disturbing stimuli (hunger, fatigue, noise, excessive handling)
Crying	Increased motor activity, with color changes	Eyes may be tightly closed or open	Grimaces	More irregular	Extreme response to unpleasant external or internal stimuli

From Barnard KE, Blackburn S, Kang R, and Spietz AL: Early parent-infant relationships, Series 1: The first six hours of life, Module 3. White Plains, NY: The National Foundation/March of Dimes, 1978, p. 21, with permission of the copyright holder and the authors.

Table 4-5 *Infant Behavioral Patterns and Sensory Capabilities*

Pattern/Capability	Parameters of Normal	Deviations From Normal/Probable Conditions
Behavioral Patterns	Cortical control and responsiveness	CNS disorders
Feeding	Variations in interest, hunger; usually feeds well within 24 hours of birth	Lethargic, tires easily or may perspire while attempting to feed; poor suck, poor coordination with swallow, cyanosis, choking
Social	Cry is lusty, strong; soon indicative of hunger, pain, attention seeking	Weak or absent; high pitched
	Smiling, focusing evident within first week	Absence; no focusing on person holding him; unconsolable
	Responds by quietness and increased alertness to cuddling, voice	
Sleep-wakefulness	Transitional period with 2 periods of reactivity: at birth and 6-8 hours later	Lethargy; drowsiness
	Stabilization with wakeful periods about every 3-4 hours	Disorganized pattern
Elimination	Develops own pattern within first 2 weeks:	See "Elimination behaviors"
	Stooling: see "Elimination behaviors"	
	Urination:	
	First few days: 3-4 times daily	Diminished number: dehydration
	End of first week: 5-6 times daily	
	Later: 6-10 times daily with adequate hydration	
Reflex response	Brainstem development and musculoskeletal intactness	Present in anencephalic neonates also
	See "Assessment of newborn's reflexes," p. 125	Absence; hyperreactive; incomplete; asynchronous
Sensory Capabilities		
Vision	Limited accommodation with clearest vision within 18-20 cm (7-8 in)	Absence of these responses may be caused by absence of or diminished acuity or by sensory deprivation
	Detects color by 2 months but attracted by black-white pattern at 5 days or less	
	Focuses and follows by 15 min of age	
	Prefers patterns to plain surfaces	
	Prefers changes in patterns by 2 months	
	At birth, can gaze intently	
Hearing	By 2 min of age, moves eyes in direction of sound	Absence of response: deafness
	Responds to high pitch by "freezing," followed by agitation; to low pitch (crooning) by relaxation	
	Can hear beginning in last trimester of fetal life	
Touch	Sensitivity to pain may be diminished (because of β-endorphins present prenatally)	
	Soothed by massaging, warmth, weightlessness (as in warm water bath)	Unable to be comforted; possible drug dependence
Smell	By days 2 to 7 can distinguish between own mother's used breast pads and those of another woman	
Taste	By 3 days of age, can distinguish between sucrose and glucose and grimaces in response to drop of lemon juice on tongue	
Motor	Coordinates body movement to parent's voice and body movement; imitates parent's actions by 2 weeks of age	Absence

NURSING CARE OF THE NORMAL NEWBORN

During the neonatal period the prenatal and postnatal characteristics of the infant merge. Gradually the former disappear as the infant grows and matures outside the womb. Although most infants make the necessary bio-psychosocial adjustment to extrauterine existence without undue difficulty, their well-being depends on the care they receive from others.

The nurse in the various roles as teacher and support person acts as an advocate for the vulnerable infant. The nurse's skills in caring for the newborn and teaching these skills to parents are of paramount importance. Nurses are present during the formative stages of parent-child interac-tions. From their unique perspective they can do much to help both parents and child.

Procedures

The practitioner working in the newborn nursery must be proficient in performing procedures specific to new-born care. This section presents step-by-step explanations and scientific rationales for routine procedures, such as the heel stick and suctioning, as well as for the nursing inter-ventions that are performed in emergency situations. The nurse should always check the policy of the institution re-garding each procedure, since minor variations exist.

Procedure 4-1

HEEL STICK

DEFINITION

Collection of a capillary sample of blood by puncturing the outer aspect of the infant's heel.

PURPOSE

To obtain blood for the determination of the infant's blood glucose level and hematocrit.
To test for phenylketonuria (PKU), galactosemia, and hy-pothyroidism.

EQUIPMENT

Bard-Parker Number 11 or Redi-Lance blade; 70% alcohol; sterile cotton pledget or gauze square; capillary tube; plastic bandage; lab slip and label.

NURSING ACTIONS	RATIONALE
Wash hands before and after touching infant and equip-ment. Apply gloves.	To prevent nosocomial infection and implement universal precautions and precautions for invasive procedures.
Identify infant.	To ensure procedure is done on correct infant.
Wrap foot selected for heel stick.	To increase blood flow to extremity.
Select correct site on heel, lateral, plantar aspect.	To avoid residual scars and corn formation that may result if procedure is not done in proper area of heel.
Cleanse heel by rubbing with 70% alcohol.	To prevent infection.
Dry with sterile cotton pledget or gauze square.	To avoid introduction of contaminants into puncture.
Use blade to puncture heel deep enough to obtain free flow of blood.	To obtain sufficient blood for test.
Discard first drop.	To minimize contamination.
Quickly collect blood in appropriate capillary tubes.	To prevent coagulation of blood.
Cover puncture site with plastic bandage.	To prevent further bleeding and infection.
Send specimen with completed laboratory slip for analysis.	To allow ongoing evaluation and adjustment of care plans.
Record time, site of puncture, infant response.	To ensure communication with other caregivers.
Cuddle and comfort infant when procedure is completed.	To promote feelings of safety.

ASSISTING WITH VENIPUNCTURE

DEFINITION

Collection of venous blood.

PURPOSE

To obtain sample of venous blood for laboratory analysis.

EQUIPMENT

Restraint blanket; sterile syringe and needles; labeled specimen tubes; laboratory slips; sterile alcohol wipes.

NURSING ACTIONS	RATIONALE
Wash hands before and after touching infant and equipment.	To prevent nosocomial infection and implement universal precautions and precautions for invasive procedures.
Identify infant.	To ensure procedure is done on correct infant.
For *external jugular venipuncture:* "Mummy" the infant as necessary. Lower the infant's head over rolled towel, edge of table, or your knee, and stabilize.	To ensure safety and expose insertion site.
For *femoral venipuncture:*	To ensure safety and expose insertion site.
Position the infant in frog posture.	To prevent occlusion of vein in this area.
Place hands over infant's knees.	
Avoid pressure of fingers over inner aspect of thigh.	
Handle the infant gently and talk quietly to her or him during the procedure.	
When procedure is completed, apply pressure over the area with sterile gauze for 1 to 3 minutes.	To prevent leakage of additional blood into tissues or formation of hematoma, which may result in hyperbilirubinemia when the trapped RBCs break down.
Observe infant for 1 hour.	To detect further bleeding (oozing, hematoma). Any enclosed bleeding could lead to hypovolemic shock, hyperbilirubinemia, or both.
Send specimen with completed laboratory slip for analysis.	To allow ongoing evaluation and adjustment of care plans.
Record time, site of puncture, amount of blood taken, reason for specimen, and infant's response.	To ensure communication with other caregivers.
Cuddle and comfort infant when procedure is completed.	To promote feelings of safety.

Procedure 4-3

SUCTIONING OF UPPER AIRWAY: ASPIRATION OF MOUTH AND NOSE

DEFINITION

Use of a blunt-tipped, flexible rubber syringe for removal of secretions from mouth and nose.

PURPOSE

To remove mucus from mouth and nose.

EQUIPMENT

Sterile bulb syringe (intact and fairly firm).

NURSING ACTIONS	RATIONALE
Wash hands before and after touching baby and equipment.	To prevent nosocomial infection and to implement universal precautions.
Position infant:	
Support the wrapped infant on the arm or on the hip (in a football hold), positioning the child's head downward.	To assist gravity drainage.
NOTE: *Never* suspend infant by ankles in head-down position.	To avoid raising cerebral venous pressure, increasing the risk of accidently dropping the infant, hyperextending and stretching the spine, and causing pain to the baby.
Suction mouth first.	To avoid stimulation of sensitive receptors around the nares that respond to stimuli by initiating gasp. Any mucus present could be pulled into lower airway.
NOTE: Compress the bulb *before* insertion, expelling air.	To prevent blowing secretions deeper into mouth and nose.

NURSING ACTIONS	RATIONALE
Insert syringe into space between cheek and gums, release compression gradually, and create suction (to suck out mucus).	To prevent tissue trauma and remove secretions.
Remove syringe from mouth. Compress syringe to empty it and to create new vacuum to repeat procedure.	To prevent secretions from being forced into respiratory tract.
Repeat these last two steps as needed in mouth, then in nose. Stop suctioning when cry is clear (infant cry does not sound as though there were mucus or a bubble in the mouth).	To assess for patent airway. If cry is clear, infant's airway is patent.
Cuddle and reassure infant once episode is over.	To comfort infant since discomfort and fear and subsequent crying increases need for oxygen.
Demonstrate care of gagging or choking infant to parents.	To teach procedure since learning to meet this emergency in the hospital increases parental self-confidence and self-esteem and prepares parents for this activity at home.
Supervise parents in this technique.	To permit correction of any parental errors.

Procedure 4-4

SUCTIONING OF MIDAIRWAY (NASOPHARYNX AND OROPHARYNX) AND STOMACH ASPIRATION USING THE DELEE MUCUS TRAP

DEFINITION

Use of a mucus-trap catheter for removal of secretions.

PURPOSE

To remove mucus or meconium from the nasopharynx and oropharynx.
To remove amniotic fluid from the stomach.

EQUIPMENT

Sterile DeLee mucus-trap catheter (available in reusable glass or disposable plastic) with two-hole tip.
Sterile water. A 120 ml (4 oz) bottle of sterile water for feeding is convenient, already in a sterile container, and decreases risk of contamination possible with large stock bottles.

NURSING ACTIONS	RATIONALE
Wash hands before and after touching baby and equipment. Apply gloves.	To prevent nosocomial infection and to implememt universal precautions and precautions for intrusive procedures.
Place infant in supine position.	To facilitate suctioning.
Lubricate catheter in sterile water.	To facilitate passage of tube and prevent infection.
Aspirate mouth and throat first, then the nose.	To prevent infant's inhalation of pharyngeal secretions.
Insert catheter:	To decrease risk of laryngeal spasm and reflex.
Orally along base of tongue.	
Nasally horizontally into nares, then raising it to advance it beyond bend at back of nares.	
Avoid forcing catheter.	**Hazard:** To prevent direct tissue trauma or perforation in presence of congenital anomalies such as choanal, esophageal, or intestinal atresia.
Suction is applied by user.	To provide sufficient negative pressure to withdraw mucus or other substances.
Limit suctioning to 10 times or less.	To avoid prolonged suctioning that stimulates laryngo spasm and reduces oxygen (O_2) content in airway.
Apply suction only as tube is withdrawn.	To prevent direct tissue trauma.
Rotate catheter when suctioning.	To prevent tissue trauma consequent to tissue's being drawn into eye of catheter.
Discontinue suctioning when:	To pass the catheter correctly: Gagging indicates entrance into esophagus; coughing indicates entrance into trachea.
The cry is clear.	
Air entry into lungs is heard by stethoscope.	
Cuddle infant.	To reassure infant.
Detach mucus trap and send the enclosed specimen to the laboratory for examination and culture as necessary.	To allow ongoing evaluation of infant's condition.
Record the amount of mucus or amniotic fluid removed.	To ensure communication with other caregivers.

Procedure 4-5

SUCTIONING OF MIDAIRWAY (NASOPHARYNX AND OROPHARYNX) USING A NASOPHARYNGEAL CATHETER WITH MECHANICAL SUCTION APPARATUS

DEFINITION

Use of mechanical suction apparatus and external suction source for removal of secretions.

PURPOSE

To remove excessive or tenacious mucus from the nasopharynx and oropharynx in resuscitating an infant.

EQUIPMENT

Catheters:
  French, rubber (moderately firm); sizes 10, 12, and 14; whistle tip; two-hole tip French; plastic disposable: sizes 8, 10, and 12; finger control; two-hole tip.
External suction source.
Sterile water. A 120 ml (4 oz) bottle of sterile water for feeding is convenient, is already in sterile container, and reduces risk of contamination possible with large stock bottles.

NURSING ACTIONS	RATIONALE
Wash hands before and after touching baby and equipment. Glove.	To prevent nosocomial infection and to implement universal precautions.
Position the infant:	To (1) separate tongue from pharyngeal wall and (2) to prevent obstruction of newborn's normally low palate and macroglossia. (Some physicians prefer to work with the baby on a flat surface with no towel.)
Place the infant in supine position.	
Place a folded towel under the head to move it slightly forward from the neck (as in sniffing).	
Adjust negative pressure on portable or wall gauges.	To prevent excessive suctioning.
Keep deep suctioning to a minimum.	**Hazard:** To prevent direct trauma to mucosa with edema formation, bleeding, or increased secretions.
	To prevent stimulation of vagal reflex: bradycardia, cardiac arrhythmias, laryngospasm, and apnea, especially if this type of suctioning is done within a few minutes of infant's birth.
Limit each suctioning to 10 seconds or less.	To prevent laryngospasm and oxygen depletion.
If infant is active, an attendant may be needed to stabilize infant's head. Or if there is time, restrain infant by mummy technique before this procedure.	To prevent trauma and facilitate suctioning. Both hands are needed to manipulate catheter and finger control of suction pressure.
Lubricate catheter in sterile water.	To facilitate passage of tube and prevent infection.
Turn suction **off** as tube is put into position.	To prevent direct tissue trauma.
Avoid forcing catheter.	**Hazard:** To prevent direct tissue trauma or perforation in presence of congenital anomalies such as choanal, esophageal, or intestinal atresia.
Insert catheter:	To decrease risk of laryngeal spasm and reflex apnea.
Orally along base of tongue.	
Nasally horizontally into nares, then raising it to advance it beyond bend at back of nares.	
With catheter in place, put thumb over finger control to create suction. Rotate tubing between fingers while withdrawing catheter.	To prevent direct trauma caused by drawing mucosa into eye of catheter.
Apply suction only as tube is withdrawn.	To prevent direct tissue trauma.
Rotate catheter when suctioning.	To prevent tissue trauma consequent to tissues being drawn into eye of catheter.
Observe infant's response.	To prevent gagging, which indicates entrance into esophagus; coughing indicates entrance into trachea.
Withdraw tube to suction posterior nasopharynx.	
Comfort infant.	To prompt feelings of safety.
Record procedure.	To ensure communication with other caregivers.

DANGER SIGNS

Respiration

1. Bradypnea—respirations ≤ 25 per min
2. Tachypnea—respirations ≥ 60 per min
3. Abnormal breath sounds—rales, rhonchi, wheezes, expiratory grunt
4. Respiratory distress—nasal flaring, retractions, chin tug, labored breathing

EMERGENCY PROCEDURE

ABNORMAL NEWBORN BREATHING

DEFINITION

The assessment and treatment of abnormal or difficult breathing patterns in the newborn infant.

PURPOSE

To recognize difficult respiratory effort in the newborn.
To clear mucus and secretion from infant's airway.
To resuscitate infant if respirations have stopped.
To prevent cardiac arrest.
To provide more available oxygen to the infant.

EQUIPMENT

Bulb syringe, sterile DeLee catheter, oxygen source, stethoscope, external suction source, sterile water.

NURSING ACTIONS	RATIONALE
Wash hands before and after touching newborn or equipment.	To prevent nosocomial infection and implement universal precautions.
Assess infant's skin color.	*To identify abnormal newborn breathing:* pallor and cyanosis signal poor tissue perfusion.
Observe infant's respiratory effort.	Flaring of the nares and expiratory grunt are early signs of respiratory distress.
Watch for retractions: subcostal, xiphoid, intercostal, suprasternal, or clavicular.	Infant is using secondary muscles to breathe; using maximum effort to overcome respiratory distress.
Listen to respirations and lung sounds with a stethoscope.	Rales, rhonchi, and wheezes can be heard if they are present.
Position infant with head down.	To allow for gravity drainage.
If lung sounds are clear, use a bulb syringe to clear mouth and nose of secretions.	*To identify obstruction:* When lung sounds are clear, obstruction may be in nares or mouth. Mucus may be obstructing nasopharynx and oropharynx.
When bulb syringe doesn't work, employ a DeLee mucus-trap catheter to clear midairway or a mechanical suction apparatus.	*To apply suction:* Mechanical suction apparatus may be more easily available than a DeLee mucus-trap catheter. To prevent pushing mucus and debris farther down the airway.
If respirations have ceased, start mouth-to-mouth resuscitation after suctioning is complete.	
When respirations are reestablished and fairly regular, start oxygen therapy.	To increase level of available oxygen to the infant to aid tissue perfusion.

EMERGENCY PROCEDURE

MOUTH-TO-MOUTH AND MOUTH-TO-NOSE RESUSCITATION

DEFINITION

Artificial resuscitation performed when respirations have ceased.

PURPOSE

To reestablish respiration.

EQUIPMENT

None needed. If available: rolled towel, plastic airway, oxygen, suction.

NURSING ACTIONS	RATIONALE
Wash hands before and after touching infant and equipment. Glove.	To prevent nosocomial infection and to implement universal precautions.
Clear airway of any mucus or debris.	To prevent blowing debris down airway.
Position infant in "sniffing" position by putting rolled towel under head to move it slightly forward from neck, or leave infant on flat surface.	To open airway by straightening trachea and permitting back of tongue to fall away from posterior pharynx.
Insert plastic airway if available.	To provide unobstructed airway (especially from tongue if infant is flaccid).
Place your mouth over infant's nose and mouth to create seal.	To permit insufflation under pressure.
Repeat the word *ho* as you gently *puff* volume of air *in your cheeks* into infant. *Do not* force air.	To prevent injury to lung tissue (e.g., pneumothorax, pneumomediastinum).
Repeat puffs at rate of 30 per minute.	To approximate normal respiratory rate.
Infant's chest should rise slightly with each puff; keep fingers on chest wall to sense air entry.	To determine if air is reaching alveolar level.
Allow chest to fall by passive recoil.	To allow removal of insufflated air.
If available, place tubing of oxygen in your mouth as you inhale quickly between puffs.	To increase O_2 content in insufflated air.
Consider airway obstruction. Prepare for laryngoscopy and endotracheal intubation aspiration. See your hospital procedure manual.	To assess for obstruction; note if chest wall does not rise and the infant's vital responses do not improve in 30 sec.
Record procedure.	To ensure communication with other caregivers.

EMERGENCY PROCEDURE

CARDIOPULMONARY RESUSCITATION (CPR)

DEFINITION

A basic emergency procedure for life support consisting of artificial respiration and manual external cardiac massage.

PURPOSE

To prevent cardiac arrest following cessation of respirations (apnea extending beyond 15 sec).
To restore cardiac function.
To restore respiratory function.

EQUIPMENT

Resuscitation equipment should be readily available in areas in which respiratory arrest might take place, and the status of this equipment should be checked regularly, at least once a day.

NURSING ACTIONS	RATIONALE
Wash hands before and after touching infant and equipment. Glove.	To prevent nosocomial infection and to implement universal precautions.

EMERGENCY PROCEDURE—cont'd

NURSING ACTIONS	RATIONALE

Resuscitation

Observe color; tap, or gently shake shoulders. — To determine unresponsiveness or respiratory difficulty.

Yell for help; if alone, perform CPR for 1 min before calling for help again. — To bring help.

Turn infant to back, supporting head and neck — To protect neck.

Place on firm, flat surface. — To support infant's spine; prevents injury during compression of sternum.

Clear airway, prn (below). — To provide unobstructed ventilation.

Tilt head back gently to "sniffing" or neutral position; use head-tilt/chin-lift maneuver. — To open airway.

Do not hyperextend neck. — To prevent kinking of airway.

Assess for evidence of breathing: — To avoid unnecessary intervention.

Observe for chest movement.

Listen for exhaled air.

Feel for exhaled air flow.

Breathe for infant. — To assist ventilation.

Take a breath.

Open mouth wide and place over mouth and nose of infant to create seal. (See Emergency Procedure, "Mouth-to-Mouth Resuscitation," p. 134). — To provide mouth-to-mouth and mouth-to-nose resuscitation.

NOTE: Repeat the word *ho* as you gently puff volume of air *in your* cheeks into infant. *Do not* force air. — To permit insufflation under pressure. To reduce risk of gastric distension, regurgitation, and subsequent aspiration.

Infant's chest should rise slightly with each puff; keep fingers on chest wall to sense air entry.

Give two slow breaths (1.0 to 1.5 seconds per breath) pausing to inhale between breaths.

Check pulse of brachial artery while maintaining head tilt. — To determine need for intervention.

If pulse is present, initiate rescue breathing. Continue until spontaneous breathing resumes at rate of every 3 seconds or 20 times per minute. — To avoid unnecessary intervention.

If pulse is not present, initiate chest compressions and coordinate with breathing. — To restore cardiac function.

NOTE: When two people are present, breathing and compressions are shared. — To prevent fatigue!

Provide compressions/breathing: — To coordinate compressions/breathing.

Pause at end of every fifth compression to allow chest to fall by passive recoil. — To allow removal of insufflated air.

Maintain 5:1 ratio for 1 or 2 rescuers.

Reassess after 10 cycles, and every few minutes thereafter. — To maintain arterial P_{O_2} level.

Chest compressions:

Maintain head tilt. With other hand, position fingers for chest compressions. — To restore cardiac function.

Place index finger of hand farthest from infant's head just under imaginary line drawn between nipples.

Move index finger to a position one fingerbreadth below this intersection. — To identify compression area.

Using 2 or 3 fingers, compress sternum to depth of ½ or ¾ inch. — To minimize the chance of damage that might occur to the liver or spleen.

Release pressure without moving fingers from the position.

Repeat at a rate of at least 100 times per minute; 5 compressions in 3 seconds or less. — To approximate normal neonatal rate.

Perform 10 cycles of 5 compressions and 1 ventilation. (If possible, compressions are accompanied by positive-pressure ventilation at a rate of 40 to 60 per minute). Use this mnemonic: one-two-three-four-five-pause-head tilt-chin lift-ventilate- continue compressions. After cycles, check the brachial pulse to determine pulselessness (Nursing '87 Books). — To assist recall of correct ratio and timing.

Continued.

EMERGENCY PROCEDURE—cont'd

NURSING ACTIONS	RATIONALE
Discontinue compressions if the infant's spontaneous heart rate reaches or exceeds 80 beats per minute (Hazinski, 1987).	To prevent disrupting cardiac rhythm that has resumed.
Relieving airway obstruction	
Use no blind finger sweeps.	To avoid pushing obstruction deeper.
Initiate back blows and chest thrusts.	**Hazard:** To avoid the risk of injury to abdominal organs; Heimlich maneuver (abdominal thrusts) should not be used for infants of 1 year of age or less.
Position child prone over forearm with head down and with infant's jaw firmly supported.	To employ gravity to help remove obstruction.
Rest supporting arm on thigh.	To prevent rescuer's fatigue.
Deliver four back blows forcefully between infant's shoulder blades with heel of free hand.	To move obstructive materials outward.
Place free hand on infant's back to sandwich her/him between both hands: one hand supports the neck, jaw, and chest; the other supports the back.	To avoid injury to infant while turning infant.
Turn infant over and place head down, supporting head and neck. Apply four chest thrusts to same location as chest compressions but use a slower rate.	To force obstruction outward.
Open the airway with a head-tilt chin-lift maneuver and attempt to ventilate.	To ventilate infant.
Repeat the sequence until it is effective.	
ALTERNATIVE POSITION: Place infant face down on your lap with head lower than trunk and head firmly supported. Apply back blows, turn infant, and apply chest thrusts as above.	To employ gravity to remove obstruction.
Continue emergency procedures until signs of recovery occur, as indicated by palpable peripheral pulses, return of pupils to normal size and responsiveness, and the disappearance of mottling and cyanosis.	To continue ventilation. To meet standards of care.
Record time and duration of procedure and effects of intervention.	To ensure communication with other caregivers.
Teach procedure to parents or other caregivers.	To increase parents' knowledge and skill in self-care measure.

Procedure 4-6

WARMING INFANT USING SERVO-CONTROL INCUBATOR

DEFINITION

Use of infant's skin temperature, rather than circulating air to provide point of control.

PURPOSE

To maintain or restore infant's body temperature if it has not returned to normal within 2 hours using a radiant overhead heater.

EQUIPMENT

Servo-Control incubators or their equivalents employ the same principle as the thermostat in maintaining an even temperature in an oven or a room.

NURSING ACTIONS	RATIONALE
Wash hands before and after touching infant and equipment. Glove, prn.	To prevent nosocomial infection and to implement universal precautions.

Procedure 4-6—cont'd

NURSING ACTIONS	RATIONALE
Set the incubator control panel at the predetermined physician-ordered level, usually between 36° and 37° C (96.8° and 98.6° F).	To maintain a skin temperature of 36.5° C (97.6° F)
Tape a thermistor probe (automatic sensor) from the control panel to the right upper quadrant of the abdomen immediately below the right intracostal margin, never over a bone.	To ensure detection of even minor changes resulting from peripheral vasoconstriction, dilation, or increased metabolism long before a change in deep (core) body temperature develops.
Check the sensor periodically for its continued firm application to skin; check and record the core temperature with a clinical thermometer; record incubator temperature readings.	To ensure proper functioning of the equipment.
Record skin temperature reading and ambient temperature inside the incubator every 2 to 4 hours after the infant's temperature is stabilized.	To help in assessing the maintenance of adequate body temperature.
Record the infant's general appearance and behavior.	To ensure communication with other health care workers.

Procedure 4-7

WARMING INFANT USING OVERHEAD RADIANT HEATER

DEFINITION

Use of an overhead radiant heat source to prevent cold stress in an infant.

PURPOSE

To maintain or restore infant's body temperature.

EQUIPMENT

Overhead radiant heater. The heater thermostat must be kept plugged into an electrical outlet at all times. It is set to maintain an abdominal skin temperature of 36.5° C (97.6° F). The set point of 36.4° C (97.5° F) is usually chosen for activation of the heater. A probe may be attached to the infant's skin by a heat-deflector sticker.

NURSING ACTIONS	RATIONALE
Wash hands before and after touching infant and equipment. Glove, prn.	To prevent nosocomial infection and to implement universal precautions.
Turn radiant heater on.	To allow a few minutes for heater to warm up.
With warm, absorbent blanket, dry and place newborn under radiant heat shield.	To reduce heat loss by evaporation, conduction, convection, and radiation.
Adjust bassinet in head-down position (about 10 degrees).	To allow for gravity drainage of mucus in respiratory tract. If infant is suspected of having intracranial hemorrhage, keep head on same level as body or slightly elevated if mucus is not excessive.
Remove gross soiling (e.g., meconium, blood).	To facilitate observation of skin coloring and any changes.
Check thermostat setting for accuracy.	To prevent overheating or underheating.
Apply thermistor probe (metal side next to the infant) with paper tape or nonirritating plastic tape to anterior abdominal wall between navel and xiphoid process; do not place over bony rib cage. Thermistor, after it is taped to abdominal wall, must be covered by small plastic-foam square insulator. Optimally, it has a cover of aluminum foil.	To improve accuracy of skin temperature reading. Sensors respond more quickly to change.
	To provide foam insulation to thermistor. To prevent warming thermistor more quickly than baby is warmed (mechanism would respond to heated probe rather than to warmed baby).

Continued.

Procedure 4-7, cont'd

NURSING ACTIONS	RATIONALE
Check frequently to ensure that probe retains skin contact.	To prevent overheating or underheating.
Observe infant for color change; crying and restlessness; increased respiratory rate.	To determine if abnormal behavior is caused by cold stress or other factors (e.g., debility, sepsis).
Note previous symptoms; recheck probe, thermostat setting, and heater contact.	Rules out equipment malfunction.
Record findings. Note time and duration of procedure.	To ensure communication with other health care workers.

Procedure 4-8

INTRAMUSCULAR INJECTION

DEFINITION
Administration of medication by injecting it into the muscle fibers for absorption.

PURPOSE
To administer medication to the newborn.

EQUIPMENT
Syringe and needle, alcohol swab, medication, bandage.

NURSING ACTIONS	RATIONALE
Wash hands before and after touching infant and equipment. Glove, prn.	To prevent nosocomial infections and to implement universal precautions.
Recheck physician's order. Identify infant.	To ensure procedure is done on correct infant.
Restrain infant if necessary.	Newborn infants offer little, if any, resistance to injections. Although they squirm and may be difficult to hold in position if they are awake, they can usually be restrained without assistance from a second person if the nurse is skilled.
Use filter needle to withdraw medication. Replace filter needle with short, small-gauge tuberculin needle.	To avoid drawing small glass shards into the syringe, which could cause injury to the infant.
Select site for injection.	Selection of the site for injection is important. Injections must be placed in muscles large enough to accommodate the medication, yet major nerves and blood vessels must be avoided. The muscles of newborns may not tolerate more than 0.5 ml. The preferred site for newborns is the vastus lateralis, although the rectus femoris muscle can also be used. These two muscles, except for the femoral artery on the medial aspect of the thigh, are free of important nerves and blood vessels. The vastus lateralis muscle is the larger of the two and is well developed in the newborn.
NOTE: The posterior gluteal muscle is very small, poorly developed, and dangerously close to the sciatic nerve, which occupies a larger proportion of space in infants than in older children. Therefore it is not recommended as an injection site until the child has been walking for at least 1 year.	
Prepare injection site with alcohol cleansing. Grasp the muscle mass of the thigh to be injected firmly in one hand and compress the muscle mass for injection with the other hand.	To prevent infection. To stabilize the limb.
Inject the medication: Poise the needle just over the site (without touching the skin) and insert the needle with quick flexion of the wrist.	The dart method for injection is inappropriate when aiming at such a small target.
Comfort the infant and settle in crib.	To allay tension.
Discard equipment	
Record medication, amount, route, and site of injection.	To ensure communication with other caregivers.

SERUM BILIRUBIN TEST

Normal values:
    Direct bilirubin: 0.1 to 0.3 mg/dl
    Indirect bilirubin: 0.2 to 0.8 mg/dl
    Total bilirubin: 0.1 to 1.0 mg/dl
    Total bilirubin in newborns: 1 to 12 mg/dl
Phototherapy is usually started if total bilirubin is between
    5 and 9 mg/dl in less than 24 hours, or between 10 to 14
    mg/dl in 24 to 48 hours.

Procedure 4-9

PHOTOTHERAPY

DEFINITION

The treatment of neonatal hyperbilirubinemia and jaundice by exposing infant's bare skin to intense fluorescent light. The blue range of light accelerates the removal of bilirubin in the skin.

PURPOSE

To reduce levels of unconjugated bilirubin and prevent kernicterus.

EQUIPMENT

Phototherapy unit, eye patches, diaper—a face mask with wire support removed works effectively (some institutions use disposable diapers).

NURSING ACTIONS	RATIONALE
Wash hands before and after touching infant and equipment. Glove.	To prevent nosocomial infection and to implement universal precautions.
Identify infant.	To ensure procedure is done on correct infant.
Undress infant.	To expose as much skin area as possible to light.
Protect infant's eyes with eye patches.	To prevent possible injury to conjunctiva or retina.
Be sure eyes are closed.	To prevent corneal abrasions.
Check eyes for drainage each shift.	To prevent or allow prompt treatment of purulent conjunctivitis, should it occur.
	Research evidence suggests that exposure of the eyes to the phototherapy light units may injure the retina.
Diapering may be accomplished by using a "string bikini," paper face mask with the metal strip removed, or a disposable diaper.	To allow optimum skin exposure, yet sufficient to protect genitals and bedding. Metal strip is heated by light and can burn baby's skin.
After placing baby under light, monitor skin temperature. If infant is in incubator, temperature dial on control panel may need to be turned to maintain proper temperature.	To prevent hyperthermia or hypothermia.
	To prevent serious injury, all electric equipment should be grounded, free of defects, and operationally sound to maximize therapeutic effectiveness and to prevent electric shock or burn to the infant or the nurse.

Client Teaching

Teaching parents about their newborn and how to provide necessary care is an important function for the nurse. The following pages include guidelines for teaching parents about hyperbilirubinemia and bathing the infant. Also presented are medications commonly administered to newborns along with their side effects and instructions for parents. This section concludes with a summary of nursing actions for care of the normal newborn.

Guidelines For Client Teaching

HYPERBILIRUBINEMIA

ASSESSMENT

1. Infant, female term newborn, 8 lb 4 oz, 3 days old.
2. Infant bilirubin level is 13.5 mg/dl.
3. Infant breast-feeding.
4. Physician's orders: serial total bilirubin levels; photo-therapy.
5. Parents unaware of causes of jaundice and what photo-therapy is.

NURSING DIAGNOSIS

Knowledge deficit (parental) related to hyperbilirubinemia and phototherapy.

GOALS
Short-term

To teach parents what hyperbilirubinemia is and why pho-totherapy is ordered.

Intermediate

To increase parents' ability to evaluate their newborn at home for hyperbilirubinemia.
To reduce parents' anxiety.

Long-term

To provide knowledge of hyperbilirubinemia that can be used to prompt treatment for older infants, subsequent infants, and other family members.

REFERENCES AND TEACHING AIDS

Charts, phototherapy equipment, eye mask, paper diaper (or face mask with wire support removed), and printed pamphlets provided by hospital or formula companies for parents to take home and refer to later.

CONTENT/RATIONALE	TEACHING ACTIONS
To review meaning of terms parents will hear: Hyperbilirubinemia: higher levels of bilirubin than normal. Bilirubin: end product of red blood cells when they mature and break down. Jaundice: yellow color of whites of eyes, skin, and mucous membranes caused by circulating bilirubin. Phototherapy: the use of fluorescent light to break down bilirubin in the skin into substances that can be excreted in the feces (stool) or urine.	Seat parents in a quiet place, where they can see charts and talk easily to the nurse. Have chart made with terms spelled out. If possible, have parents hold their wrapped infant for this part of the class.
To review process of excreting bilirubin: When red blood cells (RBCs) break down they release bilirubin. Bilirubin circulates in the blood. In the liver it is combined with another substance. In the combined form it goes by way of the blood to the kidneys and the intestines. It gives the yellow color to urine and the brown color to the stool.	Point to chart depicting process as you explain. Ask for questions. Remind parents this is a process difficult for nurses and physicians to learn, so therefore many questions and repeated explanations are expected.
Before the baby was born, her RBCs were more numerous than ours. They also had a shorter life span, 70 to 90 days instead of 120 days. When the RBCs broke down, the baby's blood carried most of the bilirubin by way of the placenta to the mother's liver to be excreted.	Show picture of baby in utero. Trace route of blood from baby to mother's liver.
After the baby was born, her liver began to take care of all the bilirubin. Even though the baby's liver functions well, it cannot handle the whole load. Bilirubin seeps out of the blood and into the tissues, staining them yellow. The blood level of bilirubin rises quickly up to the fifth day, and then goes down; the jaundice usually clears up by the end of the week.	Point out yellowness of baby's skin. Show chart with approximate amounts of bilirubin and location. Prepare graph illustrating rise and fall of bilirubin over the first week of life.
If the baby is breast-feeding, a certain amount of the jaundice may be caused by the free fatty acids, which interfere with the conjugation of bilirubin.	Show chart with contents of breast milk and point out the level of free fatty acids. Refer back to chart depicting process of conjugation.
Some babies seem to have extra bilirubin to excrete. The amount in the tissues becomes too great when the blood level reaches 12 mg/dl. There is a danger that the bilirubin at high levels will cause damage to the brain. So your doctor wants the baby to be placed under the Bililight for phototherapy. This will help the baby handle the extra bilirubin and prevent damage to the baby's brain.	Show Bililight equipment. Let parents feel warmth of the light.

Guidelines For Client Teaching—cont'd

CONTENT/RATIONALE	TEACHING ACTIONS
We put eye masks on the baby to keep the light from her eyes.	Demonstrate use of eye mask. Bring infant and place in crib away from Bililight. Apply the eye mask.
We keep the baby undressed so as much light as possible can reach her skin.	Undress baby. Place under Bililight.
We use a paper diaper or the face mask as a small diaper (a "string bikini").	Diaper the infant.
We will take her temperature often so she will not become too hot or too cold.	Take and record temperature. Settle baby comfortably.
We will give her extra water to drink because she will have watery, green stools from the extra bilirubin being excreted.	Return to seats and review care. Distribute pamphlets.
We will be taking her out of the Bililight for feedings and cuddling. We will let you know when to come for feedings and to hold her.	
We will be taking blood tests to check the amount of bilirubin and we will let you know the results.	
To reassure parents that they can have questions answered after discharge.	Leave parents with infant. Tell them they can touch her, but not shield her skin from the light.
If you have any questions, ask us any time. We will give you our phone number and you can call at any hour. It is hard not being able to take her home with you.	Demonstrate stroking baby's hand. Return in about 10 minutes to see if there are any questions. Arrange feeding schedule with mother. Mother can continue to breast-feed or bring breast milk for feedings she will miss.

EVALUATION Woman (couple) verbalizes understanding of what has been taught and asks appropriate questions.

Guidelines For Client Teaching

BATHING AN INFANT

ASSESSMENT
1. Woman has just delivered her first child, a boy.
2. She has little experience with the care of children.
3. Woman exhibits a readiness to learn by asking many questions.
4. Woman's culture does not have specific prescriptions or proscriptions for this activity.

NURSING DIAGNOSES
Knowledge deficit related to bathing an infant.
Anxiety, mild, related to care of newborn infant.

GOALS
Short-term
To have woman learn infant bathing technique.

Intermediate
To have woman become skilled in bathing and handling infant.

Long-term
To have woman adjust bathing technique to developing child.

REFERENCES AND TEACHING AIDS
Texts; hospital or clinic-prepared instructions; film or video of parent bathing a baby; and parent's class on bathing a baby.

Continued.

Guidelines For Client Teaching—cont'd

CONTENT/RATIONALE	TEACHING ACTIONS
To review the purposes for bathing: It provides opportunities for (1) a complete cleansing of the infant, (2) observing the infant's condition, (3) promoting comfort, and (4) parent-child-family socialization.	Introduction: Set tone. Have mother seated comfortably (she may need a pillow or doughnut to sit on). Make sure she can see demonstration. Welcome father (or other family member) if present, and include in the process.
To help woman fit baths into her schedule: Initial bath: The initial bath is postponed until the infant's skin temperature stabilizes at 36.5° C (97.6° F) or core temperature stabilizes at 37° C (98.6° F) for 2 hours. Daily bath: a daily bath may be given at any time convenient to the parent but not immediately after a feeding period, since the increased handling may cause regurgitation of the feeding.	Ask mother when father and siblings would be available for infant bath. To prevent cold stress.
To prevent heat loss: The temperature of the room should be 24° C (75° F), and the bathing area should be free of drafts. Heat loss in the infant is greater than in the adult because of the relatively large ratio of skin surface to body mass in the newborn. Heat loss must be controlled during the bath period to conserve the infant's energy. Bathing the infant quickly, exposing only a portion of the body at a time, and thorough drying is therefore part of the bathing technique.	Review material pertinent to care before beginning bath to prevent heat loss. Explain that infants do not shiver to increase body temperature, as adults do. Explain mechanism of burning fat for heat maintenance in the infant and the amount of energy it requires. Show a chart depicting this mechanism simplified.
To prevent skin trauma: The fragile skin can be injured by too vigorous cleansing. Vernix, the white, cheesy-looking material on the skin is not removed, since it is attached to the upper layer of the skin. Too vigorous removal results in removal of the protective skin layer. Vernix may be left on for 48 hours; if it persists beyond that time, it may be washed off gently. If stool or other debris has dried and caked on the skin, soak the area to remove it. Do not attempt to rub it off because abrasion may result. Gentleness, patting dry rather than rubbing, and use of a mild soap without perfumes or coloring are recommended. Chemicals in the coloring and perfume can cause rashes in sensitive skin.	Review material pertinent to skin care before beginning bath to prevent heat loss. Review possible sources of skin damage (for all members of family): dyes, perfumes.
Supplies and clothing are made ready. Clothing suitable for wearing indoors: diaper, shirt; stretch suit or nightgown optional. Unscented, mild soap. Baby lotion not powder. Baby powder can be inhaled by the infant. Pins, if needed for diaper, are placed well out of baby's reach.	Arrange work area while explaining process. Comment on equipment and clothing so that mother sees importance of preparing area before child is brought in. Sticking them in a bar of soap both lubricates them and keeps them away from the infant.
Cotton balls. Towels for drying infant and a clean washcloth. Receiving blanket. Bring infant to bathing area when all supplies are ready. The infant is never left alone on bath table or in the bath water, not even for a second. If the mother or nurse has to leave, the infant is taken along or put back in the crib. Test temperature of the water. It should feel pleasantly warm to the inner wrist (about 98 to 99° F). The infant's head is washed before unwrapping and undressing to prevent heat loss. Cleanse the eyes from the canthus outward, using a **clean** washcloth. For the first 2 to 3 days a discharge may result from the reaction of the conjunctiva to the substance	Model holding of infant and protecting him with hand. Review major cause of death in small children: drowning. Demonstrate testing water. Let mother feel. Explain that the infant is washed from head to toe starting with the eyes and ending with the genitals. Demonstrate cleansing the eyes and washing the face. Teach general hygiene measure to prevent spread of infection.

Guidelines For Client Teaching—cont'd

CONTENT/RATIONALE	TEACHING ACTIONS

(erythromycin) used as a prophylactic measure against infection. Any discharge should be considered abnormal and reported to the physician. When removing eye discharge avoid contamination of one eye with the discharge from the other by using a separate cotton swab and water source (running water from a tap is best) for each eye.

The **scalp** is washed daily with water and mild soap. It must be rinsed well and dried thoroughly. Scalp desquamation, called **cradle cap**, can often be prevented by removing any scales with a fine-toothed comb or brush after washing. If condition persists, the physician may prescribe an ointment to massage into the skin.

    Demonstrate washing and drying head. Use football hold. Teach mother now (or later) to use football hold.

Creases under the chin and arms and in the groin may need daily cleansing. The crease under the chin may be exposed by elevating the infant's shoulders 5 cm (2 in) and letting the head drop back.

    Demonstrate washing creases. Teach potential of warmth, moisture, and unwashed areas for providing an excellent condition for skin breakdown and infection.

Cleanse the **ears** and **nose** with twists made of moistened cotton.

    Demonstrate cleansing of ears and nose. Review reason for the saying, "Do not put anything smaller than your elbow into your ear."

Undress baby and wash body and arms and legs. Pat dry gently. Baby may be tub bathed after the cord drops off.

    Demonstrate sponge bath of infant. Rinse well. Pat dry.

To teach care of the cord:

Use a cotton swab. Dip swab in solution the physician has ordered and cleanse around base of the cord, where it joins the skin. Notify your physician of any odor, discharge, or skin inflammation around the cord. The clamp is removed when the cord is dry (about 24 to 48 hours). When you diaper the infant, the diaper should not cover the cord. A wet or soiled diaper will slow or prevent drying of the cord and foster infection. When the cord drops off in a week to 10 days, small drops of blood can be seen when the baby cries. This will heal itself. It is not dangerous.

    Demonstrate care of cord.
    Ask mother what she would report.
    Ask mother what she has heard about the cord and cord care.

To teach care of hands and feet:

Wash and dry between the fingers and toes daily.

    Check between fingers and toes.

Fingernails and toenails are not cut immediately after birth. The nails have to grow out far enough from the skin so that the skin is not cut by mistake. Before the nails can be cut, if the baby scratches himself, you can apply loosely fitted mitts over each hand. Do so as a last resort, however, since it interferes with the baby's ability to console himself. When the nails have grown, the **fingernails** and **toenails** can be cut more readily with manicure scissors (preferably with rounded tips) when the infant is asleep. Nails are kept short.

    Show picture of mitts.
    Review safety measures.

To cleanse genitals:

Cleanse the **genitals** of infants daily and after voiding and defecating. For girls, cleansing of the genitals may be done by separating the labia and gently washing from the pubic area to the anus. For uncircumcised boys, gently pull back (retract) the foreskin. Stop when resistance is felt. Wash the tip (glans) with soap and warm water and replace the foreskin. The foreskin must be returned to its original position to prevent constriction and swelling. In the majority of newborns, the inner layer of the foreskin adheres to the glans. By the age of 3 years, in 90% of boys the foreskin can be retracted easily without pain or trauma. For others, the foreskin is not retractable until

    Demonstrate cleansing of genitals.
    Review foreskin—purposes, cultural factors, anatomy and physiology—as necessary.
    Demonstrate technique and explain rationale while doing it.

Continued.

Guidelines For Client Teaching—cont'd

CONTENT/RATIONALE	TEACHING ACTIONS
the teens. As soon as the foreskin is partly retractable, and the child is old enough, he can be taught self-care.	
To review dressing the infant:	Demonstrate technique and explain rationale while doing it.
When dressing the child, do not pull shirts roughly over the face or catch fingers in shirt sleeves. Bunch up the shirt in both hands and expand the neck opening before placing the neck opening over the face; then slip the shirt over the rest of the head.	
Diapering the infant may be done before and after feeding. It is not necessary to wake the infant for changing.	
If cloth diapers are used, absorbency can be increased by bringing the bulk of the diaper in the front for a boy and in the back for a girl. This will help absorb urine so that skin is protected. The diaper between the infant's legs should not be bulky because it can cause outward displacement of the hips. A soaker pad can be placed under the infant as a protection for the blanket. The continued use of plastic or rubber pants may lead to diaper rash.	
Store infant's towels, washcloths, and supplies apart from the family for 4 to 4 months to prevent infection.	Clean and tidy area. Reassure mother you will be with her when she gives the bath tomorrow.

EVALUATION Woman gives return demonstration that shows competence.

MEDICATIONS FOR NORMAL NEWBORN

Phytonadione (Vitamine K) (prescription)
Brand names: AquaMEPHYTON, KonaKion, Mephyton
Dosage form: IM
Use: Given to neonate to assist clotting mechanism. (vitamin K is manufactured in the gut; the neonate's gut is sterile at birth.)
Side effects: Headache, nausea, decreased liver function, hyperbilirubinemia, hemoglobinuria, hemolytic anemia, rash, urticaria
Drug interactions: None given to neonate
Patient education: Tell mother to observe site for bleeding or hematoma.

Erythromycin Ophthalmic (prescription)
Brand name: Ilotycin Ophthalmic
Dosage form: Ophthalmic ointment
Use: Administered immediately after delivery to stop opthalmia neonatorum caused by *Neisseria gonorrhea and Chlamydia* organisms
Side effects: Hypersensitivity, overgrowth of nonsusceptible organisms
Drug interactions: None for the neonate
Patient education: Tell mother to report lacrimation, itching, redness, swelling.

Summary of Nursing Actions

NURSING CARE OF THE NORMAL NEWBORN

I. Goals
  A. Infant
   1. To provide support for infant's transition from in-trauterine to extrauterine life
   2. To provide freedom from trauma, infection, and injury
   3. To provide opportunities for continued bonding with primary caretakers
  B. Family
   1. To provide opportunities to acquire and increase knowledge, skill, and confidence in child-care activities
   2. To provide opportunities for parents to recognize knowledge already obtained
   3. To provide opportunity for parents to ask questions and increase data base
   4. To provide opportunities for parents to intensify bonding with their newborn

II. Priorities
  A. Physiologic functions
   1. Establish and maintain respirations
   2. Maintain stable body temperature
   3. Establish and maintain feeding and elimination patterns
  B. Nursing functions
   1. Protect infant from infection and trauma
   2. Protect infant from injury
   3. Promote infant-family attachment

III. Assessment
  A. Admission to nursery
   1. Check infant's ID with delivery room nurse.
   2. Assess for signs of problems:
     a. Gestational history (mother's age, psychosocial status, expected date of confinement, physical problems)
     b. Birth experience (labor status, maternal medications, anesthesia, type of delivery, nuccal cord, Apgar score)
     c. Care at birth (eye prophylaxis, vitamin K injection, cord clamp)
     d. General condition and activity (infant's alertness, respirations, voiding, meconium, number of cord vessels)
     e. Color (signs of jaundice or cyanosis)
   3. Physical assessment (see Table 4-2)
   4. After temperature is stabilized:
     a. Weigh on admission and at 8 hours.
     b. Check length.
     c. Check chest circumference and head circumference (repeat head circumference after caput succedaneum and molding have resolved.
   5. Assess respiratory function (see "Danger Signs, Respiration," p. 133; Emergency Procedure, "Abnormal Newborn Breathing," p. 133).
   6. Maintain patent airway (see Procedures 4-5 and 4-6 and Emergency Procedures, "Mouth-to-Mouth and Mouth-to-Nose Resuscitation," p. 134).

   7. Assess fluids and nutrients.
     a. Feeding capabilities
     b. Intake and output
   8. Assess cardiovascular system (see Table 4-1)
   9. Assess behavioral characteristics, e.g., cuddliness, sleep-wake cycles (see Tables 4-4 and 4-5).
   10. Safety: assess family provisions in relation to:
     a. Caretaking activities
     b. Social interactions
     c. Transportation of infant
     d. Professional assistance for health maintenance or illness
   11. Parental and family bonding with newborn (see Tables 4-4 and 4-5).
  B. Days 2 to 5
   1. Respiration: Observe respirations and breath sounds, recording every 8 hours while infant is in the hospital.
   2. Nutrition: Observe and record feeding behavior, amount of formula, water taken, any regurgitations.
   3. Cardiovascular system: Assess rate and rhythm of heartbeat (apical) every 4 to 8 hours while infant is in the hospital. Note its regularity and presence of murmurs.
   4. Temperature: Take and record body temperature every 8 hours while infant is in the hospital.
   5. Cord: Note healing of cord; apply povidone-iodine or triple dye as prescribed.
   6. Circumcised penis (day 3): Check healing process. Incised area of penis should appear clean. Check for infection, odor, or discharge.
   7. Urination: Record number of voidings. Note color and consistency of urine; record if abnormal.
   8. Defecation: Note and record changes in stool color and consistency and in pattern infant establishes while in the hospital.
   9. Integumentary system: Assess for
     a. Rashes
     b. Excoriations
     c. Color; by second day, jaundice
     d. Dehydration, peeling and cracking, skin turgor
     e. Wounds
     f. Cleanliness
   10. Weight: Weigh daily while infant is in the hospital.
   11. Review findings of blood tests.
     a. Phenylketonuria test 48 hours after ingestion of protein (formula or breast milk)
     b. Galactosemia
     c. Hypothyroidism
   12. Other physical findings: Assess
     a. Reflexes, Table 4-3
     b. Behavioral states, Table 4-4
   13. Safety: Assess parental competence in caring for their newborn.

Continued.

Summary of Nursing Actions—cont'd

15. Parent and family response and interaction with newborn
    a. Mother interactions: Note mother's responses when caring for and holding her infant.
    b. Father interactions: Note father's responses as he holds or cares for his infant. Assess his knowledge of and skill in caring for the infant.
    c. Grandparent
    d. Siblings: Note sibling's reactions with the infant. Note mother and father's reaction to the sibling response.

IV. Potential nursing diagnostic categories
    1. Potential for injury
    2. Potential altered nutrition: less than body requirements
    3. Ineffective airway clearance
    4. Ineffective breathing pattern
    5. Potential altered body temperature
    6. Pain
    7. Potential for infection
    8. Altered peripheral tissue perfusion
    9. Decreased cardiac output
    10. Knowledge deficit: parenting
    11. Impaired gas exchange
    12. Potential fluid volume deficit
    13. Altered patterns of urinary elimination
    14. Potential ineffective breast feeding
    15. Potential for trauma
    16. Potential altered family processes
    17. Ineffective family coping: compromised
    18. Ineffective individual coping
    19. Altered growth and development
    20. Anxiety

V. Plan implementation
    A. On admission to nursery
       1. Receive reports of newborn progress to date.
       2. Maintain ambient temperature.
       3. Perform initial admission assessment per hospital protocol.
       4. Notify physician of admission.
       5. Provide for:
          a. Skilled personnel and adequate facilities to ensure continuous assessment, protection against infection or trauma, and emergency care if needed
          b. Consideration of needs of high-risk newborn or one with special needs
          c. Complete medical or nursing records
       6. Respirations
          a. Perform procedures as necessary for clearing airway of mucus (Procedures 4-4, 4-5, and 4-6)
          b. If abnormal symptoms occur, institute interventions indicated (see Emergency Procedure, "Mouth-to-Mouth and Mouth-to-Nose Resuscitation," p. 134).
          c. Inform parents of infant's breathing pattern.

7. Feeding
   a. Provide or supervise initial feeding before the sixth hour. Note newborn's feeding behavior.
   b. Inform parents of infant's feeding behavior.
   c. Assist with breast-feeding or bottle-feeding (see Guidelines for Client Teachings, "Breast Feeding," pp. 154-155, and "Formula Feeding," pp. 156-157, and Table 4-8 and 4-9).
   d. Demonstrate and supervise practicing of care that is required if newborn chokes or regurgitates at feeding time.

8. Cardiovascular system: Prevent stress by providing warmth, fluids, nutrients and comfort as needed; protect newborn from infection and trauma.

9. Temperature: Stabilize newborn's temperature by one of the following methods:
   a. Remove blood and excessive vernix from newborn, dress in shirt and diaper, wrap snugly in blanket, and give to parent to hold.
   b. Position newborn on side in bassinet, cover with light blanket, and then place under heat lamp until temperature is stabilized. Check body temperature every hour to prevent hyperthermia.
   c. Place thoroughly dried infant under radiant panel without clothing until the temperature has stabilized. Check body temperature every hour to prevent hyperthermia. Then bathe newborn; if body temperature drops, place infant under heat panel until temperature is stabilized.
   d. Minimize heat loss by performing examinations under heat panel, and postpone initial bath (if given) until newborn's temperature reaches 36.5 C (97.6 F).

10. Cord and circumcised penis
    a. Administer prescribed dose of vitamin K and preparation AquaMEPHYTON, intramuscularly.
    b. Position infant so that no pressure is exerted on the cord or the circumcised penis.
    c. Clean routinely and as needed after soiling

11. Urination: Instruct parents as to number of times newborns void (six to ten times per day), color of urine (pale, strawcolored), and need for diaper changes.

12. Defecation
    a. Instruct parents about characteristics of their newborn's stool and stooling pattern.
    b. If necessary teach parents how to diaper their infant.

13. Integumentary system
    a. Bathe infant quickly to prevent loss of loss of heat; use mild soap and water.
    b. Remove only surface excess vernix and blood (mats the hair).

Summary of Nursing Actions—cont'd

    c. Dress, diaper, and wrap snugly.

14. Infant-family relationships
   a. Allow mother or father to hold infant as soon after birth as possible.
   b. Examine infant in presence of parents. Discuss normality of infant's condition, appearance, and behavior.
   c. Inform parents of infant's progress and characteristics.
   d. Discuss parental-family responses to child. Review plans of care.

B. Days 2 to 5.
1. Respirations: Maintain open airway
2. Feeding: Parent becomes adept at feeding infant and assessing fluid and nutritional needs.
3. Cardiovascular system: Inform parents of normality
4. Temperature
   a. Dress infant in clothing suitable to maintain warmth in varying temperatures.
   b. If baby's temperature is elevated, rule out dehydration, fever, and overheating. Give up to 120 ml (4 oz) of sterile water; remove some of infant's coverings. Recheck temperature in 1 hour. If elevation persists, call pediatrician.
5. Cord
   a. Prevent infection; clean routinely.
   b. Remove clamp when cord is dry.
   c. Demonstrate care of cord; supervise mother's care of cord.
6. Circumcised penis: Circumcision is a surgical procedure and requires routine precautions related to postsurgical care.
   a. Control excessive bleeding by use of pressure (4 × 4-inch gauze). If bleeding is not controlled, vessel may need to be ligated. Notify physician and prepare equipment (circumcision tray and suture). Maintain pressure intermittently until physician arrives.
   b. Prevent infection. Change soiled diapers and wash penis and glans with soap and water.
   c. Demonstrate care of circumcised penis to parents. Supervise mother's care the first few times.
7. Genitalia
   a. Demonstrate care and supervise mother if necessary.
   b. Wash penis with soap and water. Do not attempt to retract the foreskin with force. Replace foreskin after bathing if retracted.
   c. Wash labia from front to back. Instruct mother on washing female genitalia.
   d. Instruct parents in care of diapers and how to recognize rashes. Supervise parents changing diapers the first few times.
8. Urination: Instruct mother that diapers need to be changed frequently but it is not necessary to waken newborn for diaper change.

9. Defecation: Instruct parents on appearance of stool and changes to expect. Suggest they assess infant for pattern of stooling.
10. Weight: Report weight to physician if loss exceeds 10% of birth weight. Report weight to parents and its significance.
11. Integumentary system
   a. Inform parents of significance of jaundice and of tests if ordered.
   b. Perform heel sticks for blood specimens for bilirubin tests (see Procedure 4-1; Guidelines for Client Teaching; "Hyperbilirubinemia, pp. 140-141; and Procedure 4-10).
12. Appearance and behavior: Help parents become aware of infant's normal responses (see Table 4-4, "Behavioral States and State Behavior").
13. Bathing
   a. Give sponge bath as indicated. Wash scalp every day. Use mild, nonperfumed soap if needed. Baby lotion may be used; do not use powder and oil.
   b. Substitute tub bath for sponge bath when cord falls off.
   c. Select area for bathing—out of drafts and large enough so infant does not fall off.
   d. Organize equipment and clothing before bringing infant to area.
   e. Form habit of keeping instruments, pins, scissors, etc, closed and out of reach of infant.
   f. Cut infant's nails with manicure scissors or infant scissors while infant sleeps.
   g. Provide care for genitals.
   h. Teach parents how to bathe their infant (see Guidelines for Client Teaching; "Bathing an Infant," pp. 141-144).
14. Infant-family relations: Promote healthy infant-family bonding.
15. Safety
   a. Instruct parents in safety measures.
   b. Provide parents with written information on where to call and what to report for newborn illness or other problems.
   c. Perform heel stick on infant for necessary blood tests before discharge, i.e., for PKU, galactosemia, and hypothyroidism.
   d. If parents refuse tests before discharge, they can be performed at a later date by a physician or public health nurse. However, parents must understand that serious damage can be done in the first few weeks of life if these diseases are not diagnosed and treated.

VI. Evaluation
A. Admission to nursery
1. Report from labor room nurse is complete, and records are up-to-date.
2. Newborn is admitted to unit per hospital protocol.

Continued.

Summary of Nursing Actions—cont'd

3. Newborn is placed in crib and protected from cold stress.
4. Assessment of newborn by 24th hour by professional personnel reveals satisfactory adjustment of newborn and a normal physical status. Newborn's appearance and activity (reflexes and behavior patterns) are within normal limits.
5. Environment provides for protection and safety of infant.
6. Respirations: Airway is open, and by 6 to 10 hours, respirations are stabilized at 30 to 60 per minute with short periods of apnea (e.g., periodic breathing, apneic periods no longer than 15 seconds). Breathing is quiet, no grunting or wheezing. Chest and abdomen rise in synchronized motions, and there is no sternal retraction. Infant breathes through nose; nares do not flare on inspiration. Cyanosis may be present in hands and feet.
7. Feeding
   a. Initial feeding of newborn is done by the sixth hour. Mother begins breast-feeding at birth (first wakeful period), or newborn is given water by nursery personnel.
   b. Acceptance and swallowing of nutrients and fluids (water, formula, or colostrum) is satisfactory by twelfth hour. Amount of regurgitation of mucus or nutrients and fluids is within normal limits by 24th hour.
8. Cardiovascular system
   a. Heart rate: between 120 and 160 beats/minute; regular in rhythm by the twelfth hour; rate may drop to 100 beats/minute in deep sleep but returns immediately with activity. It increases with stress and activity. Most soft murmurs heard during neonatal period are functional and without pathologic significance.
   b. Blood pressure: Systolic pressure is 60 to 80 mm Hg; diastolic pressure is 40 to 50 mm Hg.
9. Temperature: Newborn's axillary temperature is stabilized by twelfth hour and maintained between 36.5° and 37° C (97.6° to 98.6° F).
10. Cord: Healing of cord is adequate (i.e., no oozing of blood or evidence of inflammation).
11. Penis: Healing of penis is adequate if circumcision was performed (i.e., no excessive bleeding or evidence of inflammation).
12. Urination: Some infants void at birth; most void 12 to 24 hours after birth.
13. Defecation: Meconium stool may be passed at birth or any time thereafter until 24th hour.
14. Integumentary system: Initial bath is given once newborn's temperature is stabilized. Routine care is established for hygiene.
15. Infant-family relationship: Parents interact with infant as soon as possible after birth. Parents' responses reflect their style of care, ethnic background, and energy level. Initial and subsequent contacts between parents and infant promote close parent-child ties.
16. Circumcised penis: Healing continues. Yellowish exudate forms over glans; incised site remains tender for 2 to 3 days.
17. Genitalia
    a. Female: no excoriation, may be some mucus discharge
    b. Male: clean; foreskin not retracted
18. Urination: Infant voids 6 to 10 times in 24 hours; urine is pale, straw-colored.
19. Defecation. Number and type of stools vary, depending on type of feeding. Stools go through a transitional process from meconium to greenish-yellow. Stool is more formed if infant is bottle fed.
20. Weight: Newborns lose up to 10% of birth weight in first few days (if birthweight was over 4256 g, or 9 lb 9 oz, infant may lose up to 15%). Birthweight is regained by the end of the second week.
21. Integumentary system: Icterus neonatorum begins 24 hours or later after birth in more than half of infants, reaches peak on fourth or fifth day, then subsides within 7 days of onset.
    b. Melanin in skin responds to light; color tone changes depending on amount in skin.
    c. Rashes are transitory; skin may peel, especially in folds.
22. Appearance and behavior
    a. Molding of head subsides and appears rounder by second or third day.
    b. Infant sleeps about 17 hours a day, wakes for feedings, and is alert and responsive. Cry is lusty, sustained, and demanding in tone. Muscle tone is good.
23. Daily hygiene
    a. Parents are aware of and practice necessary daily hygiene.
    b. Mother is aware of normal characteristics and behavior of her infant.
    c. Parent practices safe techniques for bathing and changing infant.
    d. Parent is knowledgeable about dressing infant and care of clothing.
    e. Parent is aware of measures used to control discomfort (diaper rash, prickly heat, and so forth).
    f. Parents become adept at caretaking activities.
24. Infant-family relationships
    a. Parent's become aware of infant's behavior and "cues" for type of care needed.
    b. Parents become knowledgeable as to what is normal or abnormal behavior.

Summary of Nursing Actions—cont'd

c. Siblings are helped to accept newborn.
d. Grandparents are willing to act as assistants to parents without taking over.
25. Safety
   a. Sources of readily available emergency care are known to parents.

b. Protection against infection and trauma is continued.
c. Parents agree to blood tests for protection of infant from metabolic diseases.
d. Plans are made for fourth week check-up and continued health supervision.

NEWBORN NUTRITION AND FEEDING

Skillful health supervision of infants requires knowledge of their nutritional needs. The nurse, one of the most important contributors, can assist with nutrition assessment and provide education and counseling. Nurses can help interpret dietary prescriptions and make appropriate referrals of more complicated problems to nutritional personnel.

Readiness for Feeding

The mechanics of digestion and muscular development are basic to the infant's success in receiving and absorbing the nutrients necessary for growth. This section presents information on the infant's digestive process and how it is affected by neuromuscular development from birth to 3 months. The relationship between feeding and psychosocial development is also included.

Table 4-6 *Digestion in Infancy: Birth to 3 Months*

Location	Function	Effect on Feeding
Salivary	Lactose is not produced in salivary secretions; amylase not available in significant quantities.	Salivary enzymes play no role in digestion of milk.
Gastric	Hydrochloric acid (HCl) and pepsin precipitate casein into curds; separate and acidify whey protein.	Protein digestion begins; lactose ($C_{12}H_{22}O_{11}$) digestion partly begins; fat is not digested in stomach.
Pancreatic and intestinal	Pancreatic and intestinal enzymes digest proteins into amino acids, reduce carbohydrate to monosaccharides, and split fatty acids from triglycerides in the small intestine.	Protein from human milk is 95% digested, and a similar percentage of protein is digested from commercial formulas that are heat treated and sufficiently dilute to produce a soft curd.
	Disaccharidases are present in border of the intestinal mucosa.	Lactose in human milk and lactose or other carbohydrates in commercial formulas are digested in intestinal mucosa.
	Pancreatic amylase is present in small quantities.	Complex carbohydrates are poorly used.
	Pancreatic lipase is present in sufficient quantity.	A total of 80% of human milk fat is digested at birth, and almost 95% is digested by 1 month.
	Lipase, naturally found in human milk, is activated by bile salts.	Digestion of fats from commercial formulas equals that of human milk; fat from other sources (butterfat) is poorly digested.

Modified from Willis NH: Infant nutrition, birth to 3 months: a syllabus, Philadelphia, 1980, JB Lippincott Co.

Table 4-7   *Neuromuscular and Psychosocial Development: Birth to 3 Months*

Neuromuscular	Psychosocial	Implication for Feeding
Month 1		
Sucking and swallowing reflexes are present at birth; stimulus in mouth leads to rhythmic sucking and swallowing pattern; tongue protrusion predominates.	Early emotional, psychologic, and social attachment of mother and infant may determine future aspects of infant's personality. Mother's feeding practices determine exposure to tactile stimulation, which is essential to infant's physical and emotional growth.	Oral reflex is a definite adaptive food-seeking reflex for survival. On reaching satiety, infant withdraws head from breast or bottle and falls asleep. If infant's needs are satisfied through food and love, trust is developed between child and mother. Feedings are main means by which infant establishes human relationship with mother.
Month 2		
Corners of mouth are well approximated but not active in sucking; open gap separates lateral portions of lips. Tonic grasp is disappearing.	Strong emotional bond develops between mother and infant and can be viewed as beginning of social interaction of infant.	Infant is individual who shapes her or his own behavior and feeding schedule. Infant learns to equate mother with food. Infant eats about 5 times each day and may sleep through night.
Month 3		
Lip movement begins to refine; lower lip pulls in; infant may smack lips. Tongue protrusion still present, but infant may swallow with less protrusion. Infant can hold onto object without focusing on it. By end of third month, control of head and eyes is achieved.	More tactile stimulation exists with breast-fed infant. Basic trust factor (if established) is manifested in infant's responses to mother. Infant ceases to cry with hunger when mother approaches. Infant stares into mother's face while feeding and shows response to human voice.	Infant recognizes bottle or breast as source of food. Milk runs out of sides of mouth when nipple is withdrawn. Infant still does not readily accept cup.

Modified from Owen AL et al: Infant feeding guide, Bloomfield, NJ, 1980, Health Learning Systems, Inc.

Feeding Methods

The decision to breast-feed or to use formula for feeding is personal, and the nurse must respect and support the mother's choice. The initiation and continuation of breast-feeding often requires assistance from health care providers. Some mothers have an easy time, whereas others experience problems and become anxious. The nurse must have a working knowledge of this form of infant feeding to provide support and guidance. For mothers who choose formula feeding, the nurse takes an active role in counselng and guidance, assisting her in obtaining knowledge and skill in this area. The information in the following pages provides the nurse with the necessary tools to assist the mother to feed her infant successfully, regardless of the method chosen. This section concludes with a sample nursing care plan and a summary of nursing actions for newborn nutrition and feeding.

Table 4-8 *Infant-Related Concerns in the Initiation of Breast-feeding*

Concern	Nursing Action
The infant does not open wide enough to grasp the nipple.	Help the mother depress the infant's lower jaw with one finger as she guides the nipple into the mouth.
The infant grasps the nipple and areolar tissue correctly but will not suck.	Help the mother stimulate sucking motions by pressing upward under the baby's chin. Expression of colostrum results, and the infant is stimulated by the taste to begin sucking.
The infant makes frantic rooting, mouthing motions but will not grasp the nipple and eventually begins to cry and stiffen her or his body in apparent frustration.	Help the mother interrupt the feeding, comfort the infant, and take time to relax herself, and then she may begin again.
The infant may suck for a few minutes and then fall asleep.	Help the mother interrupt the feeding and take time to awaken the infant. Stimulation may include loosening the wraps, holding the baby upright, talking to the baby, or gently rubbing her or his back or the soles of the feet. A sleepy infant will not nurse satisfactorily. If it is impossible to wake the baby, it is better to postpone the feeding.
The infant starts by sucking vigorously and, as the milk flows freely, develops a long, slow, rhythmic sucking. The sucking then changes to a short, rapid sucking with frequent rest periods. This behavior indicates a slowing of the flow of milk.	Help the mother massage the breasts toward the nipple. This starts the milk flowing freely again, and the infant will revert to the slow, rhythmic sucking. As soon as sucking resumes, the massage is discontinued so that the infant will not be overwhelmed and choked by the milk flowing too rapidly.

TABLE 4-9 *Mother-Related Problems in Breast-Feeding*

Problem	Nursing Action
Engorged Breasts If feeding has been on demand since birth, painful engorgement of the breasts is not likely to occur. However, because of the lag between the production of milk and the efficiency of the ejection reflexes, engorgement of the breasts may occur for up to 48 hours after the milk comes in. The mother often complains that the breast is tender and that the tenderness extends into the axilla. The breasts usually feel firm, tense, and warm as a result of the increased blood supply, and the skin may appear shiny and taut. The unyielding areolae makes it difficult for the infant to grasp the nipple. Breast-feeding can be uncomfortable to the mother and frustrating for both mother and infant.	1. Application of moist heat: apply wet cloths as hot as can be endured to the whole breast and, at the same time, express milk from the nipple. As the wet cloth cools, replace with another one. Shower and direct the hot water to the breasts. 2. Breast massage: **A,** Begin by placing one hand over the other above the breast. **B,** Gently, but firmly, exert pressure evenly with the thumbs across the top and fingers underneath the breast. **C,** Come together with the heel of the hand on each side and release at the areola, being careful not to touch the areola and nipple. **D,** Then gently lift the breast from beneath and drop lightly. Repeat 4 to 5 times with each breast. 3. Manual expression of milk: **A,** Place the thumb and forefinger on opposite sides of the breast just outside the areola, press downward into the rib cage, and then, **B,** gently squeeze together and downward; the nipple should not be pulled outward. Repeat the procedure moving the thumb and forefinger around the nipple until as much milk as desired has been expressed. If the milk is to be used later, *it should be expressed into a sterile bottle and frozen.** Milk expression is not easy for some women at first, but persistence usually brings success if the mother takes the time.
Sore Nipples The nipples may become sore during the early days of breast-feeding. Soreness may be prevented or limited by using a correct position and avoiding undue breast engorgement. If soreness occurs, it is always temporary until the nipples become accustomed to the baby's sucking (Borovies, 1984).	1. Expose the nipples to air. 2. Use a heat lamp to dry the nipples after the feeding (40-watt bulb in a desk lamp, positioned 45 cm [18 in] from breast). 3. If soreness occurs, limit sucking time to 5 minutes on each breast, the time it takes to empty the breasts of milk. 4. Use a pacifier if the infant's sucking needs have not been met. 5. Use a nipple shield. 6. Discontinue breast-feeding for 48 hours. During this time the milk is expressed manually or with a breast pump, collected in a sterilized glass, and given to the baby by bottle. Precautions for maintaining the milk in a safe condition must be followed. Bottles and nipples must be sterilized by immersing them in water and boiling for 10 minutes; any milk not immediately consumed must be refrigerated or frozen.
Plugged Ducts Occasionally a milk duct will become plugged, creating a tender spot on the breast, which may appear lumpy and hot. This might result from inadequate emptying of the milk ducts or from wearing a brassiere that is too tight.	1. Offer the sore breast first so that it will be emptied more completely. 2. Nurse longer and more often; if the breast gets too full, the plugged duct becomes worse and infection may develop. 3. Change positions at every feeding so that the pressure of the feeding will be applied to different places on the breast. 4. Apply warm compresses to the breasts between feedings to reduce the risk of infection by keeping the ducts open.
Increased Lochial Flow The breast-feeding mother may note an increase in lochial flow once feeding begins. At times afterpains are intensified to such a degree that the mother becomes uncomfortable, and her tension interferes with feeding the infant.	Offer a mild analgesic for pain 40 minutes before the feeding period. The mother may be reassured that this discomfort is transitory and will be gone in about 2 days.
Sexual Sensations For some women the rhythmic uterine contractions occurring while breast-feeding are akin to those experienced during orgasm. These unexpected sexual sensations within the context of child care may be disturbing.	Reassure as to normalcy of such feelings.

*Freeze milk that will not be used within a few hours.

TABLE 4-9, cont'd *Mother-Related Problems in Breast-Feeding*

Problem	Nursing Action

Relactation

Occasionally a mother starts breast-feeding late or discontinues it but decides at a much later date that she would like to begin again. After adopting an infant, a minority of women decide to attempt lactation even though they have never done so before or, at best, have breast-fed a previous baby of their own. With much sucking stimulus, lactation can be induced but only with great perseverance and in most cases only if a woman has once carried a pregnancy well into the second trimester. Since the mammary glands complete their development for lactation during the first 6 months of pregnancy, a woman who has never been pregnant or never carried a pregnancy beyond the first trimester is a poor candidate for successful induction of lactation.

Instruct the mother to attempt relactation or induced lactation through providing the infant substantial opportunities to suck at the breast. With much sucking stimulus over several days' time many patient and persistent women can initiate the lactation process late or once again. Their volume of milk production may be less than the infant demands, in which case a supplemental feeding following breast-feeding may be necessary. Alternatively, some women find the Lact-Aid Nursing Trainer to complement their own milk production. While the baby sucks at the breast, she or he also obtains milk via suction through a small tube leading to a bag of fresh formula that is clipped to the mother's brassiere. While the infant sucks, the mother's milk supply is built up and the infant receives adequate nutrition through the Lact-Aid feeding device.

Breast Pumping

For a number of reasons, mothers may wish to remove milk from their breasts and save it for a later feeding, take it to their hospitalized newborn, or donate it to a milk bank. Under such circumstances, milk can be expressed by hand and for some women this method is satisfactory. For many women, however, a manual or electric breast pump provides a better stimulus for milk flow and a more efficient mode of milk collection.

Instruct the mother in the use of the breast pump.

Failure of Infant to Thrive

Insufficient milk supply is rarely a problem for the well-nourished mother. Since sucking stimulates the flow of milk, feeding on demand for adequate duration should supply ample amounts of milk. Occasionally, however, an infant will fail to thrive while seemingly feeding properly.

1. Assist in the explanation of potential problems.
2. Encourage mother to turn to commercial infant formula for at least partial nutritional support of the infant, if the cause of the problem cannot be identified or the defined problem cannot be corrected.
3. Refer the mother to a pediatrician if condition continues, or prn.

Maternal Infection

If breast tenderness is accompanied by fever and a general flulike feeling, a breast infection is probably present.

Instruct the mother to notify her physician immediately.

Guidelines for Client Teaching

BREAST-FEEDING

ASSESSMENT
Primipara planning to breast-feed her infant girl who weighs 3360 g (7 ½ lb).

NURSING DIAGNOSIS
Knowledge deficit related to breast-feeding and lactation.

GOALS
Short-term

To have infant breast-feed successfully.

Intermediate

To establish a feeding pattern satisfactory to infant and mother.

Long-term

Mother able to adjust feedings to needs of newborn daughter by recognizing the infant's cues for hunger and satiety. Mother able to breast-feed successfully while maintaining chosen life-style.

REFERENCES AND TEACHING AIDS
Hospital pamphlets about infant nutrition, films on breast-feeding, posters, booklets, etc.
Text such as:
Pyle, M, RNC: Breast feeding, a family affair, Costa Mesa, Calif, 1985, Life circle.
Riordan, J: St Louis, 1983, The CV Mosby Co.
Pamphlets and books available through the La Leche League.

CONTENT/RATIONALE	TEACHING ACTIONS
To review general content tell mother: Before putting the baby to breast, I want to review some facts with you:	Fill in gaps in knowledge.
You can assume any comfortable position. Let the breast fall forward without tension. Leave one hand free to guide the nipple into the child's mouth.	Have mother experiment with positions. Have her assume the position that feels most comfortable.
I'll review the structure of the breast. The nipple can be made more prominent by gently rolling it between your fingers. The areolar area will be put in the baby's mouth with the nipple. This prevents bruising the nipple.	Have woman expose her breast. Have woman prepare her nipple. Point out areolar tissue.
Colostrum is the yellow fluid you can express from your breasts now. It is good for the baby. It contains some fat and protein and helps baby resist infections.	Demonstrate technique for expressing milk from the breast. Have woman express some colostrum.
Milk may be expected to appear 48 to 96 hours after delivery. Before the milk comes in, the breasts feel soft to the touch. After the milk comes in, the breasts feel full and warmer.	Have woman touch breasts to feel softness.
To teach breast-feeding technique: Have mother hold the baby so that her cheek touches the breasts. The pressure against the outer angle of the lip begins the rooting reflex. The baby will turn toward the nipple. She can smell the colostrum and milk and this will also make her turn toward the nipple.	Demonstrate rooting reflex by touching finger to infant's lips and cheek.
Have woman put the baby to breast by guiding the nipple and areolar tissue into the infant's mouth and over the tongue. Compress breast with thumb above and fingers below areola to permit infant to latch on effectively.	Have the woman practice. Tell her to avoid holding the breast like a cigarette.
To teach expected infant responses and maternal sensations tell woman: At first the baby sucks in short bursts of three to five sucks followed by single swallows. In 1 to 2 days a sucking pattern evolves. This consists of 10 to 30 sucks followed by swallowing. The infant's lips and jaws exert pressure on the areola and the tongue "cradles" the nipple so that the tip is not eroded. The pressure combined with negative intraoral pressure brings milk into the mouth.	Bring infant to mother. Have her assess her baby's suck by placing her finger in the baby's mouth with the finger pad touching and stroking the palate. She should be able to feel the tongue cushioning the joint of the finger and stroking the finger, while keeping the gum covered. She should not feel an insecure or loose suction on the finger, or a tapping of the gum on the finger alone or combined with the tongue slipping back and forth across the gum (licking).
When the baby is sucking properly, there is no "clicking" noise. This clicking noise means she is sucking on her own tongue in the back of the throat, past the nipple. You should hear the rhythmic suck-swallow breathing	Have mother suck her own tongue at the back of the throat to hear the clicking sound.

Guidelines For Client Teaching—cont'd

CONTENT/RATIONALE	TEACHING ACTION
pattern that indicates milk is flowing. Some mothers can sense if the infant has drawn the areolar tissue into the mouth along with the nipple.	
Now let's get the baby ready and put her to breast; first making sure she is awake.	If necessary, waken the baby by stroking her cheek, rubbing her feet, and talking to her.
Now put her to breast by bringing the baby to the breast not the breast to the baby. The baby's face, chest, genitals, and knees should all be facing your body. Touch her upper lip with your nipple: see how she turns toward you and opens her mouth. Pull baby as close to you as you can.	Help mother position baby so that the head is directly facing the breast and the nipple is not pulled to one side. Guide woman through feeding. Point out and explain sensations she is feeling.
Feel how the baby's jaws fit behind the nipple and the nipple is deep in her mouth?	
If infant needs more breathing space, lift your breast; or make a "dimple" in your breast for breathing space.	Caution woman that making a "dimple" may be done too vigorously and the nipple will be dislodged.
You may need to hold your nipple throughout the entire feeding for a few weeks.	Observe technique, degree of relaxation, offer praise.
I will be back to help you put her to the other breast. It is a good idea to use both breasts at each feeding. Once the milk has come in you can tell which breast to start with next time by feeling the weight. The heaviest one has the most milk, so start with that one. In the meantime, put a safety pin on your bra on the side that you finished, so you will know which side to start out with next time.	Review need to empty both breasts since an empty breast signals woman's body to produce more milk.
To remove the baby from the breast, place a finger in the corner of the baby's mouth until the suction is broken. The breast can then be comfortably removed. I will be back in about 15 minutes or use your call bell if you need help. Leave mother to enjoy her baby.	Return in about 15 minutes to supervise mother removing baby from the breast. Remind her that breast-feeding time is not limited.
Before putting the baby to the other breast I will show you how to burp her. Some babies never burp, others do frequently. Gently rub or pat the baby's back.	Demonstrate burping. Supervise mother putting baby to other breast.
After feeding, place the baby on her right side. This allows air in stomach to come up and not bring the milk with it.	Show woman a picture of an infant on right side.

EVALUATION Mother demonstrates competency in breast-feeding.

Guidelines For Client Teaching

FORMULA FEEDING

ASSESSMENT

Sharon, age 17, delivered her daughter 6 hours ago. The infant is a healthy term baby weighing 2912 g (6 1/2 lb). The nurse fed the infant (sterile water) initially at 2 hours of age. Her sucking and swallowing reflexes were normal. The mother is anxious about bottle-feeding her infant. Up to now she has had no contact with babies.

NURSING DIAGNOSES

Knowledge deficit related to bottle-feeding an infant. Anxiety, mild, related to being a new parent.

GOALS

Short-term

To teach Sharon how to bottle-feed her baby.

Intermediate

To help Sharon assess the amount of feeding her daughter requires.
To teach Sharon how to prepare the formula.

Long-term

To increase Sharon's awareness of her infant's needs.

REFERENCES AND TEACHING AIDS

Posters, films, and hospital and commericial booklets from formula companies related to formula/bottle-feeding an infant. Bottle, nipple; cork and needle.
Cans of formula; ready to feed, and that which has to be mixed with water.

CONTENT/RATIONALE	TEACHING ACTIONS
To review general content tell mother:	Give baby to the mother to hold while the discussion goes on.
Before starting to feed the baby I'll go over a few points that will help you feed her.	Show Sharon picture of baby.
Baby needs to be wide awake, like the one in the picture.	Show Sharon a sample bottle of formula.
These are hospital bottles of formula. They can be stored at room temperature. You may use this brand or the one your pediatrician recommends. They contain 4 oz of formula (120 ml). Your baby will probably drink 2 to 3 oz (60 to 90 ml) at a feeding for a few days and then increase. If you do not use all the formula, throw the remainder away, since it spoils once opened.	
You can keep track of how many ounces the baby drinks in 1 day by writing it down. When you take the baby for a check-up, your physician or nurse will ask you the amount of intake.	Show Sharon how to note time and amount.
Your baby will probably be hungry every 2 1/2 to 3 hours. If she fusses or cries in between feedings, check her diaper or her need to be picked up and cuddled. As she gets older, she may be thirsty. Check with the pediatrician concerning water supplementation.	
Test the temperature of the formula by letting a few drops fall on the inside of your wrist. If the formula feels comfortably warm to you, it is the correct temperature. If the formula is refrigerated, warm it by placing the bottle in a pan of hot water. Check it often for correct temperature.	Shake a few drops of formula on Sharon's inside writst. Dry her wrist with a facial tissue.
Test the size of the nipple hole by holding the bottle and nipple upside down. The formula should drip from the nipple. If it runs in a stream, the hole is too big. If it has to be shaken for the formula to come out, the hole is too small. To correct this you can try a softer nipple or enlarge the hole in the nipple or both. To enlarge hole, heat a needle stuck into a cork (used as a handle) and insert the hot needle into the nipple. New nipples may be softened by boiling for 5 minutes before using. If nipple collapses, unscrew bottle lid to let air in.	Demonstrate how to check nipple hole. Demonstrate with needle embedded in cork. Heat over match flame and enlarge the hole on the sample nipple.
Some babies need burping. They tend to swallow air when sucking. Burp the baby before feeding, if she has been crying, then after every ounce of formula. As she gets	Show pictures of mother burping baby. Demonstrate burping technique with Sharon's baby.

Guidelines for Client Teaching—cont'd

Content/Rationale	Teaching Actions
older and you get more experienced, you will know when to burp her.	
To feed the baby, place the nipple in the baby's mouth over her tongue. It should rest against the roof of her mouth. This stimulates sucking reflex.	Show Sharon picture of nipple in baby's mouth. Have her practice.
Hold the bottle like a pencil. Keep nipple filled with milk so baby doesn't suck air.	Point out on picture. Demonstrate.
Start out with baby away from you until nipple is in her mouth. If she is too close, she will turn toward you and not the nipple, this is the rooting reflex.	Have Sharon hold baby away from herself.
After she starts feeding, then you can hold her close.	Help Sharon start feeding.
Some infants take longer to feed than others. Slow, patient feeding, keeping the infant awake, and encouraging her to take more may be necessary.	Reassure Sharon that this is a characteristic of infant feeding and not poor mothering.
The stools of a formula-fed baby are soft but formed. They will be yellow with a characteristic odor. She will probably defecate either during the feeding or after. Change the diaper immediately since the composition of the stool is irritating to the skin.	Show picture of type of stool baby will have once meconium has passed.
To review safety measures tell mother:	
While she is feeding I will review some safety tips.	Use poster to show dangers. Ask Sharon to demonstrate what to do if baby chokes. Place bulb syringe.
Don't prop the bottle, the nipple may fall against the throat and block the air, or the baby could drown in her formula or aspirate any that was regurgitated.	
Infants should never be left alone while feeding until they are old enough to remove bottle from their mouth.	
Bottles taken to bed can lead to early dental problems in young children (baby bottle syndrome).	
Let's practice how to hold baby and use the bulb syringe in case she should choke.	
I will be back in 10 minutes if you have any questions.	Check amount of formula for hospital record.
After baby is finished, place the baby in her crib on her right side so air can come up easily.	Supervise burping the baby. Show picture of baby on right side.

EVALUATION Sharon demonstrates competence and skill in formula/bottle-feeding her infant and asks appropriate questions.

Sample Nursing Care Plan

NEWBORN NUTRITION AND FEEDING

ASSESSMENT	NURSING DIAGNOSIS (ND)/ PLAN (P)/GOAL (G)	RATIONALE/ IMPLEMENTATION	EVALUATION

Prenatal:
    Prenatal assessment of infant feeding preferences.
    Cultural, religious, social, and financial considerations influencing feeding choice.
    Practices of woman's friends and her mother.
	ND: Knowledge deficit related to infant feeding.
	 P: Establish a comprehensive data base.
	 G: Client will make an informed decision about breast- or formula-feeding her infant.
		To aid a woman in choosing a method of feeding her infant, the nurse will:
		 Evaluate woman's (couple's) goals and preferences for feeding.
		 Discuss pros and cons of both methods of feeding.
			Client chooses a method of infant feeding suitable to her needs and life-style.

Continued.

Sample Nursing Care Plan—cont'd

Assessment	Nursing Diagnosis (ND)/ Plan (P)/Goal (G)	Rationale/ Implementation	Evaluation
Personal (and father's) goals and preferences.		Encourage questions, concerns, or feelings surrounding newborn nutrition and feeding. Dispel misconceptions surrounding the feeding choice. Encourage the woman to discuss her decision with those members of the family who will be active in child care.	
First day of life: Assess infant's ability to breast- or formula-feed. 1. Reflexes—suck, swallow, gag. 2. No structural abnormalities (e.g. choanal atresia). Assess infant's readiness for feeding (e.g., rooting reflex, infant's responsiveness). Assess amount and frequency of feeds.	ND: Ineffective airway clearance related to poor suck, swallow, or gag reflexes. ND: Altered nutrition: potential for less than body requirements, related to infant's lack of interest in feeding or regurgitation. P: Perform comprehensive physical assessment. G: Infant will possess readiness to feed and demonstrate intact reflexes.	*To evaluate the infant's ability to feed, the nurse will:* Have infant suck on finger. Remove excess mucus from nose and mouth, burp prn. Feed infant initial feeding of sterile water. Initiate and evaluate mother's preferred choice of feeding as soon as possible.	Reflexes (root, suck, swallow, and gag) are present and sufficiently developed to permit feeding by breast or bottle. Infant accepts, swallows, retains, and assimilates feeding.
Assess woman's ability to feed infant.	ND: Knowledge deficit related to infant feeding. P: Provide information, demonstrate, and observe return demonstration. G: Client will learn how to successfully feed her infant.	*To aid in successful feeding efforts by the mother, the nurse will:* Encourage the use of wakeful periods for feeding infant. Assist the mother with the feeding technique she has chosen. Instruct as to feeding techniques and nutritional needs of the infant. Demonstrate and supervise care needed if infant chokes, gags, or spits up. Record amounts of formula or time at breast and note infant's response.	Client successfully feeds her infant.
Assess infant's ability to defecate and urinate.	ND: Constipation related to a structural or mechanical defect. P: Perform a complete physical examination and monitor pattern of elimination daily. G: Infant will demonstrate a normal pattern of elimination	*To evaluate infant elimination, the nurse will:* Record urine amounts and time. Record character of stool and time. Notify physician if no urine within the first 8 hours of life or no stool within the first 24 hours of life.	Infant demonstrates normal pattern of elimination.

Sample Nursing Care Plan—cont'd

ASSESSMENT	NURSING DIAGNOSIS (ND)/ PLAN (P)/GOAL (G)	RATIONALE/ IMPLEMENTATION	EVALUATION
		Report and record any structural defects noted (e.g., imperforate anus).	
Parity. First breast-feeding experience? Knowledge about breast-feeding. Support system for breast-feeding experience. Assess breast-feeding problems—mother-related and infant-related.	ND: Knowledge deficit related to breast-feeding and its complications. P: Provide information, demonstrate, and observe return demonstration. G: Client will breast-feed successfully and comfortably and will establish a pattern satisfactory to infant and herself.	*To teach breast-feeding techniques, the nurse will:* See Guidelines for Client Teaching: Breastfeeding," p. 154. See Table 4-9, Mother-related concerns in breast-feeding.	Client successfully and comfortably breast-feeds with a pattern that is satisfying to her and her infant.
Parity. Has she bottle-fed previously? Knowledge about bottle-feeding and amounts of formula required. Financial status (WIC Program).	ND: Knowledge deficit related to preparation of formula and bottle-feeding an infant. P: Provide information, demonstrate, and observe return demonstration. G: Client will learn how to prepare formula and bottle-feed her infant and assess the amount of feeding the child requires.	*To teach client to bottle-feed and assess the amount of formula an infant requires, the nurse will:* See guidelines for client teaching: formula feeding.	Client successfully prepares formula and bottle-feeds her infant and demonstrates an awareness of the infant's needs (formula, frequency of feeds, etc.).
Follow-up care: Assess weight gain. Assess growth pattern. Assess hydration status (weight, skin, turgor, sunken eyes or fontanels, moistness of mucous membranes). Assess frequency of feeds, amounts of formula, or breast-feeding time. Assess child's satisfaction between feeds. Assess elimination pattern.	ND: Altered health maintenance related to poor nutritional patterns or elimination problems. ND: Altered nutrition: less or more than body requirements related to infant feeding pattern. ND: Knowledge deficit related to growing infant's nutritional needs. P: Provide information, demonstrate, and observe return demonstration. G: Client will be adept at adjusting feeding process to meet infant's nutritional needs. G: Infant will grow and gain weight within the normal limits for age. G: Infant will establish a regular elimination pattern.	*To evaluate infant's nutritional status the nurse will:* Weigh and measure length. Evaluate growth according to age. Note and report poor or excessive growth. Note, report, and seek treatment for dehydration. Discuss feeding pattern and amounts with mother and evaluate child's satisfaction. Encourage client to verbalize feeding problems. Evaluate and report problems with elimination. Teach client infant satisfaction signs.	Client adjusts feeds according to child's needs. Child receives adequate nutrition to grow within the normal limits for age. Child establishes a regular elimination pattern. Child sleeps well between feedings, exhibits no problems (colic, gas pains, regurgitation) with feedings; child gains weight.

Summary of Nursing Actions

NEWBORN NUTRITION AND FEEDING

I. Goals
  A. For the infant
    1. To provide the levels and types of nutrients to support the infant's body composition, activity, growth and development
    2. To minimize the physiologic stress associated with digestion, metabolism, and excretion of nutrients
    3. To supply sufficient water to maintain adequate body water control
  B. For the mother
    1. To provide knowledge that can be used for sound decision making for nutrition and feeding practices
    2. To assist her to become skilled in the feeding method of her choice
    3. To foster mother-child bonding and pleasure

II. Priorities
  A. Confirm newborn's ability to ingest nutrients (i.e., vomiting, swallowing, presence of gag reflex, absence of structural abnormalities).
  B. Confirm newborn's ability to digest nutrients (i.e., infant thrives).
  C. Confirm infant's ability to eliminate wastes.
  D. Ensure that mother (caretaker) has the necessary knowledge and skill to provide nutrition needed by the infant.
  E. Ensure that mother has necessary income to obtain needed nutrients for her and her infant.

III. Assessment
  A. First day of life
    1. Assess infant's ability to breast- or bottle-feed.
      a. Reflexes: vomit, swallow, gag
      b. No structural abnormalities (e.g., choanal atresia, cleft palate)
    2. Assess infant readiness for feeding (e.g., rooting reflex readily elicited, infant alert and responsive).
    3. Assess infant's ability to defecate and urinate.
    4. Assess mother's level of knowledge of nutrition and feeding, and observe the skills she possesses.
    5. Assess condition of nipples if mother is breast-feeding
    6. Assess any high-risk situations that may be harmful if mother were to breast-feed (e.g., drug or alcohol dependence, antibiotic usage, HIV infection, etc.)
  B. Days 2 to 5
    1. Examine general condition of infant as part of routine care.
    2. Obtain reports from mother (family) concerning satisfaction of infant (e.g., whether infant sleeps soundly between feedings, regular routine for feeding established, infant appeased by nourishment).
    3. Observe mother while she is feeding infant to determine skills and areas where assistance is needed.
    4. Observe infant during and after feeding to note any irregularities in sucking or swallowing or problems in retention of feeding.
    5. Assess condition of mother's breasts.
    6. Assess mother's knowledge of breast care if she is breast-feeding.
    7. Assess mother's knowledge of diet for lactation and ability to obtain necessary nutrients.

IV. Potential nursing diagnostic categories
  A. First day of life
    1. Ineffective airway clearance
    2. Diarrhea
    3. Knowledge deficit
    4. Impaired verbal communication
    5. Anxiety
    6. Pain
    7. Potential alteration in skin integrity
    8. Potential ineffective breast feeding
  B. Days 2 to 5
    1. Ineffective airway clearance
    2. Diarrhea
    3. Knowledge deficit
    4. Impaired verbal communication
    5. Anxiety
    6. Pain
    7. Potential alteration in skin integrity
    8. Potential ineffective breast feeding
    9. Altered nutrition: less or more than body requirements
    10. Noncompliance
    11. Potential for trauma
    12. Impaired swallowing
    13. Potential fluid volume deficit
    14. Altered health maintenance
    15. Potential for infection
    16. Potential for aspiration
    17. Potential for constipation
    18. Ineffective individual coping
    19. Potential altered parenting

V. Plan/implementation
  A. First day of life
    1. Test infant's abilities.
      a. Have infant suck on finger.
      b. Remove excess mucus.
      c. Feed infant sterile water.
      d. Initiate feeding of infant by mother (breast or bottle) as soon as possible (e.g., put to breast at birth, if feasible).
    2. Use wakeful periods for feeding infant. Wake infant before attempting to feed; otherwise baby might choke.
    3. Assist mother with the feeding technique she has chosen.
    4. Instruct as to nutritional needs of infant during first few days of life.
    5. Instruct as to feeding abilities of infants (e.g., their sucking needs, burping technique, varia-

Summary of Nursing Actions—cont'd

tions in appetite. Learning to nurse requires practice for mother and infant).

6. Demonstrate or supervise care needed if infant gags, chokes, or spits up during feeding process.
7. Record amounts of formula taken, times of breast- or bottle-feeding, and response of infant.
8. Record character of stool and urine and time.
9. Instruct breast-feeding mother on care of her breasts to prevent erosion and cracking of nipples, to augment supply of milk, and to prevent infection of breast or infant

B. Days to 2 to 5
1. Share findings of infant's nutritional state with mother.
2. Make mother or care providers aware of infant's nutritional needs for growth.
3. Assist mother in becoming skillful and adept at breast- or bottle-feeding (see Table 4-9, "Mother-Related Problems in Breast-Feeding," Guidelines for Client Teaching, "Breast Feeding, pp. 154-155; Guidelines for Client Teaching, "Formula-Feeding," pp. 156-157).
4. Establish relaxed environment in which mother undertakes feeding process (free from pain, comfortable position, assistance from interested, supportive, and knowledgeable nurse, and privacy).
5. For breast-feeding mother, provide adequate diet (additional protein and fluids) and daily routine for care of breasts.
6. For bottle-feeding mothers, provide information on preparation and storage of formulas.
7. Assist mother (caretakers) in recognizing cues infant uses and pattern of hunger and satiety each infant develops. Assist mother in dealing with concern as to her ability to provide adequate nourishment for her newborn.
8. Provide information regarding community resources.
9. Instruct family as to symptoms that indicate gastrointestinal disturbances. Provide family with information as to whom to call for assistance and what symptoms to report.

VI. Evaluation
A. First day of life
1. Reflexes (rooting, sucking, swallowing, gagging) are present and sufficiently developed to permit infant to feed by breast or bottle.
2. Periods of wakefulness when infant is alert and hungry are used to facilitate initiation of the feeding process and to promote a satisfactory mother-child interaction.

3. Mother begins to feed her infant by breast or bottle.
4. Regurgitation or vomiting episodes are controlled, and the mother is able to care for the infant so that an open airway is maintained.
5. Infant accepts, swallows, retains, and assimilates feeding.
6. Infant passes meconium and urinates.
7. Mother cares for breasts.

B. Days 2 to 5
1. Infant's nutritional state is satisfactory evidenced by weight gain, adequate skin turgor, soft skin; non depressed fontanels; active and alert infant when awake; good muscle tone; infant sleeping contentedly 2 to 5 hours between feedings; appropriate voiding and stooling; crying from stress of hunger appeased by feeding
2. Mother is aware of infant's nutritional needs for growth.
3. Mother is adept at breast- or bottle-feeding techniques.
   a. Breast-feeding
      (1) Initiating and terminating session
      (2) Enhancing supply of milk
      (3) Protecting nipples from erosion or fissures
      (4) Adjusting number of feedings to meet infant's changing needs
      (5) Using alternative methods of feeding infant to free mother to take part in other activities
   b. Bottle-feeding
      (1) Preparing formula
      (2) Initiating and terminating feedings
      (3) Adjusting schedule and formula to meet infant's changing nutritional needs
      (4) Mother knowing not to prop bottles or to leave infant alone with a bottle
      (5) Mother adopting practices that ensure infant-mother contact
4. Mother and family have knowledge of infant's cues for feeding and elimination patterns.
5. Mother and family are aware of and use community resources for procuring adequate nutrients.
6. Mother is aware of symptoms that indicate gastrointestinal disturbances: depressed fontanels, dry skin, eyes lacking in luster, diarrhea with green, curdy stools, fever, refusal of feedings and fluids, lethargy, irritability, and a diminished number of voidings of urine.
7. Mother is aware of need to obtain medical care promptly to arrest lethal processes of dehydration and acid-base imbalance.

Bibliography

Fanaroff A and Martin R: Behrman's neonatal-prenatal medicine, St Louis, ed 2, 1987, The CV Mosby Co.

Korones SB: High-risk newborn infants: the basis for intensive nursing care, ed 4, St Louis, 1986, The CV Mosby Co.

Owen, AL, et al: Infant feeding guide, Bloomfield, NH, 1980, Health Learning System.

Pritchard JA, MacDonald DC, and Gant NF: Williams obstetrics, ed 17, New York, 1985, Appleton-Crofts.

Standards for Cardiopulmonary Resuscitation (CPR) and Emergency Cardiac Care (ECC): Part IV. Pediatric basic life support, JAMA 255(21):2954, 1986.

USP-DI: Drug information for the health care provider, ed 6, Rockville, Md, 1986, United States Pharmacopeial Convention, Inc.

Whaley, LF and Wong DL: Nursing care of infants and children, ed 3, St Louis, 1987, The CV Mosby Co.

Willis NH: Infant nutrition: birth to 6 months: a syllabus, Philadelphia, 1980, JB Lippincott Co.

UNIT
5

Normal Postpartum Period

The maternity nurse needs a solid understanding of normal physiologic responses during the postpartum period. This will enable the nurse to provide quality nursing care. Knowledge of normal findings will allow the nurse to plan for care and encourage client participation. Women and their families will be better able to anticipate and adjust to postpartum changes if they have been provided with adequate health information. The nurse is in a key role to provide health education to women and their families. The nurse can help ease the transition from pregnancy to motherhood.

The nurse who makes pertinent assessments, plans and implements client-centered care, and evaluates the effectiveness of the care is playing an important role in the health of the child-bearing family.

This unit focuses on the anatomic, physiologic, and emotional changes during the postpartum period and the nursing care needed during this time. Sample nursing care plans and a summary of nursing actions encompass and deal with the early postpartum period, when the nurse has the most contact with the client.

POSTPARTUM ASSESSMENT

Sharp assessment skills are paramount during the postpartum period. The nurse must continually observe the client for signs and symptoms that signal potential problems. This section presents the basic assessment data and parameters with which the nurse must be familiar to evaluate each client.

Table 5-1 *Lochia and Nonlochia Bleeding*

Lochia	Nonlochia Bleeding
Lochia usually trickles from the vaginal opening. The steady flow is greater as the uterus contracts.	If the bloody discharge spurts from the vagina, there may be cervical or vaginal tears in addition to the normal lochia.
A gush of lochia may result as the uterus is massaged. If it is dark in color, it has been pooled in the relaxed vagina, and the amount soon lessens to a trickle of bright red lochia (in the early puerperium).	If the amount of bleeding continues to be excessive and bright red, a tear may be the source.

Table 5-2 *Vital Signs and Blood Pressure After Delivery*

Normal Findings	Deviations from Normal Findings and Probable Causes
Temperature	
During first 24 hours, may rise to 38° C (100.4° F) as a result of dehydrating effects of labor. After 24 hours the woman should be afebrile.	A diagnosis of puerperal sepsis is suggested if a rise in maternal temperature to 38° C (100.4° F) is noted after the first 24 hours after delivery and recurs or persists for 2 days. Other possibilities are mastitis, endometritis, urinary tract infections, and other systemic infections.
Pulse	
Bradycardia is a common finding for the first 6 to 8 days after delivery. Bradycardia is a consequence of increased cardiac output and stroke volume. The pulse returns to nonpregnant levels by 3 months after delivery. A pulse rate of between 50 and 70 beats/min may be considered normal.	A rapid pulse rate or one that is increasing may indicate hypovolemia secondary to hemorrhage.
Respirations	
Respirations should fall to within the woman's normal predelivery range.	Hypoventilation and hypotension may follow an unusually high subarachnoid (spinal) block.
Blood Pressure	
Blood pressure is altered *slightly* if at all. Orthostatic hypotension, as indicated by feelings of faintness or dizziness immediately after standing up, can develop in the first 48 hours as a result of the splanchnic engorgement that may occur after delivery.	A low or falling blood pressure may reflect hypovolemia secondary to hemorrhage. However, it is a late sign, and other symptoms of hemorrhage usually alert the staff. An increased reading may result from excessive use of vasopressor drugs or oxytocic drugs. Since pregnancy-induced hypertension (PIH) can persist into or occur first in the postpartum period, routine evaluation of blood pressure is needed. If a woman complains of headache, hypertension must be ruled out as a cause before analgesics are administered. If the blood pressure is elevated, the woman is confined to bed and the physician notified.

Table 5-3 *Comparison of Postpartum Headaches*

	Postsubarachnoid Anesthesia	Stress Headache	Meningeal Irritation	Pregnancy-Induced Hypertension (PIH)
Cause	Leakage of cerebrospinal fluid through puncture in dura into extradural space	Anxiety, muscle tension especially in neck, shoulders; fatigue, hunger	Aseptic chemical meningeal irritation	Etiologic factors of PIH (e.g., vasospasm)
Onset	Days 1-2	Variable		Late in the development of PIH; a frequent forerunner of eclampsia (convulsions)*
Location	Forehead, deep behind eyes; radiates to both temples and to occipital area	Band around head; occipital		Frontal or occipital, or generalized
Intensity	Severe to mild	More or less constant ache		Severe, constant throbbing or "splitting"
Modifiers	Increased intensity in sitting or standing position; eases in supine position	Relieved by physical and psychologic rest, food	Not relieved by lying down	Resistant to relief from analgesics
Duration	1-3 days to several weeks	Variable	1-3 days	Duration of severe PIH

Table 5-3, cont'd.   *Comparison of Postpartum Headaches*

	Postsubarachnoid Anesthesia	Stress Headache	Meningeal Irritation	Pregnancy-Induced Hypertension (PIH)
Therapy	Increase oral fluids Supplement oral fluids with at least 1000 ml 5% dextrose in normal saline solution Administer analgesics Assist physician in establishing extradural "blood patch" wtih client's own blood Tight abdominal binder	Implement good communication techniques to help her identify concerns, to ventilate feelings regarding labor/delivery experience; facilitate rest; offer food and fluids; administer medications as necessary; utilize comfort measures (e.g., back rubs, etc.).	Administer analgesics, fluids, and other supportive measures	Treatment for PIH

Table 5-4   *Progression of Puerperal Changes: Days 1 Through 3*

Assessment	2-24 Hours (Day 1)	25-48 Hours (Day 2)	49-72 Hours (Day 3)
Temperature	Elevated (38° C [100.4° F])	Within normal range	Within normal range
Pulse	Bradycardia: 50-70 beats/min	Bradycardia may persist or rate may return to within normal range	Bradycardia may persist or rate may return to within normal range
Blood pressure	Within normal range	Within normal range	Within normal range
Energy level	Euphoric, happy, excited, or fatigued; may show need for sleep	Often tired, slow moving	Anxious to go home; level within normal range, but variable
Uterus	At umbilicus or just below	1 cm or more below umbilicus	2 cm or more below umbilicus
Lochia	Rubra; moderate; few clots, if any; fleshy odor of normal menstrual flow	Rubra to serosa; moderate to scant; odor continues to be "fleshy" or absent	Rubra to serosa; scant; odor continues to be "fleshy" or absent
Perineum	Edematous; clean, healing	Edema lessening; clean, healing	Edema lessening or absent; clean, healing
Legs	Pretibial or pedal edema; Homans' sign negative	Edema lessening; Homan's sign negative	Edema minimal or absent; Homans' sign negative
Breasts	Remain soft to palpation Colostrum can be expressed	Begin to feel firmer Occasionally feel lumpy	Increase in vascularity and initiation of swelling Feel firmer and warmer to touch Milk expected within 2-4 days after delivery
Appetite	Excellent; may ask for double helpings, snacks	Usually remains excellent	Varies; appetite may have returned to normal range or may lessen (especially if client is constipated)
Elimination Voiding Defecation	 Up to 3000 ml None expected	 Large amounts None expected	 Amount/24 hours is lessening Usually defecates; may need enema, etc.
Discomfort	Generalized aching; perineal area: episiotomy, hemorrhoids	Muscle aches; perineal area: episiotomy, hemorrhoids	Possible tension headache, perineal area: usually lessening; breasts, nipples

GENERAL CARE

Although the plan of care should be tailored for each individual client, several conditions and problems are common to most partpartum women. This section provides tabular information, step-by-step procedures, decision trees, and medication data for these commonly occurring conditions.

Table 5-5   *Summary of Measures to Stimulate Uterine Tone*

Nonpharmacologic Measures	Rationale
Massage	Causes reflex contraction of muscles. Overstimulation could lead to muscle fatigue and atony.
Remove clots, if present	Keeps uterus empty to allow muscle fibers to contract completely.
Keep bladder empty	Prevents bladder distension, which elevates and displaces uterus, resulting in uterine atony.
Stimulate breasts or nipples (manually or by suckling infant)	Causes release of oxytocin from posterior pituitary.

Pharmacologic Interventions	Action, Uses During Puerperium	Onset of Effect, Duration, Usual Dose	Contraindications, Precautions	Comments
Oxytocin injection, USP (10 U/ml) (Pitocin, Syntocinon, Uteracon), oxytocic, synthetic posterior pituitary hormone	Stimulates phasic uterine muscle contraction, promotes milk-ejection (let-down) reflex, facilitates flow of milk during engorgement.	IV injection, 10 U; onset in 1 min. IV infusion, 10-40 U/1000 ml 5% dextrose or physiologic electrolyte solution. IM injection, 3-10 U; onset in 3-7 min; duration 30-60 min.	Hypersensitivity; return of atony when effect wears off. May cause severe hypertension if client is also receiving ephedrine, methoxamine, or other vasopressors.	**Alert:** Assess for return of atony; store in cool place.
Ergonovine maleate, USP, NF (Ergotrate maleate); oxytocic, ergot alkaloid	Stimulates prolonged, nonphasic uterine contractions.	Oral: 0.2-0.4 mg every 6-12 hr for 48 hr; onset in 6-15 min. IM injection: 0.2 mg (1 ml) if nausea precludes oral preparation, onset "in a few minutes." Initial response: firm, titanic contraction. Subsequent response: alternating minor relaxations and contractions for 1½ hr; then vigorous rhythmic contractions for 3-4 hr after injection.	Severe hypertensive episodes may occur if given to hypertensive clients or those receiving vasoconstrictors; hypersensitivity; nausea, vomiting; sudden change in blood pressure or pulse.	**Alert:** Assess for changes in blood pressure, pulse; store in cool place.
Methylergonovine maleate, NF (Methergine); oxytocic, ergot alkaloid and congener of lysergic acid (LSD)	Stimulates rapid, sustained titanic uterine contractions; used in treatment of subinvolution; has only minimum vasoconstrictive effect.	Oral: 0.2 mg tab, every 6-8 hr for maximum of 1 wk; onset in 5-10 min. IM injection 0.2 mg (1 ml) every 2-4 hr; onset in 2-5 min. IV infusion (*emergency only*): 0.2 mg (1 ml) *slowly over 60 sec;* onset immediate.	Nausea, vomiting; transient hypertension; dizziness, headache; tinnitus; diaphoresis; palpitations; temporary chest pains.	**Alert:** Do not administer with Percodan—may result in hallucinations; assess blood pressure; store in cold place, away from light.

Procedure 5-1

NURSING ACTIONS FOR UTERINE ATONY (BOGGY UTERUS)

DEFINITION

Loss of uterine muscle tone causing the blood vessels at the site of previous placental attachment to bleed profusely. Also known as "boggy uterus."

PURPOSE

To prevent hemorrhage by maintaining muscle tone.

EQUIPMENT

None required.

NURSING ACTIONS	RATIONALE
Wash hands before and after touching woman or linens and equipment.	To prevent nosocomial infection and to implement universal precautions.
Assess uterine fundus for tone (firmness).	No further action must be taken if firm, and lochial discharge is appropriate.
Assess lochial bleeding.	
If uterus is not contracted, massage gently.	To stimulate muscle contraction without causing muscle fatigue.
	To encourage self-care.
Teach woman to locate and expel clots; reassess in 15 minutes.	To empty uterus so that "living ligature" can function.
	To verify cessation of bleeding.
Prevent bladder distension:	Distended bladder can cause uterine relaxation:
Encourage spontaneous voiding; give rationale.	Spontaneous voiding helps woman maintain sense of control over her body.
	Knowing why bladder needs to be emptied completely adds to woman's knowledge base and encourages self-care.

DECISION TREE: BOGGY UTERUS

Assessment

Uterus is relaxed.

Steps in Decision Making

Gentle massage of fundus

- Firm contraction*; bladder empty
  - Remains firm; no clots
  - Becomes firm; clots expelled
    - Reassess in 15 min; give physician-ordered oxytocic‡ prn
    - Remains firm*; no clots
- Firm contraction†; bladder full
  - Firm contraction with massage
  - Empty bladder: (1) assist with voluntary voiding or (2) catheterize
  - Remains firm*; no clots
- Remains atonic†
  - Immediately expel any clots; empty bladder; and reassess
  - Remains atonic
  - Stay with client, applying manual compression to uterus while another staff member notifies physician
  - Implement physician's orders; follow-up care depends on problems diagnosed and medical or surgical protocol of care.

> No further physical action is needed.
> Teach client importance of voiding and emptying bladder completely at least every 3 to 4 hours.
> See Procedure 5-1.

---

*Fundus is in midline, at level appropriate for time since delivery.
†Fundus is above umbilicus or at level higher than appropriate for time since delivery; uterus may or may not be displaced to right (usually by full bladder or full rectum).
‡See Table 5-4.

Procedure 5-2

CARE AFTER REPAIR OF EPISIOTOMY OR LACERATION

DEFINITION

Treatment of the surgical incision of the perineum, done electively to facilitate delivery of the baby and prevent perineal lacerations (a torn, jagged wound).

PURPOSE

To promote healing, increase comfort, teach mother self-care techniques, and identify and treat complications.

EQUIPMENT

Ice pack with cover; squeeze bottle; sitz bath and thermometer, or surgi-gator (if available); towels, as necessary; anesthetic cream or spray; witch hazel pads (Tucks).

NURSING ACTIONS	RATIONALE
Wash hands before and after touching woman and equipment. Glove, prn.	To prevent nosocomial infection and to implement universal precautions.
Gather equipment.	To improve efficiency.
Explain procedure to woman.	To decrease anxiety and elicit cooperation.
ICE PACK	
Apply a covered ice pack to perineum.	To decrease chance of "burn" from cold pack.
1. During first 2 hours after delivery.	To decrease edema formation at this time and increase comfort later.
	To provide anesthetic effect.
2. After the first 2 hours after delivery.	To provide anesthetic effect.
SITZ BATH	
Built-in type	
Prepare bath by thoroughly scrubbing with cleaning agent and rinsing.	To decrease possibility of infection from another woman; prevents irritation from cleaning agent.
Pad with towel before filling.	To promote comfort and keep woman from slipping (padding before filling keeps towel from floating).
Fill ½ to ⅓ full with water of correct temperature 38° to 40.6° C, or 45° C (100.4° to 105° F, or 113° F)	To provide temperature soothing to some women. The increased blood flow to area is thought by some to facilitate healing; others think that this causes swelling and adds to discomfort.*
Encourage woman to use twice a day or more often once she is ambulating, for 20 minutes.	To provide comfort and aid healing.
Place call bell within easy reach.	To ensure safety since the warm water and other factors (i.e., increased blood supply to perineum, lochial discharge, weakness) may cause woman to feel faint and need assistance.
Teach woman to enter bath by tightening gluteal muscles and keeping them tightened and then relaxing them after she is in the bath.	To decrease perineal discomfort while sitting down.
	To allow water to reach perineum.
Place dry towels within reach.	To increase comfort and ensure safety.
Ensure privacy.	To show respect for woman.
Check woman in 15 min; assess pulse as needed.	To ensure safety. Increased or irregular pulse may indicate cardiovascular stress; assist woman back to bed.
Apply anesthetic cream or spray.	To decrease perineal discomfort, use sparingly 3 to 4 times per day.
Use witch hazel pads (Tucks) after voiding or defecating; woman pats perineum dry from front to back, then applies witch hazel pads.	To decrease swelling and promote healing
Disposable type:	
Clamp tubing and fill water bag.	To prevent spillage.
Raise toilet seat, place bath in bowl with overflow opening directed toward front of toilet.	To allow water to drain into toilet bowl.
Place container above toilet bowl.	To drain water bag by gravity.

*Other authors propose cool sitz bath.

Procedure 5-2 cont'd

Nursing Actions	Rationale
Attach tube into groove at front of bath.	To situate tubing below level of water.
Loosen tube clamp to regulate rate of flow; fill bath to about ½ full; continue as above for built-in sitz bath.	See rationale for built-in sitz bath.

SQUEEZE BOTTLE

Nursing Actions	Rationale
Demonstrate for and assist woman; explain rationale.	To cleanse perineum after voiding.
	To encourage self-care.
Fill bottle with tap water warmed to approximately 38° C (100° F) (comfortably warm on the wrist).	To provide comfortable temperatures.
Instruct woman to position nozzle between her legs so that squirts of water reach perineum as she sits on toilet seat.	To cleanse and soothe perineum.
Explain that it will take several squirts of water over perineum.	To cleanse perineum well.
Remind her to blot dry with toilet paper or clean wipes (provided by the agency).	To avoid tissue trauma and promote comfort.
Remind her to avoid contamination from anal area.	To prevent infection.

SURGI-GATOR

Nursing Actions	Rationale
Assemble Surgi-Gator.	To cleanse and provide comfort to perineum.
Instruct woman regarding use and rationale.	To encourage self-care.
Explain that each woman is issued her own applicator.	To prevent infection.
Follow package directions.	To promote maximum benefit of appliance.
Instruct her to sit on toilet with legs apart and to put nozzle so tip is just past the perineum, adjusting placement as needed.	To provide the jets of water to the perineal area.
Remind her to return her applicator to her bedside stand.	To prevent loss or cross infection.

DRY HEAT

Nursing Actions	Rationale
Inspect lamp for defects.	To prevent fires or burns.
Cover lamp with towels.	To prevent burns if lamp touches skin.
Position lamp 50 cm (20 in) from perineum; use three times a day for 20-minute periods.	To provide comfortable warmth.
	To promote comfort. For some women, keeps area dry and thereby promotes healing.
Teach regarding use of 40-watt bulb at home.	To provide effective "heat" lamp in the home.
Provide privacy by careful draping over woman since knees must be kept up and separated for benefit.	To promote privacy.
	To demonstrate respect and caring.
If same lamp is being used by several woman, clean it carefully between uses.	To prevent cross infection.

TOPICAL APPLICATIONS

Nursing Actions	Rationale
Teach regarding use of sprays, ointments, or witch hazel pads (Tucks) that are applied directly to sutured area.	To add to woman's knowledge base and encourage self-care.

CLEANSING SHOWER

Nursing Actions	Rationale
Wash perineum with mild soap and warm water at least once daily.	To minimize fear of "breaking the stiches" or pain which deters women from washing perineum.
Cleanse from symphysis pubis to anal area.	To prevent contamination of the vagina and urethra with fecal material.
Apply peripad from front to back, protecting inner surface of pad from contamination.	To prevent infection from contamination.
Wrap soiled pad and place in covered waste container.	
Change pad every time she voids or defecates or at least four times per day.	To prevent infection.
Wash hands before and after changing pads.	To prevent infection.
Assess amount and character of lochia with each pad change.	To identify possible complications early.

DECISION TREE: FULL URINARY BLADDER

Assessment

Uterine fundus is well above umbilicus on the right; full bladder is palpated; I&O record indicates intake is considerably greater than output; client states no urge to void or has urge to void but cannot; last voiding, 4 hours ago.

Steps in Decision Making

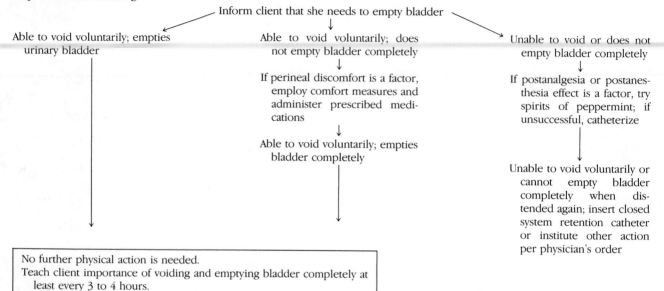

Inform client that she needs to empty bladder

Able to void voluntarily; empties urinary bladder

Able to void voluntarily; does not empty bladder completely

↓

If perineal discomfort is a factor, employ comfort measures and administer prescribed medications

↓

Able to void voluntarily; empties bladder completely

Unable to void or does not empty bladder completely

↓

If postanalgesia or postanesthesia effect is a factor, try spirits of peppermint; if unsuccessful, catheterize

Unable to void voluntarily or cannot empty bladder completely when distended again; insert closed system retention catheter or institute other action per physician's order

No further physical action is needed.
Teach client importance of voiding and emptying bladder completely at least every 3 to 4 hours.

Procedure 5-3

NURSING ACTIONS FOR FULL URINARY BLADDER

DEFINITION
Emptying urinary bladder.

EQUIPMENT
Catheter tray, as needed.

PURPOSE
To prevent bladder distension to decrease potential for bladder wall atony, infection, and uterine hemorrhage.

NURSING ACTIONS	RATIONALE
Facilitate spontaneous voiding	
If woman is ambulatory, assist her to bathroom.	To verify woman's ability to walk without difficulty.
Assist her onto bedpan; provide privacy, pour warm water over the vulva, sound of running water, and provide call bell.	To facilitate spontaneous voiding.
Provide ordered medications if discomfort of the perineum is hindering spontaneous voiding.	To minimize discomfort that increases difficulty of spontaneous voiding.
Some women can void spontaneously if they know it is permissible to void in the sitz bath (then follow the bath with a shower) or while squirting water over perineum (see Procedure 5-2).	To relax woman, and dilute the urine, thus increasing woman's comfort.
Teach techniques to facilitate spontaneous voiding (e.g., void immediately when the urge is present; straddle the toilet seat facing the tank or sit on toilet in regular fashion and lean forward; push all the urine out even if it "makes noise").	To assist natural response to physiologic event. To direct the flow of urine away from repair of episiotomy and lacerations. To give woman permission to "make noise" (many learned to "pee quietly" as little girls to be more "ladylike"). Urinating with force is more likely to empty the bladder completely.
Expose the urinary meatus to fumes from peppermint spirits.	To help woman void spontaneously if at all possible to decrease possibility of infection from catheterization and to give her a sense of control over her body functions.
Verify that woman knows rationale for need to empty bladder.	To add to her knowledge base and encourage self-care.
Catheterize, if needed, per physician's order	To overcome the swelling, pain, and residual effects of analgesia/anesthesia that may prevent spontaneous voiding.
If spontaneous voiding has not occurred by 6 hours after delivery, catheterization is usually ordered.	To ensure emptying of the bladder.
Use aseptic technique.	To minimize infection.
If urinary meatus is difficult to visualize because of swelling, with a dry sterile swab, gently brush upward from the vagina to the clitoris.	To cause the meatus to gape so that catheter can be inserted with the least amount of trauma.
Observe for symptomatology of infection: pain or burning on voiding, fever.	
Provide catheter care.	To minimize infection.
Obtain urine specimen to send for culture, sensitivity, and routine urinalysis.	To identify infection or other complication early.
If urinary antibiotic is started, counsel woman to continue to take antibiotic for the full time it is prescribed (usually 1 week).	To prevent infection that may flare up again if antibiotic is stopped too early.
If a drug such as sulfisoxazole (Gantrisin) is ordered, caution woman to avoid drinking cranberry juice.	To ensure safety. Cranberry juice and sulfisoxazole (Gantrisin) combine to form a precipitate that causes considerable discomfort and requires therapy for about a week to clear out of the urinary tract.
After catheterization, assess for adequacy of spontaneous voiding (e.g., record times and amounts).	To ensure bladder functioning and adequacy of emptying.
Report retention with overflow.	
Teach woman symptomatology of urinary tract infection.	To provide identification and therapy to reduce morbidity. To prevent bladder infections that reduce the body's ability to fight other infections.

Procedure 5-4

SUPPRESSION OF LACTATION

DEFINITION

Process of inhibiting the synthesis and secretion of milk from the breasts.

PURPOSE

To discourage lactation by mechanical suppression or pharmacologic suppression, increase comfort, teach mother self-care techniques.

EQUIPMENT

Tight compression "uplift" breast binder or well-fitted supporting brassiere, covered ice packs.

MEDICATIONS

Analgesics, bromocriptine mesylate (Parlodel), other antilactogenics and consent forms.

NURSING ACTIONS	RATIONALE
Wash hands before and after touching woman and equipment. Glove, prn.	To prevent nosocomial infection and to implement universal precautions.
Assess woman and inquire as to whether she wants to breast- or bottle-feed.	Infant feeding is a personal choice.
Mechanical suppression	
Apply a tight compression "uplift" binder for about 72 hours; advise woman to use a snug brassiere after 72 hours (some hospitals do not use binders, women are told to wear a snug brassiere from the very beginning).	Treatment of choice. To give body message that milk production is not needed. Stimulus for lactation and discomfort usually ease after 72 hours.
Avoid any stimulus that could support lactation (e.g., breastfeeding the infant, expression of colostrum, pumping of the breast, using warm water on the breasts).	Nipple stimulation releases prolactin from posterior pituitary. Emptying breast is the primary stimulus for lactation.
Use covered ice packs or analgesics as necessary.	To promote comfort.
Do *not* restrict fluid intake or use diuretics.	These methods do not suppress lactation.
Remind mother that breast firmness, tenderness, and distension (engorgement) are temporary.	Symptoms usually decrease starting about the third day.
Administration of bromocriptine mesylate (Parlodel)	To suppress lactation by preventing the secretion of prolactin.
Confirm physician's explanation of drug to woman.	This nonhormonal, nonestrogenic agent does not act on mammary tissues.
Begin medication after vital signs and blood pressure have stabilized but no sooner than 4 hours after delivery	*One side effect is hypotension in some women.*
Remain with woman when she ambulates for the first time. Assess blood pressure every 4 hours for 72 hours.	Precautionary measure against injury from fainting. Identifies hypotension.
Instruct woman:	To encourage self-care.
Recommended therapeutic dosage is 1 2.5-mg tablet twice daily with meals.	To teach accepted method of taking medication.
Medication is continued for 14 days, or if necessary, for 21 days.	
A rebound of breast secretion, congestion, or engorgement is experienced by a percentage of women.	To prepare woman for possible breast tenderness and need to start mechanical suppression methods.
Breast symptoms are usually only mild to moderate in severity.	To relieve anxiety by knowing that this occurrence is normal.
Use mechanical suppression method to suppress symptomatology.	To encourage self-care.
Administration of other antilactogenics	To add to woman's knowledge base.
Follow hospital protocol for obtaining an informed consent.	The administration of estrogens or androgens is not used often today and is not recommended to suppress lactation. Research has implicated the use of estrogens or
Administer medication per physician's directions.	other hormones as lactation-suppressant drugs in the
Observe woman for thrombus formation.	cause of endometrial cancer. The woman must give informed consent to the use of these drugs. Estrogens have also been implicated in the occurrence of thromboembolism after delivery, particularly after cesarean delivery or complicated vaginal delivery.

POSTPARTUM MEDICATIONS

Bromocriptine Mesylate (Prescription)

Brand names: Parlodel
Dosage form: pO
Use: Prevention of postpartum lactation
Side effects: Blurred vision, diplopia, burning eyes, headache, convulsions, anxiety, nervousness, frequency of urination, incontinence, diuresis, nausea, vomiting, anorexia, cramps, rash, orthostatic hypotension, lowered blood pressure shock, dysrhythmias.
Drug interactions:
Decreased action of these drugs: phenothiazines, methyldopa, imipramine, haloperidol, droperidol, amyltriptyline, oral contraceptives.
Increased action of antihypertensives, levodopa.
Patient education: Change position slowly, use contraceptives (other than oral) because new pregnancy is possible.

Benzocaine (Prescription and Over The Counter)

Brand names: Americaine, Dermoplast
Dosage form: Topical and aerosol spray
Uses: Rectal (hemorrhoidal) and episiotomy pain
Side effects: Rash, sensitization, irritation
Interactions-None known
Patient Education-Report rash, irritation, redness, swelling. Do not inhale spray or get in eyes.

Docusate Calcium/Potassium/Sodium (prescription and over the counter)

Brand names: Surfack, Colace, Kasof, Bu-lax, Docinate D.S.S., Laxinate, Regutol, Roctate
Dosage form: pO and enema (potassium)
Uses: Stool softener
Side effects: Nausea, vomiting, anorexia, and cramps
Interactions: None known
Patient education: Swallow whole; normal bowel movements do not always occur daily; do not use for nausea and vomiting or constipation

CLIENT TEACHING BEFORE DISCHARGE

With postpartum clients being discharged only a few days after delivery, teaching has become one of the nurse's most important responsibilities. The nurse must make certain that the client is aware of symptoms that signify the need for immediate care, such as hemorrhage, as well as how best to deal with routine problems, such as hemorrhoids. The client also should be provided information on exercise, resumption of sexual intercourse, and contraception. The nurse is in a unique position to assist the woman in focusing on self-care as well as care of the new infant. The information in this section will assist the nurse in performing this aspect of care.

This section concludes with a sample nursing care plan and a summary of nursing actions for the early postpartum period, when the nurse has the most contact with clients who have experienced normal delivery without complications.

DANGER SIGNS

Postpartum (Physical)

1. Fever, with or without chills
2. Foul-smelling or irritating vaginal discharge
3. Excessive lochia or vaginal discharge
4. Recurrence of bright red vaginal bleeding after the lochia has changed to rust color
5. A swollen area on the leg that is painful, red, or hot to the touch
6. Localized swelling or a painful, hot area on the breast
7. A burning sensation during urination or an inability to urinate
8. Pelvic or perineal pain

Guidelines for Client Teaching

CARE OF HEMORRHOIDS

ASSESSMENT

1. Multipara 12-hours-postpartum. Large painful hemorrhoids protruding from anal opening.

NURSING DIAGNOSES

Pain, related to swollen hemorrhoids.
Knowledge deficit related to the care and treatment of hemorrhoids.
Bathing/hygiene self-care deficit related to hemorrhoid care.

GOALS
Short-term
To reduce hemorhoidal swelling and promote comfort.

Intermediate
To reduce or eliminate pain and itching.

Long-term
To teach mother self-care techniques.

REFERENCES AND TEACHING AIDS
Charts and pamphlets explaining what hemorrhoids are.
List of instructions for woman to take with her explaining symptoms and treatments.

CONTENT/RATIONALE	TEACHING ACTIONS
To provide content about hemorrhoids: Hemorrhoids are anal varicosities that are precipitated by pregnancy and constipation. The pressure on the pelvic floor by the presenting part and the act of expulsion causes them to protrude and become inflamed.	Show woman picture of chart explaining this.
To provide information for self-care: I will show you what to use to reduce the swelling and decrease the discomfort. First, try a covered ice pack, Leave the pack in place for 20 minutes, repeat every 4 hours. This will reduce the swelling. Cover the ice pack to avoid possibility of a cold "burn."	Show woman the witch hazel pads (Tucks), an ice pack, ointments prescribed by her physician, sitz bath, and rubber glove or finger cots.
Next, apply the cold witch hazel pads, using each one once and discarding after you urinate or defecate. Always wipe from front to back. This stops contamination of episiotomy and open vaginal orifice.	Demonstrate this technique.
A sitz bath will provide an anesthetic effect. If the hemorrhoids are still bothersome, put on a glove or a finger cot, lubricate it with water-soluble lubricant and push the hemorrhoid back inside the anus. This may have to be repeated after a bowel movement. Anal reflex will extrude the hemorrhoid again.	Teach woman sitz bath procedure. Teach woman how to replace the hemorrhoid after putting on a glove and applying lubricant. Once the hemorrhoid is reduced maintain digital pressure for 1 to 2 minutes.
Unless the condition was present before pregnancy, it will correct itself once the increased blood supply and pressure symptoms of pregnancy are diminished and regular bowel habits are reestablished.	Reassure woman and encourage self-care.

EVALUATION Woman establishes self-care and discomfort is diminished.

Guidelines for Client Teaching

POSTPARTUM EXERCISES

ASSESSMENT

1. Woman has just completed a full-term pregnancy.

NURSING DIAGNOSES

Knowledge deficit related to postpartum exercises.
Knowledge deficit related to diastasis of rectus abdominus muscle.
Potential body image disturbance related to postpartum body changes.

GOALS

Short-term

Woman verbalizes understanding of exercise program.
Woman begins exercise recommended for the first postpartum day.

Intermediate

Woman follows exercise program without problems or untoward responses (i.e., fatigue, increased pain).

Long-term

Woman continues with a balance between rest and exercise or activity.
Woman verbalizes satisfaction with way she feels and looks.

REFERENCES AND TEACHING AIDS

Handout with illustrations and descriptions of exercise program.
Filmstrip.
Demonstration of exercises by the nurse.

CONTENT/RATIONALE	TEACHING ACTIONS
To inform the woman about exercise and help her define realistic expectations, the nurse presents the following content: Rigorous exercise may initiate uterine bleeding, fatigue, or discomfort. Toning of the abdominal muscles takes time. Program progresses slowly from easy to more demanding exercises (Ketter and Shelton, 1983).	Caution woman against too rigorous and taxing exercises, regardless of the physical fitness of the woman. Review exercise program per physician's orders. Encourage woman not to rush.
Girdles or other abdominal supports tend to make the woman "forget" to keep abdominal muscles contracted and therefore delay regaining tone. Fatigue or discomfort drain energy needed for recovery and care of newborn and of self. Kegel's exercises begun soon after delivery, or as soon as anesthesia has worn off, aid in the recovery of the pubococcygeal muscle, which is stretched during vaginal delivery.	Discourage woman from wearing girdles or other abdominal supports. Remind woman to stop if exercise makes her too tired. Assess woman's knowledge of Kegel's exercises and review as needed.
To counsel the woman who has diastasis (separation) of the rectus abdomini muscle, reinforce the fact that there is no known therapy to prevent or treat the condition.	Encourage discussion of woman's feelings about the facts that the separation usually lessens with time, but if the separation is quite wide, it may not return to pre-pregnant state; and exercise or girdles have not been known to speed the rate of recovery.

EVALUATION Teaching has been effective when the nurse observes that the woman learns how to do the exercises and, at the follow-up visit to the physician or clinic, she indicates she has followed the exercise program and verbalizes she is pleased with the way she looks.

Guidelines For Client Teaching

RESUMPTION OF SEXUAL INTERCOURSE

ASSESSMENT

1. Couple needs information on how and when to resume sexual intercourse after delivery.
2. Couple states they would like to resume sexual intercourse by third or fourth postdelivery week if bleeding has stopped and the episiotomy is healed.
3. Couple has heard that the first experience with intercourse following delivery may be uncomfortable.
4. Couple has heard that response to sexual stimulation may be altered for a short time after delivery.
5. Couple needs to keep the lines of communication open to remain close and not hurt each other's feelings.

NURSING DIAGNOSES

Knowledge deficit related to resumption of sexual intercourse following delivery:

1. Timing of first intercourse.
2. Need for contraception if pregnancy is not desired.
3. Need for understanding the woman's emotional status at this time.

Anxiety related to knowledge deficit of postdelivery physiology and healing.

Pain related to dryness of vaginal mucosa.

Potential pain related to healing abdominal incision (after cesarean delivery).

Potential pain related to newly healed episiotomy.

Ineffective family coping related to lack of knowledge of:

1. Timing for resumption of sexual intercourse.
2. Measures needed to promote comfort.
3. Precautions to prevent unplanned pregnancy (see Guidelines for Client Teaching, "Postdelivery Contraception," p. 178).

Potential for infection related to lack of understanding of hygienic measures.

GOALS

Short-term (within 3 to 4 weeks)

Woman or couple verbalizes understanding of instructions and content.

Couple discusses subject freely between them and mutually agree to their course of action.

Couple learns to discuss subject with regard to each other's feelings.

Intermediate

Couple resumes sexual intercourse by mutual agreement.

Experience is without discomfort.

No pregnancy results.

Couple continues to communicate effectively with one another.

Long-term

Couple maintains open lines of communication.

Couple mutually agrees on choice of fertility management for present time.

Couple maintains closeness and sexual satisfaction that was part of their lives before the baby arrived.

REFERENCES AND TEACHING AIDS

Printed instructions.
Illustrations.
Texts relevant to subject.

CONTENT/RATIONALE	TEACHING ACTIONS
To provide information about postdelivery physiology and its effects on resumption of sexual intercourse:	Share information with woman and couple.
The couple can safely resume sexual intercourse by the third or fourth postdelivery week if bleeding has stopped and the episiotomy has healed. For the first 6 weeks to 6 months the vagina does not lubricate well because steroid depletion inhibits the vasocongestive response to sexual tension.	Encourage open discussion between couple. Lead discussion by being candid and using open-ended questions. Encourage the couple to ask questions. Encourage couple to problem-solve the situation together.
Physiologic reactions to sexual stimulation for the first 3 postdelivery months are marked by a reduction in both rapidity and intensity of response. Vasocongestion of the labia majora and minora is delayed well into the plateau phase. The walls of the vagina are thin and pink, a condition similar to senile vaginitis. This results from the hormonal starvation of the involutional period. Finally, the size of the orgasmic platform and strength of the orgasmic contractions are reduced.	Suggest slowly building up to the act of intercourse by allowing for caressing, kissing, and shared tenderness.

Guidelines for Client Teaching—cont'd

CONTENT/RATIONALE	TEACHING ACTIONS
A water-soluble gel, cocoa butter, or a contraceptive cream or jelly might be recommended for lubrication. If some vaginal tenderness is present, the partner can be instructed to insert one or more clean, lubricated fingers into the vagina and rotate them within the vagina to help relax it and to identify possible areas of discomfort. A coital position in which the woman has control of the depth of the penile penetration is also useful. The side-by-side or female-superior position is often recommended.	Provide as many alternatives as possible to serve as a basis for discussion and to provide choices. Acknowledge that this may be a difficult area for some people to talk about freely. Provide pictures and explanations of these alternatives.
The presence of the baby influences postdelivery lovemaking. Parents hear every sound made by the baby; conversely they may be concerned that the baby hears every sound they make. In either case any phase of the sexual response cycle may be interrupted by hearing the baby cry or move, leaving one partner or both frustrated and unsatisfied. The amount of psychologic energy expended by the parents in child care activities may lead to fatigue. Newborns require a great deal of attention and time, not to mention what is necessary to take care of twins or triplets, and older children as well (Fischman et al., 1986).	Validate that although these responses are within normal expectations, it still may be difficult to deal with frustration at times. Suggest that the woman take a rest during the day when the baby sleeps.
Some women have reported sexual stimulation to plateau and orgasmic levels when nursing their babies. Although nursing mothers have a longer delay in ovarian steroid production, they are often interested in returning to sexual activity before nonnursing mothers. Nursing mothers also report higher levels of postdelivery eroticism.	Validate that these feelings are normal and that the woman should not be upset or alarmed.
In the event of fetal or newborn death or the birth of an infant that is small, sick, or deformed, the emotional energy required of the woman and her partner, the mother's depleted physical state, and the stress of burying the dead child or of visiting the hospitalized child strain all relationships. Professional caregivers can only speculate about the effect on sexual relationships during these stressful times as a result of little definitive data.	Help parents cope with grief. Provide information on support groups. They can be of tremendous help at a time like this; lending a sympathetic ear and offering advice and comfort to the couple.
The woman should be instructed to follow the Kegel's exercises to strengthen her pubococcygeal muscle. This muscle is the major sphincter of the pelvis. It is associated with bowel and bladder function and with vaginal perception and response during intercourse.	Teach Kegel's exercises. Provide written instructions for the woman to take with her.

EVALUATION This is a private subject, the nurse must use tact when speaking to the woman or the couple about the attainment of goals. The nurse's care and teaching was effective if the couple's goals were met: sexual intercourse has been resumed to the satisfaction of the couple and without physical or emotional discomfort; the couple confirm continued effective communication.

Guidelines For Client Teaching

POSTDELIVERY CONTRACEPTION

ASSESSMENT

1. Woman or couple request information regarding contraception after delivery.
2. Woman has idea that she cannot become pregnant while breast-feeding.

NURSING DIAGNOSES

Knowledge deficit related to the many methods of contraception.

Potential for ineffective breast-feeding related to the resumption of hormonal contraception.

Potential for ineffective family coping related to the stress of an unplanned pregnancy.

GOALS

Short-term

Woman or couple verbalizes understanding of content discussed.

Couple discusses postdelivery contraceptive methods available to them.

Intermediate

Couple mutually agrees on and employs simple barrier methods of contraception: (i.e., condoms, contraceptive gels or foams, diaphragm).

Couple discusses any problems they may have with these methods of contraception.

Long-term

Couple discusses and mutually agrees on a choice of fertility management.

Couple maintains open lines of communication.

Couple will reevaluate method of contraception as time goes on, or if there are any adverse effects from the one they are employing.

REFERENCES AND TEACHING AIDS

Inserts from packages of chosen contraceptive.

Hospital/clinic teaching materials.

Flip chart showing anatomy of pelvic structures or total body plastic medical models.

Hospital or clinic audiovisual teaching materials.

Samples of contraceptive device, basal body temperature charts, and thermometer.

Fresh egg white (for teaching about cervical mucus).

Handouts of printed information.

CONTENT/RATIONALE	TEACHING ACTIONS
To provide content about contraception.	Discuss and outline a tentative plan on discharge from hospital.
	Continue discussion of fertility management at the first postpartum visit.
	Share information with woman and couple.
Women *may* not ovulate while they successfully breast-feed their infants because ovarian functions are *usually* suppressed by a high level of serum prolactin.	Encourage questions.
	Promote open discussion between couple.
	Encourage couple to problem-solve the situation together.
Follicle formation is usually suspended, and ovulation usually does not occur.	Provide as many alternatives as possible to provide choices and serve as a basis for discussion.
Women who do not breast-feed frequently or on demand (e.g., every 3 to 4 hours) or *who supplement the infant's feeding* do not maintain an effectively high level of serum prolactin. If these women do not employ contraceptives, they may conceive again, sometimes without having a menstrual period following the previous pregnancy.	Teach woman (couple) cervical mucus and symptothermal method as one means of determining resumption of ovulatory menstrual cycles.
If the mother is not breast-feeding, she may resume use of oral contraceptives (after delivery) under the physician's direction. If she is breast-feeding, barrier contraception, such as a diaphragm, condom, gel, or foam, should be employed until the first postdelivery examination, at which time the desired method can be instituted.	Acknowledge that this may be a difficult area for some people to talk about.

EVALUATION Teaching actions have been effective when the couple's goal of preventing unwanted pregnancy has been achieved. The couple states they discussed and mutually agreed on a choice of fertility management. They consult the clinic or physician when they have questions.

Sample Nursing Care Plan

EARLY POSTPARTUM

ASSESSMENT	NURSING DIAGNOSIS (ND)/ PLAN (P)/GOAL (G)	RATIONALE/ IMPLEMENTATION	EVALUATION

Vital signs
  Temperature
  Increased pulse
  Record of blood loss or anemia
	ND: Potential for infection related to significant problems that can arise during labor, delivery, and postpartum.
	ND: Potential knowledge deficit related to signs and symptoms of infection.
	P: Prevention or timely identification and treatment of infection.
	P: Meet woman's information needs.
	G: Woman does not develop signs and symptoms of infection. Woman increases her knowledge about infection and fever.
	ND: Potential for hyperthermia related to infection.
	P: Identify and treat hyperthermia.
	G: Woman will learn and use temperature-reduction techniques, and temperature will return to within normal limits.
		To identify infection the nurse will assess for:
		Chills or fever of 38° C (100.4° F) or more.
		Localized redness, heat, pain anywhere on body.
		Urinary frequency, pain, or burning on urination.
		Foul-smelling lochia.
		
		To initiate measures to lower temperature the nurse will:
		Report fever to physician.
		Encourage oral fluids or continue IV fluids as ordered.
		Decrease environmental temperature, remove blankets or heavy clothing.
		Administer antipyretic medication as ordered.
			Woman reports any symptoms she experiences immediately.
			Woman is aware of normal ranges of vital signs.
			Woman does not develop infection; or if she does, identification and resolution are timely.
			
			Woman uses same temperature-reduction techniques at home.
			Woman understands information presented.
			Woman's temperature returns to within normal range.

Increased blood pressure Decreased blood pressure	ND: Potential for injury maternal, related to hypertension/hypotension. P: Monitor for signs and symptoms of deviations from normal values; monitor per hospital protocol and woman's needs. G: Woman will remain normotensive.	*To promote normotensive state in new mother the nurse will:* Give anticipatory guidance for prevention (i.e., diet, exercise, medication). Teach woman about orthostatic hypotension related to splanchnic engorgement.	Woman is aware of normal range. Woman implements preventive measures. Woman takes precautions against fainting during first ambulation; calls for assistance.
Headache	ND: Pain: headache related to stress, increased blood pressure, spinal anesthesia. P: Help woman prevent headache; monitor for headache; implement appropriate therapy.	*To prevent or decrease headache the nurse will:* Teach relaxation and stress-reduction techniques. Administer medications for increased blood pressure as ordered. Have woman lie down.	Woman knows and uses relaxation techniques. Woman knows importance of taking antihypertensive medications. Woman understands reason for headache and complies with prevention or treatment.

Continued.

Sample Nursing Care Plan—cont'd

ASSESSMENT	NURSING DIANGOSIS (ND)/ PLAN (P)/GOAL (G)	RATIONALE/ IMPLEMENTATION	EVALUATION
	G: Woman will not have headache; or, headache and its cause are identified and treated promptly.	Keep woman recovering from spinal anesthesia flat for prescribed number of hours. Administer medications as ordered. Increase fluid intake. Prepare for blood patch procedure.	
Uterus Position, size Tone Response to gentle massage Rate of involution Afterpains	ND: Potential for injury related to hemorrhage from an atonic uterus postdelivery. P: Prevent atonic uterus, prevent hemorrhage through teaching and direct care. G: Hemorrhage does not occur. ND: Pain related to uterine involution/afterpains. P: Prevent or minimize discomfort. G: Woman states that afterpains are tolerable and she is satisfied with measures used.	*To prevent hemorrhage from atonic uterus the nurse will:* Assess tone and response to gentle massage. Use nonpharmacologic or pharmacologic measures to maintain tone and relieve discomfort of afterpains. Teach woman how to assess fundus. Teach woman how to massage uterus.	Woman understands purpose of firm uterus and follows through with self-massage.
Lochia Color and character Amount Size, number of clots Odor ("fleshy")	ND: Potential for infection/ hemorrhage related to conditions causing abnormal lochia. P: Detect and prevent underlying causes of deviations from normal. G: Woman's lochia remains within normal limits.	*To prevent possible hemorrhage and infection of endometrium the nurse will:* Monitor amount and character of lochia. If heavy, reassess source of bleeding, uterine tone, and degree of bladder distension. Expelled clots should be charted as to size and amount. Teach expected regression (color and amount) during involution. Teach woman about atony of the uterus and subsequent hemorrhage, and explain that clots prevent the living ligature from working.	Woman verbalizes understanding and reports any unusual symptoms. Lochia is moderate or less with no clots or just a few small clots.
Perineum Healing of episiotomy/laceration Swelling, bruising Hematoma	ND: Impaired skin integrity related to episiotomy/ lacerations acquired during delivery.	*To ensure proper healing and prevent infection and development of other problems the nurse will:*	Perineum heals well. Hemorrhoids regress. Woman employs comfort measures.

Sample Nursing Care Plan—cont'd

ASSESSMENT	NURSING DIANGOSIS (ND)/ PLAN (P)/GOAL (G)	RATIONALE/ IMPLEMENTATION	EVALUATION
Size, number of hemorrhoids	P: Promote healing, prevent further complications. G: Woman's childbirth-related tissue trauma heals without difficulty. ND: Pain, related to episiotomy, laceration, hemorrhoids, swelling, bruising, or hematoma. P: Prevent or minimize discomfort. G: Woman's discomfort is prevented or minimized.	Monitor perineal healing. Provide comfort measures. Wash hands before and after care of perineum. Teach woman comfort measures—ice packs, sitz baths, heat lamp, anesthetic sprays or creams, witch hazel pads (Tucks). Give woman opportunity to look at perineum and its repair (if interested). Describe to woman what to expect while perineum is healing and hemorrhoids are regressing. Teach woman to prevent contamination of perineum and vulva by washing hands before and after pericare; wiping from front to back; changing peripads often; changing underwear daily and when soiled.	Comfort is maintained. Woman verbalizes understanding of information presented, uses proper pericare.

Urinary tract
  Symptoms of infection
  Distension
  Completeness of emptying
  Ability to void
  Total amount in 24 hours
	ND: Potential for infection related to bladder trauma during delivery, or retention and stasis of urine.
	P: Prevent distension and stasis of urine.
	G: Woman does not experience bladder distention.
		To prevent urinary tract infection the nurse will:
		Teach woman to wipe from front to back.
		Use strict aseptic technique when catheterization is necessary.
		Help woman void and empty bladder completely.
		Teach woman symptoms of urinary tract infection: urgency; frequency and burning on urination; and blood in urine.
			Woman does not develop urinary infection.
			Woman understands symptoms and reports development of same.

	ND: Urinary retention related to anesthesia and bladder trauma. P: Assist woman to void; catheterize if necessary. G: Woman resumes normal pattern of urine elimination.	*To assist woman in voiding the nurse will:* Encourage oral fluids. Assist to bathroom, if possible. Run water in sink for encouragement. Pour warm water down perineum or immerse in warm sitz bath. Catheterize per physician's order. Teach Crede's method (use of manual pressure on bladder to express urine).	Woman voids and empties bladder completely at least every 4 hours. Bladder distension does not occur. If catheterization is necessary, infection or loss of self-esteem does not occur.
Bowels Bowel sounds	ND: Constipation related to	*To assist woman with first*	Woman's bowel elimination

Continued.

Sample Nursing Care Plan—cont'd

ASSESSMENT	NURSING DIANGOSIS (ND)/ PLAN (P)/GOAL (G)	RATIONALE/ IMPLEMENTATION	EVALUATION
Passing flatus Abdominal distension Bowel movement Constipation Diarrhea Hemorrhoids	fear of tearing stitches or pain, medications, decreased peristalsis, hemorrhoids. P: Prevent bowel problems through teaching and direct care. G: Woman does not experience bowel problems.	*bowel movement the nurse will:* Encourage and assist with early ambulation, fluids, foods with roughage. Encourage immediate response to urge to defecate. Administer stool softeners as prescribed. Employ care of perineum. Counsel woman on fluids, foods; exercise; bowel habits; hygiene after defecation. Check chart for record of last bowel movement during labor and delivery.	pattern restored. Woman has minimum discomfort. Woman continues to use preventive and comfort measures learned during hospitalization.

Breasts
  Soft, filling, firm
  Engorged
  Painful
  Mastitis
	ND: Pain of engorged breasts related to lactation or suppression.
	
	P: Assist with comfort measures for lactation or suppression; meet information needs.
	G: Woman's goal of lactation or suppression is met with little if any discomfort.
		To assist woman with suppression of lactation the nurse will:
		Teach newborn nutrition and feeding.
		Tell woman to wear a good supporting bra or provide a binder.
		Place ice packs to breasts for engorgement as ordered.
		Give medications as prescribed:
		  bromocriptine,
		  Deladumone (use of this medication requires the woman's signed informed consent).
		To assist woman with lactation and breast-feeding the nurse will:
		Teach newborn nutrition and feeding.
		Teach hygiene: use warm water, no soap; wash breasts first with fresh washcloth.
		Tell woman to wear good supporting bra (nursing bra, if possible).
		Teach use of breast pump and manual expression.
		Teach positioning for breast-feeding.
		Give information on breast-feeding support groups (i.e., La Leche League).
			Lactation is suppressed with minimum discomfort.
			
			Lactation initiated successfully with minimal or no discomfort.
			
			Woman is satisfied with breast-feeding experience.

Sample Nursing Care Plan—cont'd

ASSESSMENT	NURSING DIANGOSIS (ND)/ PLAN (P)/GOAL (G)	RATIONALE/ IMPLEMENTATION	EVALUATION

Nipples
  Protruding
  Inverted
  Sore or tender
  Cracked or bleeding
	ND: Impaired skin integrity related to learning to breast-feed and take care of nipples.
	P: Teach feeding techniques and care of nipples.
	G: Woman learns feeding techniques and care of nipples.
		To teach care of nipples the nurse will:
		Assist woman with breast-feeding.
		Employ preventative and comfort measures: Masse' cream, rotation of newborn's position at breast, correct latching-on, correct removal of baby from breast by breaking suction with finger first.
			Woman learns feeding techniques and care of nipples.
			Nipples are not injured or uncomfortable.

Hemoglobin and hematocrit May be decreased at this time	ND: Altered cardiopulmonary tissue perfusion related to anemia. P: Detect and correct anemia to prevent complications. G: Anemia is detected if present and corrective measures are initiated. ND: Knowledge deficit related to anemia. P: Increase woman's knowledge about anemia, its cause, treatment, and prevention. G: Woman's anemia is resolved; future occurence is prevented.	*To monitor hemoglobin and hematocrit:* Order laboratory work as ordered. Retrieve information and place on chart. Alert physician to low levels and implement orders, as necessary. *To meet woman's knowledge needs, the nurse will discuss:* Rationale for tests. Range of normal values and where woman's values fit within that range. Relationship to nutrition.	Values are within normal limits. Woman learns self-care through nutrition. Woman prevents anemia in self and family.

Coagulation factors
  Thrombus formation
  Intravascular coagulation: local or disseminated (DIC)
	ND: Pain from thrombus formation related to alterations in coagulation process.
	ND: Potential for injury related to development of DIC.
	P: Monitor to detect and correct problem to prevent further complications.
	G: Woman develops no problem related to coagulation.
		To protect woman from thrombus formation or other coagulopathies the nurse will:
		Monitor for and teach woman symptomatology of thrombus formation (Homans' sign).
		Monitor for and teach woman problems with ambulation and exercise, redness or swelling of calf or leg.
		Monitor for symptoms of DIC.
		Teach woman rationale for assessment, measures to take should symptomatology of thrombus occur.
			No coagulation problems occur.
			Woman recognizes and seeks therapy for symptomatology of thrombus formation.

Summary of Nursing Actions

NURSING CARE DURING THE EARLY POSTPARTUM PERIOD

I. Goals
  A. For the mother: a successful physical recovery from childbirth and establishment of mother-child relationship
  B. For the newborn: an uncompromised adjustment to extrauterine existence and a successful incorporation into the family system
  C. For the family: a satisfying family-newborn relationship, an appropriate family participation in healthy care of themselves and the newborn, and a return to mutually satisfying family commitments

II. Priorities
  A. Prevent hemorrhage and infection.
  B. Promote comfort.
  C. Promote involution and return of nonpregnant physiologic functioning.
  D. Encourage self-care.
  E. Provide rubella vaccination and $Rh_o(D)$ immune globulin as needed.
  F. Promote mother-father-infant relationships.
  G. Promote siblings and grandparent's relationship with infant.

III. Assessment
  A. Interview
    1. Ethnic or cultural variations and nursing actions desired
    2. Knowledge of hygiene
    3. Nutrition: amounts taken, food preferences, knowledge of, for self and family
    4. Readiness for discharge from hospital:
      a. Extent of skill in self-care
      b. Clients' need for knowledge of:
        (1) Breast self-examination
        (2) Resumption of sexual intercourse
        (3) Contraception
      c. Client's need for help at home, acquisition of care seat for newborn, social assistance (e.g., food stamps)
      d. Client's knowledge of:
        (1) Danger signs and symptoms for which to call the physician
        (2) Resources for assistance (e.g., hemorrhage, infection, information such as Tel-Med)
  B. Physical examination
    1. Receive report from nurse in labor unit and review prenatal record
    2. Assess physical recovery
      a. Vital signs and blood pressure
      b. Involution: fundus, lochia, perineum
      c. Legs: Homan's sign, edema
      d. Breasts and nipples
      e. Elimination: urinary, bowel
    3. Assess for comfort
      a. General comfort and energy level
      b. Breasts: engorgement, nipples
      c. Afterpains
      d. Perineum: episiotomy and laceration repair sites
      e. Bladder and voiding
      f. Hemorrhoids
      g. Bowel evacuation
      h. Legs (calves and varicose veins)
    4. Assess ability to ambulate (both tolerance for and knowledge of need for) and plans for exercise and rest at home.
  C. Laboratory tests
    1. Hematocrit (Hct) or packed cell volume (PCV)
    2. Complete blood count (CBC) if needed
    3. Urinarlysis if needed
    4. Need for rubella vaccination
    5. Need for $Rh_0(D)$ immune globulin

IV. Potential nursing diagnoses
  A. Noncompliance (specify)
  B. Knowledge deficit
  C. Altered nutrition: more or less than body requirements
  D. Impaired verbal communication
  E. Altered health maintenance
  F. Potential for injury
  G. Powerlessness
  H. Spiritual distress
  I. Altered tissue perfusion (specify)
  J. Potential for infection
  K. Impaired skin integrity
  L. Altered patterns of urinary elimination
  M. Diarrhea
  N. Constipation
  O. Impaired physical mobility
  P. Pain
  Q. Sleep pattern disturbance
  R. Self esteem disturbance: situational low self esteem
  S. Personal identity disturbance
  T. Altered sexuality patterns
  U. Potential activity intolerance
  V. Potential ineffective breast-feeding
  W. Ineffective family coping: compromised
  X. Ineffective individual coping
  Y. Altered family processes
  Z. Fatigue
  AA. Fear
  BB. Anxiety
  CC. Potential fluid volume deficit
  DD. Parental role conflict
  EE. Altered role performance
  FF. Body image disturbance

V. Plan/implementation
  A. Orientation to room
    1. Welcome and greet by name. Orient to personnel, unit, and procedures as necessary:

Summary of Nursing Actions—cont'd

a. Check woman's understanding of use of call bell.

b. Review routine of care: infant feeding and rooming-in, visiting regulations, ordering diets, etc.

c. Arrange for interpretor or translator as necessary.

2. Record. Report as necessary. Teach mother normal limits.

3. Implement therapy for emergent problems: infection, hemorrhage pregnancy-induced hypertension (PIH).

B. Physical care

1. Assist woman with first ambulation after delivery; explain reason (e.g., splanchnic engorgement) so that woman and family remember to call for assistance to ambulate.

2. Continue to monitor for symptomatology that would indicate infection or PIH.

3. Notify physician if findings are outside of normal range. Institute prescribed therapy if needed.

4. Check with woman and her record regarding known allergies. Implement nonpharmacologic interventions first (e.g., for comfort) before using medications. Inform woman of medication and its expected effects if she does not know this. Chart medications; assess and record woman's response.

5. Meet woman's knowledge needs regarding involution: describe and give rationale for procedures to be used in assessing woman's recovery from childbirth and return of reproductive organs to nonpregnant state. Repeat and reinforce during hospital stay.

6. Keep uterus empty and contracted. Implement physician's orders regarding low hematocrit (e.g., blood replacement, nutrition counseling).

a. See Decision Tree "Boggy uterus," p. 167

b. See Procedure 501, "Nursing Actions for Uterine Atony"

c. See Table 5-5, "Summary of Measures to Stimulate Uterine Tone"

d. Institute comfort measures for woman's discomfort and teach her self-care for afterpains

7. See Procedure 5-2, "Care after Repair of Episiotomy or Laceration"

a. Institute hygienic and comfort measures

8. Teach woman and family regarding reportable findings after discharge (e.g., return of lochia rubra, foul odor to lochia, uterine tenderness, fever, and chills).

a. Implement physician's orders regarding infection (e.g., intravenous fluids, antimicrobial medications).

b. Offer printed instructions regarding reportable symptomatology and appropriate phone numbers.

c. Teach regarding expected return of menstruation.

9. Meet woman's knowledge needs for fluid intake and emptying of bladder and reporting of symptomatology of infection to physician.

10. Encourage adequate fluid intake and emptying of bladder, at least every 4 hours.

11. Provide and teach woman hygienic care.

a. See Decision Tree, "Full Urinary Bladder," p. 170.

b. See Procedure 5-3, "Nursing Actions for Full Urinary Bladder"

12. Meet knowledge needs regarding defecation during postpartum period.

a. Encourage use of fluids, food with roughage, and exercise to promote regular bowel habits.

b. Avoid use of enemas for women whose deliveries were complicated by fourth-degree lacerations or if episiotomy extended through the rectum.

c. Counsel regarding expected spontaneous reduction of hemorrhoids during the puerperium and the continued avoidance of constipation with straining at stool.

d. See Guidelines for Client Teaching, "Care of Hemorrhoids," p. 174.

13. Meet woman's knowledge needs regarding breast and nipple care, techniques of infant feeding, support of breasts, and lactation. (See Unit 4 for newborn nutrition and feeding.)

14. Meet woman's knowledge needs regarding suppression of lactation. See Procedure 5-4, "Suppression of lactation"

a. Institute measures to suppress lactation per physician's directives, e.g., administer bromocriptine, mesylate (Parlodel). See box, "Postpartum Medications," p. 173.

b. Minimize engorgement by:

(1) Application of supportive bra

(2) Avoidance of breast stimulation, e.g., manual expression, warm water to breasts

15. Meet woman's knowledge needs regarding thrombus formation, prevention, symptomatology, and urgency in notifying physician.

a. Encourage leg exercises and ambulation.

b. If symptomatology occurs, immobilize and elevate leg, avoid massage, and report to physician immediately.

c. Apply supportive stockings per physician's directives.

16. Meet nutritional needs

17. Discuss with woman and husband the resumption of sexual intercourse after healing occurs and discomfort eases.

a. Explain external changes in appearance of vaginal introitus.

b. See Guidelines for Client Teaching: "Re-

Continued.

Summary of Nursing Actions—cont'd

  sumption of Sexual Intercourse," pp. 129-130; and "Postdelivery Contraception," p. 178.

18. Teach postpartum exercises as ordered by physician (see Guidelines for Client Teaching, "Postpartum Exercises," p. 175.
19. Meet mother's knowledge needs regarding expected diuresis and weight loss.
20. Remind woman and family that she is still not able to wear prepregnant clothes and that some people might think she is still pregnant in early days after delivery.
21. Ensure adequate supply of soap, towels, etc.
22. Ensure cleanliness of bath, showers, sitz rooms, and basins.
23. Assist with hygienic measures

C. Psychosocial care and health maintenance

1. Refer to social service if family needs financial assistance for food.
2. Offer and provide written information.
3. Refer to nutritionist.
4. Meet woman's and family's knowledge and skill needs through:
   a. Discussion with her and with family members
   b. Formalized classes in hospital
   c. Illustrations and photographs
   d. Printed material and instructions
   e. Asking her and them to write down notes and questions
5. Reinforce physician's explanation for need for vaccination and precautions against pregnancy within 3 months.
6. Administer per hospital protocol.
7. Fill out card for $Rh_o(D)$ immune globulin (RHoGAM) and give to mother.
8. May consider using this opportunity to discuss vaccination schedule for infant.
9. Determine that family has infant seat by checking car when discharging mother and infant. Return mother and infant to unit if there is no infant seat. Call social worker for loan of infant seat if needed.

D. Complete recording and close the chart

VI. Evaluation

A. Orientation to room

1. Woman, family, and personnel establish a therapeutic relationship.

B. Physical care

1. Vital signs and blood pressure remain within normal limits.
2. Hematocrit: 42% ± 5%.
3. White cell mass within first 10 to 14 days may be 20,000 to 25,000/mm^3.
4. Proteinuria may be present during first week.
5. Woman receives correct medications and dosages by the correct route. Medication is effective. Woman knows medication, its purpose, and expected results. Woman experiences no allergic or other untoward responses.

6. Involution progresses normally.
   a. Size of uterus diminishes.
   b. Uterine tone is maintained by contraction and retraction of uterine muscles. Uterus feels firm and contracts readily after massage. During the first 12 hours after delivery, contractions are strong, regular, and coordinated. Thereafter intensity, frequency, and regularity decrease. Afterpains occur for 2 to 3 days and are more noticeable in multipara than in primipara and during suckling of infant.
7. Progression of lochia discharge is within normal limits.
   a. Lochia rubra contains blood, placental and decidual debris, and clots and is dark red. It persists from delivery through third day.
   b. Lochia serosa is thin, serous, and brownish and lasts from fourth to tenth day.
   c. Lochia alba, a yellowish-white discharge, contains an increased number of leukocytes and lasts from tenth day to as long as sixth week.
   d. Odor remains characteristically "fleshy" rather than foul. Amount of discharge is moderate for first 2-3 days and then is scant. Some women may have none after 2 weeks; in, others discharge persists until sixth week.
8. Perineum remains free of infection and signs of childbirth trauma. Episiotomy or laceration repair heals well. Hemorrhoids resolve.
9. Breasts and nipples remain free of infection. Engorgement is prevented or minimized.
10. Mother learns to assist infant to nurse at the breast or from the bottle.
11. Lactation begins:
   a. For 2 to 3 days after delivery breasts secrete colostrum in increasing amounts.
   b. By second day in multiparas and by third day in primiparas, breasts become engorged, firm, tense, and tender.
   c. This is caused by venous or lymphatic stasis. In 36 to 48 hours pain disappears as swelling spontaneously subsides. Fever does not accompany this process. Soon afater onset of this engorgement, true milk is formed and let-down reflex in response to suckling of infant or manual manipulation causes expression of milk.
12. Bottle feeding is begun.
   a. Suppression of lactation is successful.
   b. Engorgement is prevented or minimized.
13. Legs remain free of evidence of thrombus formation (e.g., there is no pain, warmth, localized tenderness, swollen, reddened vein that feels hard to touch). Homan's sign remains negative. If varicosities are present, they diminish in size.
14. Defecation occurs spontaneously or with the aid of laxatives, stool softeners, or enemas by the

Summary of Nursing Actions—cont'd

third day. Defecation occurs with minimal or no discomfort.

15. Woman voids spontaneously by 8 hours after delivery and thereafter voids copious amounts frequently for 48 hours as retained tissue fluids are released.
    a. Complete emptying of bladder occurs. Nurse palpates empty bladder and well-contracted involuting uterus in midline.
    b. Urination occurs without symptomatology of urinary tract infection, e.g., frequency, urgency, sensations of burning (dysuria).
    c. Urine is straw-colored and clear; odor is not foul.
16. Woman follows good handwashing technique, cleanses her perineum, and changes her pads appropriately; cleanses her breasts and nipples appropriately.
17. Woman's nutritional needs are met and she is comfortable with type and amount of prescribed diet.
18. Woman states she can and will continue to maintain good nutrition.
C. Psychosocial and health maintenance
    1. Woman and family indicate understanding of health-maintenance activities:

     a. Couple is aware of contraception techniques available, and their questions are answered to their satisfaction.
     b. Woman and family are aware of continued need for rest, exercise, and nutrition.
     c. Postdelivery immunization is completed, e.g., rubella vaccination and prevention of Rh isoimmunization, if appropriate.

2. Couple is aware of danger signals, safety measures, and phone numbers of whom to contact for:
    a. Hemorrhage
    b. Infection
    c. Thrombolism
    d. Hypertension or hypotension
    e. Depressive states
    f. Couple is aware of need for medical examination in 4 to 6 weeks for mother.
    g. Family has an approved car seat for transporting infant home.
3. Family has list of phone numbers of community resources.
4. Records are complete.
5. Discharge summary is available for the 4- to 6-week examination.

References

Fischman SH et al: Changes in sexual relationships in postpartum couples JOGN Nurs 15:58, Jan/Feb 1986.

Ketter DE and Shelton BJ: In-hospital exercises for the postpartal woman, MCN 8:120, 1983.

Bibliography

Bull M and Lawrence D: Mother's use of knowledge during the first postpartum weeks, JOGN Nurs 14:315, July/Aug 1985.

Horn M and Manion J: Creative grandparenting: bonding the generations, JOGN Nurs 14(3):233, 1985.

Lane G, Cronin K, and Peirce A: Flow charts: clinical decision making in nursing, Philadelphia, 1983, JB Lippincott Co.

Newell NJ: Grandparents: the overlooked support system for new parents during the fourth trimester, NAACOG Update Series, 1(lesson 21), Washington, DC, 1984, The Association.

Pritchard JA, MacDonald PC, and Gant NE: Williams obstetrics, ed 17, Norwalk, Conn, 1985, Appleton-Century-Crofts.

Russel TR: Managing hemorrhoids during and after pregnancy, Contemp OB/GYN 21:March 1983 (special issue).

Wong S and Strepp-Gilbert E: Lactation suppression: nonpharmaceutical versus pharmaceutical method, JOGN Nurs 14(4):302, July/Aug 1985.

Complications of Childbearing

The vast majority of pregnancies progress normally and result in the birth of a healthy infant. Each year, however, hundreds of thousands of pregnancies and births are categorized as high risk. Complications affecting pregnancy, labor, and delivery threaten the integrity of the entire family and challenge all members of the health care team to provide comprehensive, holistic care.

To identify high-risk clients effectively, nurses must be knowledgeable about the factors that place a pregnancy or birth at risk and the ways of assessing for these factors. To care competently for clients at risk, nurses need to understand the implications of various conditions and diseases on childbearing and the techniques employed to minimize negative outcomes.

ASSESSMENT OF RISK FACTORS

Early identification of the client at risk facilitates the implementation of preventive and therapeutic measures to avert or minimize the potential consequences of childbearing complications. Risk assessment begins with the interview and physical examination. If problems are suspected or identified, various diagnostic techniques should be employed to provide additional data. The nurse must know the factors that place clients at risk throughout the childbearing process, as well as how to administer and interpret various screening tests.

Risk Factors

The nurse who is conversant with factors that can place a client at risk is often the member of the health care team who alerts other health providers to the need for special screening or care. Certain factors that jeopardize the childbearing woman and her fetus or neonate are presented in this section.

CATEGORIES OF HIGH-RISK PREGNANCY

Maternal Age and Parity Factors

1. Age 16 years or under
2. Nullipara 35 years or over
3. Multipara 40 years or over
4. Interval of 8 years or more since last pregnancy
5. High parity (5 or more)
6. Pregnancy occurring 3 months or less after last delivery

Nonmarital Pregnancy

PIH, Hypertension, Kidney Disease

1. Preeclampsia with hospitalization before labor
2. Eclampsia
3. Kidney disease—pyelonephritis, nephritis, nephrosis, etc.
4. Chronic hypertension, severe (160/100 mm Hg or over)
5. Blood pressure 140/90 mm Hg or above on 2 readings 30 minutes apart

Anemia and Hemorrhage

1. Hematocrit 30% or below in pregnancy
2. Hemorrhage (previous pregnancy)—severe, requiring transfusion
3. Hemorrhage (present pregnancy)
4. Anemia (hemoglobin below 10 g) for which treatment other than oral iron preparations is required (hemolytic, macrocytic, etc.)
5. Sickle cell trait or disease
6. History of bleeding or clotting disorder at any time

Fetal Factors

1. Two or more previous premature deliveries (twins = one delivery)
2. Two or more consecutive spontaneous abortions (miscarriages)
3. One or more stillbirths at term
4. One or more gross anomalies
5. Rh incompatibility or ABO immunization problems
6. History of previous birth defects—cerebral palsy, brain damage, mental retardation, metabolic disorders such as phenylketonuria (PKU)
7. History of large infants (over 4032 g [9 lb])

Paternal Age (?) and Other Factors (?)

Dystocia (History of or Anticipated)

1. Contracted pelvis or cephalopelvic disproportion (CPD)
2. Multiple pregnancy in current pregnancy
3. Two or more breech deliveries
4. Previous operative deliveries, (e.g., cesarean or midforceps delivery)
5. History of prolonged labor (more than 18 hours for nullipara; more than 12 hours for multipara)
6. Previously diagnosed genital tract anomalies (incompetent cervix, cervical or uterine malformation, solitary ovary or tube) or problem (ovarian mass, endometriosis)
7. Short stature (1.5 m [60 in] or less)

History of or Concurrent Conditions

1. Diabetes mellitus; gestational diabetes
2. Hyperemesis gravidarum
3. Thyroid disease (hypothyroidism or hyperthyroidism)
4. Malnutrition or extreme obesity (20% over ideal weight for height; 15% under ideal weight for height)
5. Organic heart disease
6. Syphilis and TORCH infections: toxoplasmosis, rubella in first 10 weeks of *this* pregnancy, cytomegalovirus (CMV), and herpes simplex; AIDS
7. Tuberculosis or other serious pulmonary pathologic condition (e.g., emphysema, asthma)
8. Malignant or premalignant tumors (including hydatidiform mole)
9. Alcoholism, drug addiction
10. Psychiatric disease or epilepsy (documented)
11. Mental retardation

Those with Previous History of

1. Late registration
2. Poor clinic attendance
3. Home situation making clinic attendance and hospitalization difficult
4. Mothers, including minors, without family resources (including desertions, adoptions, injuries, separations, family withdrawals, sole support)

Modified from Fogel CI and Woods NF: Health care of women: a nursing perspective, St Louis, 1981, The CV Mosby Co.

Table 6-1 *Factors that Place the Pregnancy and Fetus-neonate at High Risk by Trimester and During Labor*

Category	Factors that Result in Risk	Category	Factors that Result in Risk
First Trimester		**Third Trimester**	
Anatomic	Maternal	Anatomic	Malpresentation
	Ectopic pregnancy		Cord complications
	Uterine abnormality		Placenta previa*
	Retroversion of uterus	Maternal complications	Hypertensive disease*
Physiologic	Fetal		Rh incompatibilities
	Gross chromosomal defect		Diabetes
	Hydatidiform mole		Thyrotoxicosis
	Multiple pregnancy	Infections	Viral infection*
	Poor trophoblast invasive-		Pneumonia
	ness	Nutritional	Protein lack
	Folate deficiency		Iron deficiencies
	Endocrine deficiency		Abruptio placentae*
	Hyperemesis gravidarum	Therapeutic to mother	Antibacterial drugs
	Defective sperm		Tetracycline
Psychologic	Psychologic shock		Antithyroid drugs
	Drugs		Corticosteroids
Therapeutic	Elective abortion (aspiration,		Anticonvulsants
	saline solution, prostaglan-		Anticoagulants
	din) before this pregnancy	Fetal complications	Premature rupture of membranes
	Drug therapy		Preterm labor; postmaturity
	X-ray therapy		Hydramnios or oligohydramnios
Infection	Viral infection		Multiple gestation
Genetic	Sporadic mutation	Environmental	Poverty
	Inherited characteristics		Drugs, tobacco, alcohol
	Sex-linked disease		Inadequate nutrition
Environmental	Poverty		
	Drugs, tobacco, alcohol	**Labor**	
	Inadequate nutrition	Anatomic	Fetal head compression
			Malpresentation
Second Trimester			Umbilical cord prolapse
Anatomic	Maternal		Breech presentation
	Uterine abnormality		Placenta previa; abruptio placentae
	Incompetent cervical os		Rigid soft tissues
	Fetal		Multiple gestation
	Gross abnormality		Placental or umbilical cord compression
	Acute hydramnios		Excessive or inadequate fetal size
	Multiple pregnancy	Physiologic	Dehydration
	Poor implantation		Ketosis
Maternal complications	Rh incompatibility		Fetal acidosis (pH 7.25 or less in the first
	Cyanotic heart disease		stage of labor)
	Hypertension		Meconium staining of amniotic fluid
	Renal disease		Fetal bradycardia or tachycardia (longer
	Urinary tract infections		than 30 minutes)
	Accidents		Abnormal nonstress test or oxytocin chal-
	Anoxia of hypertensive disease		lenge test
	or epilepsy		Falling urinary estriol levels
Infections	Polio, syphilis, hepatitis,		Immature fetal lungs
	TORCH,† AIDS		Severe preeclampsia-eclampsia
Genetic	Amniocentesis	Maternal complications,	Sedative depression
Environmental	Poverty, drugs, tobacco, alco-	iatrogenic	Hypotension; anesthesia; supine position
	hol		Oxytocin (Pitocin) augmentation or induc-
	Inadequate nutrition		tion of labor
			Prolonged labor; precipitous labor (less
			than 3 hours)
			Operative delivery: cesarean, forceps, vac-
			uum extraction
		Uterine and placental	Uterine hypotonicity, hypertonicity, inertia
			Placental insufficiency

Modified from Fogel CI and Woods NF: Health care of women: a nursing perspective, St Louis, 1981, The CV Mosby Co.
*Associated with intrauterine growth retardation (IUGR).
†Toxoplasmosis, rubella, cytomegalovirus, and herpes simplex.

FACTORS THAT PLACE THE POSTPARTUM WOMAN AND NEONATE AT RIGH RISK

Specific factors that place **mother in high-risk** category:
1. Hemorrhage
2. Infection
3. Abnormal vital signs
4. Traumatic labor or delivery
5. Psychosocial factors

Criteria for selection of high-risk infants for admission to neonatal intensive care units:

1. Specific factors that place **infant in high-risk** category:
   a. Infants continuing or developing signs of respiratory distress syndrome (RDS) or other respiratory distress
   b. Asphyxiated infants (Apgar score of less than 6 at 5 minutes); resuscitation required at birth
   c. Preterm infants; dysmature infants
   d. Infants with cyanosis or suspected cardiovascular disease; persistent cyanosis
   e. Infants with major congenital malformations requiring surgery; chromosomal anomalies
   f. Infants with convulsions, sepsis, hemorrhagic diathesis, or shock
   g. Meconium aspiration syndrome
   h. Central nervous system (CNS) depression for longer than 24 hours
   i. Hypoglycemia
   j. Hypocalcemia
   k. Hyperbilirubinemia

2. Factors indicating **moderate risk**:
   a. Dysmaturity
   b. Prematurity (weight between 2000 and 2500 g)
   c. Apgar score of less than 5 at 1 minute
   d. Feeding problems
   e. Multiple birth
   f. Transient tachypnea
   g. Hypomagnesemia or hypermagnesemia
   h. Hypoparathyroidism
   i. Failure to gain weight
   j. Jitteriness or hyperactivity
   k. Cardiac anomalies not requiring immediate catheterization
   l. Heart murmur
   m. Anemia
   n. Central nervous system depression for less than 24 hours

Diagnostic Techniques

Various tests of fetal status are valuable in determining and monitoring the well-being of the fetus. Although these tests have been made as safe as possible, each procedure involves some degree of risk. The status of each client must be assessed to determine if the advantages of a particular procedure outweigh its risk and expense. The nurse should keep in mind that no single test can provide comprehensive data for planning care. Each has its limitations in terms of diagnostic accuracy and applicability.

This section presents information on techniques that often require both the nurse's participation and guidelines for interpreting the results. It is often the nurse's responsibility to obtain the woman's written consent for these procedures. The nurse is legally and professionally obligated to be certain that the woman understands the reason for the test, the risks involved, and the implications of potential results.

Table 6-2 *Diagnostic Ultrasound: Operational Modes**

Modality	Product	Principal Use
Pulsed wave†		
A mode	Static image	Diagnostic evaluation of brain
B mode (gray scale)*†	Static image	Images of abdominal and pelvic structures
M mode	Dynamic imaging	Monitoring of heart and measuring of heart wall displacement
Real time*	Static image and dynamic imaging	Provides dynamic imaging and static images
Continuous wave		
Doppler mode*	Ranging mode	Fetal heart monitoring

*Used extensively in obstetrics and gynecology.
†Pulsed wave—sound emitted at intervals; continuous wave—sound emitted continuously; A mode—one-dimensional image that appears as spikes on a horizontal base; distance between spikes can be measured (e.g., biparietal diameter [BPD]); B mode (gray scale)—rough, two-dimensional image of various tissue densities for visualizing tissue texture and contour; M mode—time-related tracings showing straight lines for motionless structures and wiggly lines for structural motion (e.g., atrial septal defects and patent ductus arteriosus); static—stationary; dynamic—moving; Doppler mode—detection of change in frequency (wavelength) of structures in motion (e.g., blood flow in umbilical cord and placenta, closure of fetal cardiac valves); real time—dynamic imaging (limb and respiratory movements), as well as static images (BPD, placental location).

Table 6-3 *Major Indications for Obstetric Sonography*

First Trimester	Second Trimester	Third Trimester
Confirm pregnancy	Establish or confirm dates†	If no fetal heart tones
Confirm viability	If no fetal heart tones	Clarify dates/size discrepancy
Rule out ectopic pregnancy	Clarify dates/size discrepancy	Large for dates—rule out
Confirm gestational age*	Large for dates—rule out	Macrosomia (diabetes mellitus)
Birth control use	Poor estimate of dates	Multiple gestation
Irregular menses	Molar pregnancy	Polyhydramnios
No dates	Multiple gestation	Congenital anomalies
Postpartum pregnancy	Leiomyomata	Poor estimate of dates‡
Previous complicated	Polyhydramnios	Small for dates—rule out
Pregnancy	Congenital anomalies	Fetal growth retardation
Caesarean delivery	Small for dates—rule out	Oligohydramnios
Rh incompatibility	Poor estimate of dates	Congenital anomalies
Diabetes mellitus	Fetal growth retardation	Poor estimate of dates‡
Fetal growth retardation	Congenital anomalies	Determine fetal position—rule out
Clarify dates/sizes discrepancy	Oligohydramnios	Breech
Large for dates—rule out	If history of bleeding—rule out total placenta previa	Transverse lie
Leiomyomata	If Rh incompatibility—rule out fetal hydrops	If history of bleeding—rule out
Bicornuate uterus		Placenta previa
Adnexal mass		Abruptio placentae
Multiple gestation		Determine fetal lung maturity
Poor dates		Amniocentesis for lecithin/sphingomyelin ratio
Molar pregnancy		Placental maturity (grade 0-3)
Small for dates—rule out		If Rh incompatibility—rule out fetal hydrops
Poor dates		
Missed abortion		
Blighted ovum		

From Athey PA and Hadlock FP: Ultrasound in obstetrics and gynecology, ed 2, St Louis, 1985, The CV Mosby Co.
*Accuracy ± 3 days.
†Accuracy ± 1 to 1½ weeks.
‡Accuracy only ± 3 weeks.

Table 6-4 *Application of Sonography During Pregnancy*

Condition	Sonographic Evidence	Intervention
Impending abortion (before eighth menstrual week)	Poorly formed or "sagging" gestational sac	Eliminate time trying to save pregnancy; possibly decrease blood loss and sequelae of blood loss or of treatment for blood loss
Fetal death (after eighth menstrual week)	No cardiac activity	Empty uterus before development of *retained dead fetus syndrome*
Ectopic pregnancy	Adnexal mass	Early surgical intervention to prevent emergency situation
Molar pregnancy	"Snow storm" appearance within enlarged uterus	Terminate pregnancy to decrease morbidity from preeclampsia and begin surveillance of hCG* levels
Developmental uterine abnormalities	Resembles coexistent solid neoplasm; variable appearance	Avoid misdiagnosis with inappropriate therapy; provide time to consider type of delivery

IUD (not a rare occurrence)	Locate site
	  Imbedded in myometrial wall apart from gestational sac and placenta
	  Located partially or totally within gestational sac or within placenta
		Pregnancy usually goes to term with no IUD-related problem
		
		Pregnancy usually ends in spontaneous abortion and may be associated with generalized sepsis

*Human chorionic gonadotropin.

Table 6-5 *Biochemical Monitoring Techniques*

Test	Results	Significance of Findings
Maternal Urine Estriols	High and rising levels	General fetal well-being
	Low and falling levels	Possible fetal jeopardy
Maternal Blood		
Human placental lactogen	High levels	Large fetus; multiple gestation
	Low levels	Threatened abortion, IUGR, postmaturity
Unconjugated plasma estriol	High and rising levels	General fetal well-being
	Low and falling levels	Possible fetal jeopardy
Heat-stable alkaline phosphatase	Normally elevated during pregnancy	Poor correlation with fetal outcome
Oxytocinase	200-400 U at term	General fetal well-being
	Low levels	Associated with fetal death, postmaturity, IUGR
Coombs' test	Titer of 1:8 and rising	Significant Rh sensitization
Alpha-fetoprotein	See below	
Amniotic Fluid Analysis		
Color	Meconium	Possible hypoxia or asphyxia
Lung profile		Fetal lung maturity
L/S ratio	>2	
PGL*	Present	
Creatinine	>2 mg/dl	Gestational age > 36 weeks
Billirubin (ΔOD† 450/nm)	<0.015	Gestational age > 36 weeks, normal pregnancy
	High levels	Fetal hemolytic disease in rhesus isoimmunized pregnancies
Lipid cells	>10%	Gestational age > 35 weeks
Alpha-fetoprotein	High levels after 15-week gestation	Open neural tube or other defect
Osmolality	Decline after 20-week gestation	Advancing nonspecific gestational age

Genetic disorders
  Sex-linked
  Chromosomal
  Metabolic
	Dependent on cultured cells for karyotype and enzymatic activity	

From Tucker SM: Fetal monitoring and fetal assessment in high-risk pregnancy, St Louis, 1978, The CV Mosby Co. In an effort to summarize these studies in tabular form, generalization must be made.
*Phosphatidylglycerol.
*Delta optical density.

Procedure 6-1

AMNIOCENTESIS

DEFINITION

The removal of a small amount of amniotic fluid for laboratory analysis and prenatal diagnosis.

PURPOSE

To establish prenatal diagnosis of genetic problems, estimate gestational age, identify and monitor isoimmune disease, accomplish amniography and fetography, perform second-trimester elective abortion, estimate fetal lung maturity (L/S ratio).

EQUIPMENT

Amniocentesis tray; electronic fetal monitor; flashlight; amber-colored test tubes (or test tubes wrapped in aluminum foil); razor (to shave abdomen); bandage; antibacterial cleanser; sterile gowns, masks, and gloves; ultrasound machine and conductive gel.

NURSING ACTIONS	RATIONALE
Wash hands before and after touching woman and equipment. Glove, prn.	To prevent nosocomial infection and to implement universal precautions.
Prepare woman for procedure:	Collaborative effort facilitates procedure.
Take baseline vital signs and fetal heart rate (FHR).	To assess subsequent values.
Premedicate (if ordered).	To assist woman in relaxing.
Place woman in supine position with her hands under her head or across her chest.	To position woman in a way that facilitates procedure.
Prepare the abdomen with a shave and a scrub with povidone-iodine (Betadine), if ordered by physician.	To minimize possibility of infection.
Draw blood sample.	To compare with postprocedure blood sample for assessing probable fetomaternal hemorrhage.
	To assess levels of AFP.
Act as a support person during procedure:	As with any surgical procedure, the woman and family will be tense and anxious as to the outcome.
Explain reason for such a long needle.	The needle passes through layers of fat and muscle before reaching the uterus. Actually only a small portion of the needle enters the uterus. Show woman that the ultrasound guides the doctor in placement of the needle.
Reinforce the physician's explanation for not using local anesthetic.	The physician will not use a local anesthetic for two reasons: (1) It "stings" and (2) it would mean two needles. Once the skin is pierced, there is a sensation of pressure, but not pain.
Assist the physician:	To collaborate in the completion of the procedure accurately and with least potential for injury to maternal-placental-fetal unit.
Label three sterile tubes.	To identify specimen.
If bilirubin determination is needed, darken the room, use a flashlight, and immediately cover the filled amber-colored or aluminum foil-wrapped tube.	To prevent light from altering bilirubin, since a true reading cannot be obtained if the fluid is exposed to light.
After fluid is withdrawn, wash all povidone-iodine off the abdomen and apply a bandage.	To prevent skin burn.
Assist with or draw blood sample.	To assess for the presence of fetomaternal hemorrhage.
	To assess AFP level.
Continue monitoring the FHR for 30 minutes and assess for uterine contractions.	To identify complications.

Table 6-6 *Typical Amniotic Fluid Increase During Pregnancy*

Weeks' Gestation	Amniotic Fluid Volume (ml)
12	50
14	100
16	175
18	250
20	325

From Queenan JT: Contemp OB/GYN 15:61, Feb 1980.

ACOUSTIC STIMULATION TEST

The *acoustic stimulation* test is another method of testing antepartum FHR response. The test takes approximately 10 minutes to complete, with the fetus monitored for 5 minutes before fetal acoustic stimulation to obtain a baseline FHR. The sound source is then applied on the maternal abdomen over the fetal head. Monitoring continues for another 5 minutes, and the strip chart is assessed.

Results	*Interpretating*
Reactive acoustic stimulation test	FHR acceleration of at least 15 bpm for at least 120 seconds or two accelerations of at least 15 bpm for at least 15 seconds
Nonreactive acoustic stimulation test	Inability to fulfill either criterion for reactivity as described above within 5 minutes

CONTRACTION STRESS TEST

The basis for the CST is that a healthy fetus can withstand a decreased oxygen supply during the physiologic stress for a contraction. Contractions may occur spontaneously or be produced by nipple or oxytocin stimulation. A compromised fetus will demonstrate late decelerations that are nonreassuring and indicative of uteroplacental insufficiency.

Results	*Interpretation*	*Clinical Significance*
Negative	No late decelerations with a minimum of three uterine contractions lasting 40 to 60 seconds within a 10-minute period	Reassurance that the fetus is likely to survive labor, should it occur within 1 week; more frequent testing may be indicated by the clinical situation.
Positive	Persistent and consistent late decelerations occurring with more than half the contractions	Management lies between use of other tools of fetal assessment and termination of pregnancy; a postive test indicates that the fetus is at increased risk for perinatal morbidity and mortality; the physician may perform an expeditious vaginal delivery following a successful induction or may proceed directly to cesarean delivery
Suspicious	Late decelerations occurring with less than half the uterine contractions once an adequate contraction pattern has been established	NST and CST should be repeated within 24 hours; if interpretable data cannot be achieved, other methods of fetal assessment must be used
Hyperstimulation	Late decelerations occurring with excessive uterine activity (contractions more often than every 2 minutes or lasting longer than 90 seconds) or a persistent increase in uterine tone	
Unsatisfactory	Inadequate uterine contraction pattern or tracing too poor to interpret	

NONSTRESS TEST (FETAL ACTIVITY DETERMINATION)

The basis for the NST or FAD is that the normal fetus will produce characteristic heart rate patterns. Acceleration of fetal heart rate (FHR) in response to fetal movement is the desired outcome of the NST. This then allows most high-risk pregnancies to continue, with the test being repeated twice a week.

Results	*Interpretation*	*Clinical Significance*
Reactive	Two or more accelerations of FHR of 15 beats per minute (bpm) lasting 15 seconds or more, associated with each fetal movement in a 20-minute period	As long as twice weekly NSTs remain reactive, most high-risk pregnancies are allowed to continue
Nonreactive	Any tracing with either no FHR accelerations or accelerations less than 15 bpm or lasting less than 15 seconds throughout any fetal movement during testing period	Further indirect monitoring may be attempted with abdominal fetal electrocardiography in an effort to clarify FHR pattern and quantitate variability; external monitoring should continue, and a contraction stress test (CST) should be done
Unsatisfactory	Quality of FHR recording not adequate for interpretation	Test is repeated in 24 hours, or a CST is done, depending on the clinical situation

HYPERTENSIVE STATES IN PREGNANCY

Hypertensive states during pregnancy constitute a physiologic risk for the woman and fetus or neonate and a psychologic risk for the woman and her family. Diminished placental perfusion secondary to arteriolar vasospasm places the fetus at risk. Eclampsia (seizures) from profound cerebral effects is the major maternal hazard.

Early recognition and timely intervention are vital to arrest the progression of the disorder (if possible), to prevent eclampsia, and to ensure the safe delivery of the infant. Appropriate management depends on early recognition, accurate differentiation of various hypertensive states, and timely interventions.

Assessment for Hypertension

Pregnancy-induced hypertension (PIH) can occur without warning, or symptoms may gradually develop. It is therefore important to assess for signs suggesting the onset or presence of PIH during each prenatal visit. These symptoms include the following:

1. Rapid rise in blood pressure
2. Rapid gain in weight
3. Generalized edema
4. Quantitative increase in proteinuria
5. Epigastric pain
6. Marked hyperreflexia; especially transient or sustained ankle clonus
7. Severe headache
8. Visual disturbances
9. Oliguria with urinary output of less than 100 ml in 4 hours
10. Drowsiness, listlessness (dulled sensorium)
11. Nausea and vomiting, severe

Although eclampsia is normally preceded by various signs and symptoms, convulsions can appear without warning. Tonic-clonic convulsions can be described in the following ways:

Stage of invasion: 2 to 3 seconds; eyes fixed; twitching of facial muscles.

Stage of contraction: 15 to 20 seconds; eyes protrude and are bloodshot; all body muscles in tonic contraction (e.g., arms flexed, hands clenched, legs inverted).

Stage of convulsion: Muscles relax and contract alternatively. Respirations are halted and then begin again with long, deep stertorous inhalation. Coma ensues (2 to 3 minutes to hours).

Occurrence: During prenatal, intranatal, or postdelivery period.

Recurrence: Within minutes of first convulsion or never.

The nurse should also know about laboratory tests and other techniques, such as assessment of deep tendon reflexes.

Plasma creatinine and urea levels are determined. Urine is monitored for amount per hour and for protein. Proteinuria is defined as protein present in amounts greater than 300 mg/L (+ 1) in a 24-hour specimen or greater than 1 g/L (+ 2) in a random daytime urine sample on 2 or more occasions at least 6 hours apart (Table 6-8). The urine must be a midstream clean-catch or catheter-derived specimen if there is the possibility of contamination by vaginal discharge. The woman is assessed for the HELP syndrome—hemolysis (microangiophathic), elevated liver enzymes (AST or SGOT, ALT or SGPT), and low platelet count. The hematocrit is monitored.

Table 6-7 *Assessing Deep Tendon Reflexes (DTRs)*

Degree	Grading	Clinical Significance and Nursing Actions
Brisk with sustained clonus	5+	Woman not responding to medications as desired; may be accompanied by apprehension, restlessness, excitability; notify physician
Hyperactive response (brisk with transient clonus)	4+	Woman not responding to medications as desired; may be accompanied by apprehension, restlessness, excitability; notify physician
More than normal (brisk)	3+	Woman responding; however, important to assess frequently
Normal, active	2+	Safe dosage level, therapeutic effect
Low response (sluggish or dull)	1+	Notify physician for medical directives
No response	0	Turn off magnesium sulfate drip; change to "keep open" solution; notify physician for immediate care; prepare antidote (20 ml vial of 10% calcium gluconate) for injection

Table 6-8 *Protein Readings*

Code	Milligrams per Deciliter
0	
Trace	
+1	30 mg/dl (equivalent to 300 mg/L)
+2	100 mg/dl
+3	300 mg/dl
+4	Over 1000 mg (1 g)/dl

Classification and Differential Diagnosis

To communicate effectively with other members of the health care team, the nurse must understand the classifications that distinguish the various hypertensive states of pregnancy. The most recent classifications prepared by the Committee on Terminology of the American College of Obstetricians and Gynecologists is presented in Table 6-9.

The nurse should also understand the differences between essential hypertension and PIH, as well as the differentiation of mild and severe preeclampsia. This information is also included in this section.

Table 6-9 *Classification of the Hypertensive States of Pregnancy*

Type	Description
Pregnancy-Induced Hypertension (PIH)	
Gestational hypertension	The development of hypertension after 20 weeks of gestation in a previously normotensive woman without proteinuria; the blood pressure returns to normal within 10 postpartum days
Preeclampsia	The development of hypertension and proteinuria with or without edema in a previously normotensive woman after 20 weeks of gestation or early postpartum; in the presence of trophoblastic disease it can develop before 20 weeks of gestation
Eclampsia	The development of convulsions or coma in a preeclamptic woman
Superimposed preeclampsia or eclampsia	The development of preeclampsia or eclampsia in a woman with concurrent hypertension
Concurrent Hypertension and Pregnancy (CHP)	
Chronic hypertension	Hypertension that develops before pregnancy or before week 20 of gestation that is not pregnancy associated

Modified from Gilbert ES and Harmon JS: High-risk pregnancy and delivery: nursing perspectives, St Louis, 1986, The CV Mosby Co.

Table 6-10 *Differential Diagnosis of Essential Hypertension and Preeclampsia (PIH)*

Features	Essential Hypertension	Preeclampsia (PIH)
Onset of hypertension	Before pregnancy; during first 20 weeks of pregnancy	After 20 weeks of pregnancy (exception: trophoblastic tumors*)
Duration of hypertension	Permanent; hypertension beyond 3 months postdelivery	Hypertension absent 10 days postdelivery
Family history	Often positive	Usually negative, may be positive
Past history	Recurrent "toxemia"	Psychosexual problems common
Age	Usually older	Generally teenaged or in early 20s
Parity	Usually multigravida	Usually primigravida
Habitus	May be thin	Usually eumorphic
Retinal findings	Often arteriovenous nicking, tortuous arterioles, cotton-wool exudates, hemorrhages	Vascular spasm, retinal edema; rarely, protein extravasations
Proteinuria	Often none	Usually present; absent at 6 weeks postdelivery

Reproduced with permission, from Benson RC, editor: Current obstetric and gynecologic diagnosis and treatment, ed 5. Copyright 1984 by Lange Medical Publications, Los Altos, Calif.
*Hydatidiform mole (molar pregnancy).

Table 6-11 *Differentiation of Mild and Severe Preeclampsia*

	Mild Preeclampsia*	Severe Preeclampsia
Maternal Effects		
Blood pressure	Rise in systolic blood pressure of 30 mm Hg or more. A rise in diastolic blood pressure of 15 mm Hg or more or a reading of 140/90 mm Hg × 2, 6 hr apart.	Rise to 160/110 mm Hg or more on two separate occasions 6 hr apart with pregnant woman on bed rest.
MAP	140/90 = 107.	160/110 = 127.
Weight gain	Weight gain of more than 1.4 kg (3 lb)/mo during the second trimester, more than 0.5 kg (1 lb)/wk during the third trimester, or a sudden weight gain of 2 kg (4-4½ lb)/wk at any time.	Same.

Proteinuria
  Qualitative dipstick
  Quantitative 24-hr analysis
	Proteinuria of 300 mg/L in a 24-hr specimen or greater than 1 g/L in a random daytime specimen on 2 or more occasions 6 hr apart as protein loss is variable. With dipstick varies from trace to 1+.	Proteinuria of 5-10 g/L in 24 hours or 2+ or more protein on dipstick.

Edema	Dependent edema, some puffiness of eyes, face, fingers; pulmonary rales absent.	Generalized edema, noticeable puffiness of eyes, face, fingers. Pulmonary edema → rales.
Reflexes	Hyperreflexia 3+. No ankle clonus.	Hyperreflexia 3+ or more. Ankle clonus.
Oliguria	Output matches intake.	Oliguria: less than 100 ml/4 hr output.
Headache	Transient.	Severe.
Visual problems	Absent.	Blurred, photophobia, blind spots on funduscopy. Retinal arterial spasm.
Irritability	Transient.	Severe.
Serum creatinine	Normal.	Elevated.
Thrombocytopenia	Absent.	Present.
SGOT elevation	Minimal.	Marked.
Fetal Effects		
Placental perfusion	Reduced.	Decreased perfusion expressed as IUGR in fetus FHR: late decelerations.
Premature placental aging	Not apparent.	At birth placenta appears smaller than normal for the duration of the pregnancy. Premature aging is apparent with numerous areas of broken syncytia. Ischemic necroses (white infarcts) are numerous, and intervillous fibrin deposition (red infarcts) may be recorded.

*No preeclampsia should be considered "mild" (Danforth and Scott, 1986; Knuppel and Drukker, 1986; Lindheimer and Katz, 1985).

Nursing Care

The most effective therapy for PIH is preventing progression of the condition. Home management is satisfactory if the preeclampsia is mild and fetal growth retardation is not a problem. This section begins with guidelines for client teaching and a sample nursing care plan for home care of preeclampsia.

If the woman's condition becomes increasingly severe, hospitalization is recommended. One of the most important goals of care is preventing or controlling convulsions.

Various drugs used in controlling hypertension in pregnancy and labor are summarized in this section. The medication most commonly used is magnesium sulfate, an anticonvulsant and smooth muscle relaxant. Danger signs of magnesium sulfate toxicity and its antidote are provided.

Also included are drugs and equipment that should be readily available for the hospitalized woman with PIH, and a guide to the immediate care during a convulsion. The section concludes with a sample nursing care plan for hospital management of severe preeclampsia.

Guidelines for Client Teaching

HOME CARE OF PREECLAMPSIA

ASSESSMENT

1. Woman with two children pregnant with twins.
2. Thirty-third week of gestation.
3. Mild hypertension.
4. Generalized edema.
5. Proteinuria, +2

NURSING DIAGNOSES

Potential for injury: fetus and mother, related to edema, proteinuria, and hypertension.

Knowledge deficit related to PIH and its effects on mother and baby.

Knowledge deficit related to diet required to PIH.

Knowledge deficit related to assessment of blood pressure and edema.

Fluid volume deficit related to generalized edema.

Altered health maintenance related to activity intolerance.

Potential noncompliance related to two preschoolers at home and woman's need for bedrest.

Activity intolerance: decreased, related to minimizing effects of PIH.

Ineffective individual coping related to activity restriction.

Impaired home maintenance management related to activity restriction.

Ineffective family coping related to mother's restricted activity and concern over a complicated pregnancy.

Potential altered parenting related to family and personal stress.

Constipation, related to decreased activity, decreased gastric motility, pregnancy.

GOALS

Short-term

To increase woman's understanding of PIH and encourage her and her family's participation in her care.

To teach woman (couple) how to monitor severity of PIH.

To teach woman about diet prescribed for her by the physician.

To aid woman in maintaining adequate rest by arranging support systems.

Intermediate

To continue monitoring effects of PIH on woman and fetus.

To have woman comply with decreased activity and diet.

Long-term

To prepare for potential complications such as an early birth.

To decrease anxiety.

To keep PIH under control until delivery of the twins.

REFERENCES AND TEACHING AIDS

Pamphlets and booklets from hospital, clinic, or physician's office explaining PIH and its problems and treatments.

Diagrams or charts to be used in explanation of PIH.

Printed list of potential complications for woman to take home.

List of phone numbers to call for emergency assistance to be placed by the woman's phone.

List of community or social services that may be of assistance to the family while the woman is on bedrest.

Continued.

Guidelines for Client Teaching—cont'd

CONTENT/RATIONALE	TEACHING ACTION
To increase woman's (couple's) knowledge of PIH, share the following:	Show diagrams and charts while explaining how the condition develops, who's at risk, and what signs to look for.
How the condition can effect woman's fetuses and her.	Use simple terms and do not scare woman. It is important that she understand what could happen if treatment regimen is not taken seriously, however, it is not necessary to increase her fear and anxiety.
There is no definite cause for PIH but there are many theories that support the symptoms that occur, which are a result of changes in the functioning of body organs.	
To implement assessment and self-management of PIH:	Show woman (couple) how to assess extent of edema.
Review assessment and management	
Pitting edema.	
Protein in urine.	Demonstrate chemstrip for protein in urine.
Fetal activity.	Instruct woman how to monitor fetal activity within a certain amount of time.
Daily weight.	Instruct woman to weigh herself daily and record weight.
Intake and output.	Give woman a list of common household measures and instruct her on how to keep a record of her intake and output.
Danger signs.	Give woman a list of the danger signs of PIH that should be reported to the physician immediately.
Diet, as it pertains to sodium and protein intake.	Discuss the diet that was prescribed for her by her physician. Instruct woman as to food groups that are equivalent to 70 to 80 g of protein. Provide a printed list for her to take home with her. Instruct woman as to amounts of salt to use in preparing or serving foods. Advise her to refrain from eating salty convenience or snack foods (i.e., potato chips).
Rationale for diet:	
Helps reduce edema and blood pressure.	
Helps baby grow.	
Roughage and fluids.	Advise woman about including ample roughage and fluids, restricted exercise can aggravate constipation.
Bedrest.	Instruct woman (couple) on what is meant by bedrest. Emphasize need to spend most of the day in bed, preferably lying on her left side; ambulation for meals and to go to the bathroom are usually permitted.
	Discourage going up and down stairs.
	Restrict outings to visits to the physician's office.
Activity and the need for diversion within woman's restrictions.	Encourage the family to take part in her care and take over care of the house, younger children, cooking, etc.
To assist family in mobilizing support and coping:	
Social worker or support systems in the community may be needed if there are no family support systems.	Refer to community agencies as necessary.
Open discussion of problems is beneficial in implementing care.	To avert potential for impaired family processes, encourage open discussion and problem-solving problems with the pregnancy, younger children, and taking care of the house.
Mutual problem-solving facilitates tension reduction, supporting or improving coping skills.	
Assistance and reassurance facilitate compliance to medical regimen.	

EVALUATION The nurse can be reasonably assured that teaching is effective if woman adheres to medical regimen with family support, woman has a healthy baby, and all goals are met.

Sample Nursing Care Plan

HOME MANAGEMENT OF PIH

ASSESSMENT	NURSING DIAGNOSIS (ND)/ PLAN(P)/GOAL(G)	RATIONALE/ IMPLEMENTATION	EVALUATION
Populations at risk: Primigravida (<15 to >35) Multiple gestation Diabetes Rh incompatability Renal disease Hypertension Over 20 weeks' gestation	ND: Knowledge deficit related to PIH and those women at risk. P: Educate those women at risk to prevent or minimize PIH. G: Woman does not develop PIH.	*To teach woman about PIH the nurse will:* Assess risk factors at each prenatal visit. Take a complete nursing history including family and social history. Discuss problems with woman. Discuss rationale for treatment. Include support person or family in discussions.	Woman verbalizes understanding of information presented. Woman states she will come to all prenatal visits as scheduled.

Symptomatology of PIH:
Sudden weight gain
Generalized edema
Increase in blood pressure *over baseline:*
  Systolic: 15 mm Hg
  Diastolic: 30 mm Hg
Proteinuria
	ND: Potential for injury: fetus and mother related to hypertension, vasospasm, decreased glomerular filtration rate, and edema.
	P: Detect and control PIH.
	G: Woman's PIH remains in control.
		To teach woman how to assess for PIH the nurse will teach her to:
		Assess weight every day—watch for an increase of 2 or more pounds per week.
		Monitor fluid intake and urine output.
		Observe for pitting edema of lower extremities, tight rings, shoes, facial puffiness.
		Teach how to use dipstick for assessment of proteinuria.
			Woman reports weight, urine output, results of urine dipstick, and edema to nurse every day.

Knowledge of symptomatology
Readiness to learn
Ability to learn content (as influenced by effects of illness or medications, language barrier, age, or experience, or innate intelligence)
	ND: Knowledge deficit related to severity of PIH and effects on mother and fetus.
	P: Teach woman (family) danger signs and symptoms to look for with increasing severity of disease.
	G: Woman knows signs and symptoms and has a printed list readily available to her and her family members; promptly reports symptomatology to health care provider.
		CNS symptomatology:
		  Blurred vision.
		  Headaches.
		  Nausea and vomiting.
		  Hyperreflexia.
		  Convulsions.
		Hepatic symptoms:
		  Epigastric pain (RUQ).
		Urinary output:
		  Proteinuria >2+.
		  Oliguria.
		Fetal distress:
		  Decreased fetal activity.
		  Changes in fetal activity.
		Placentae abruptio:
		  Vaginal bleeding or spotting.
		  Uterine tenderness.
		  Change in fetal activity.
		  Abdominal pain.
			Woman (family) demonstrates understanding of information presented.
			Woman (family) tests urine several times per day.
			Woman experiences diuresis.
			Woman reports fetal activity and keeps scheduled appointments.
			Woman verbalizes understanding of information presented.
			Woman reports any problems.

Woman overweight or undernourished Excessive sodium intake Inadequate protein and caloric intake	ND: Altered nutrition: less than or more than body requirements. ND: Knowledge deficit related to diet required	*To help woman with her nutritional status the nurse will:* Provide nutrition counseling re: intake of sodium chlo-	Woman keeps a diet history. Woman verbalizes understanding of limiting salty foods and lowering sodium intake.

Continued.

Sample Nursing Care Plan—cont'd

ASSESSMENT	NURSING DIAGNOSIS (ND)/ PLAN(P)/GOAL(G)	RATIONALE/ IMPLEMENTATION	EVALUATION
Financial status Cultural/religious influences Pitting edema	in PIH. P: Provide nutrition counseling. G: Woman accepts and learns to follow diet prescribed by physician. ND: Potential intravascular fluid volume deficit related to protein loss and fluid shifts to the extravascular space. P: Provide adequate protein intake. G: Woman consumes adequate diet.	ride ("salt"), protein, calories; re: physician's orders; re: personal and family preferences, budget, and storage and preparation facilities.	Woman follows prescribed diet
Home situation: resources that would permit woman to be on bedrest and to restrict activity Woman needs help around house Knowledge of stress reduction techniques	ND: Activity intolerance related to the disease process. P: Help woman (family) arrange for home management of PIH. G: Woman (family) implements home care as prescribed.	*To assist woman to comply with bedrest the nurse can:* Teach woman importance of remaining in bed. Teach relaxation (see guidelines for client teaching). Act as a client advocate and put family in touch with community support systems. Assess family and internal support systems.	Woman remains on bedrest, left side as much as possible. Woman uses relaxation techniques with success. Arrangements are made for help with house and any other children in family.

Table 6-12 *Pharmacologic Control of Hypertension and Its Sequelae in Pregnancy and Labor*

| Medication | Target Tissue | Effects of Medication | | Nursing Actions |
		Maternal	Fetal/Neonatal	
Anticonvulsants				

Magnesium sulfate IV or IM
Dosage varies
	Myoneural junction: decreases acetylcholine, thereby depressing neuromuscular transmission
	Thyroid: decreases parathormone secretion, resulting in increased urinary excretion of calcium
	Placental perfusion dynamics not altered
		Minimum hypotensive effect
		Minimum if any direct effect on CNS because of blood-brain barrier to magnesium
		Hypocalcemia
		CAUTION: Do not give excessive dosages that tend to decrease urinary output to depress deep tendon reflexes (DTRs)
		DANGER: Muscular paralysis (cardiopulmonary)
		Antidotes: calcium gluconate, neostigmine, pentylenetetrazol (Metrazol)
		Increases duration of labor; amount of oxytocin needed to stimulate labor is higher
			Mild depression in small number (6%)
			Neonatal hypermagnesemia easily treated: calcium; exchange transfusion with citrated blood
			No effect on FHR variability in healthy term fetus; neonatal toxic effects rare (Sibai, 1987)
				Notify perinatal staff
				Decrease CNS irritability
				  Arrange environment to promote rest
				  Provide continuous nursing care
				Encourage kidney perfusion with left side-lying position and insert indwelling urinary catheter; monitor urinary output every hour
				  Under 25 ml/hr—do not repeat dose
				  Diuresis—good prognostic sign
				Repeat dose per order if:
				  DTRs present
				  Respirations of 12/min or more
				  Urinary output over 1 dl/4 hr
				Assess maternal condition
				  Hydration
				  Affect
				  Other signs or symptoms of preeclampsia
				Keep 10 ml of 10% calcium gluconate at bedside; with linen/equipment for delivery, eclamptic tray, oxygen, and suction equipment

Diazepam (Valium)	Thalamus and hypothalamus: direct depressant effect	Effective in initial management of eclamptic convulsions
		Rapid IV administration may lead to apnea or cardiac arrest
			Flattens FHR baseline (loss of beat-to-beat variability), an important criterion in assessing fetal oxygenation
			High levels in newborn:
			  Depressed sucking ability
			  Hypotonia
			  Temperature instability (decrease)
			  Decreased respiratory rate
				Notify perinatal staff
				Assess DTRs, respirations, signs of labor
				Monitor labor; see Normal labor

Barbiturates (rapid-acting) Phenobarbital sodium: 0.2-0.3 mg IV Amobarbital sodium: 0.25-0.5 g IV	CNS: depressant effect	Controls seizures	Depressant effect on fetus May minimize hyperbilirubinemia	See Diazepam

Continued.

Table 6-12, cont'd. *Pharmacologic Control of Hypertension and Its Sequelae in Pregnancy and Labor*

| Medication | Target Tissue | Effects of Medication | | Nursing Actions |
		Maternal	Fetal/Neonatal	
Antihypertensive*				
Hydralazine (Apresoline, Neopresol) (arteriolar vasodilators) 50 to 200 mg (0) per day	Peripheral arterioles: decreases muscle tone, thereby decreasing peripheral resistance Hypothalamus and medullary vasomotor center; minor decrease in sympathetic tone	Headache Flushing Palpitation Tachycardia Some decrease in utero placental blood flow	Minimum effects; some decrease in Po₂	Assess for effects of medications Alert mother (family) to expected effects of medications Assess blood pressure (precipitous drop can lead to shock and perhaps to abruptio placentae) and urinary output Maintain bedrest with side rails for safety
Methyldopa (Aldomet) (used if maintenance therapy is needed): 250-500 mg orally every 8 hr (α₂-receptor agonist)	Postganglionic nerve endings: interferes with chemical neurotransmission to reduce peripheral vascular resistance CNS: sedation	Sleepiness Postural hypotension Constipation Rare: drug-induced fever in 1% of women and positive Coombs' test in 20%	After 4 months of maternal therapy, positive Coombs' test in infant	See Hydralazine
Diuretics†				
Thiazides	Arteriolar smooth muscles: reduces responsiveness to catecholamines	Ineffective in preventing preeclampsia Further reduces already-present decreased plasma volume of preeclampsia Complications Fluid and electrolyte imbalance Pancreatitis Decrease in carbohydrate tolerance Hyperuricemia	Hyponatremia Thrombocytopenia	Arrange to have blood drawn to measure levels of Na, Cl, H₂O, K, and H+ to prevent hyponatremia, hypokalemia, hypochloremia, metabolic acidosis
Furosemide (Lasix): 40 mg IV	Loop of Henle	Relieves pulmonary edema Excessive use results in hypokalemia and hyponatremia	No abnormalities noted	See Thiazides
Ethacrynic acid (Edecrin) Mannitol (for impending renal failure, oliguria, DIC): 12.5-25 mg IV	Similar to furosemide Osmotic diuretic: pulls fluid into vascular bed (therefore not recommended for persons with congestive heart failure)	Similar to furosemide Increases renal plasma flow and urinary output Flushes out kidneys Reduces swelling in ischemic cells in kidney and myocardium	Deafness No known effect	See Thiazides See Thiazides
Blood volume expanders				
Salt-poor, serum albumin‡	Intravascular volume	Increases blood volume		

*By midpregnancy, diastolic and systolic blood pressure normally falls by 10 to 15 mm Hg. If diastolic blood pressure is 75 mm Hg or more in second trimester and 85 mm Hg or more in third trimester, statistical increase in fetal mortality occurs.
NOTE: For obese woman, use thigh cuff or ultrasound to obtain accurate readings.
†For control of chronic hypertension, pulmonary edema, renal oliguria, acute renal failure, chronic nephrotic syndrome. If used, physician must be ready to justify action.
‡May not be appropriate for woman with severe preeclampsia–eclampsia.

DANGER SIGNS

Magnesium Sulfate Toxicity

1. Sudden hypotension
2. Urinary output less than 25 ml/hr
3. Respiration less than 12/min
4. Hyperreflexia, hyporeflexia, absence of reflexes
5. Serum levels of 10 to 12 mg/dl: reflexes absent*
6. Serum levels of 15 to 17 mg/dl: respiratory arrest
7. Serum levels of 30 to 35 mg/dl: total paralysis and cardiac arrest
8. Sudden decrease in FHR

*Clear sign of toxicity. Discontinue STAT (Sibai, 1987).

Antidote for Magnesium Sulfate Toxicity

The antidote for magnesium sulfate toxicity is a calcium salt such as **calcium gluconate**. A 10 ml vial of a 10% aqueous solution of calcium gluconate should be kept at the bedside. If needed, it is administered over 3 minutes intravenously and repeated every hour until the respiratory, urinary, and neurologic depression has been alleviated. *The maximum number of injections of a calcium salt is 8 injections in a 24-hour period.*

DRUGS AND EQUIPMENT FOR PREVENTIVE TREATMENT OF CONVULSIONS OF ECLAMPSIA

DRUGS	EQUIPMENT
Magnesium sulfate: 2 ampules, 10 ml/ampule (5 g 50%); 500 mg (4 mEq)/ ml	Emergency delivery pack Ophthalmoscope Reflex hammer
Sodium bicarbonate: 50 ml (7.5%) (44.6 mEq)	Fetal monitor Padded tongue blade
Hydralazine: 5 ampules, 20 mg/ampule	Plastic airway Oxygen and suction
Heparin sodium: 10 ml, 5000 USP units/ml	Tourniquets Syringes: 2, 10, and 50 ml
Diazepam: 2 ml, 5 mg/ml	Cutdown tray
Chlordiazepoxide: 5 ml, 20 mg/ml	IV administration supplies
Epinephrine: 2:1000, 1 mg/ ml	Sphygmomanometer with an appropriate- sized cuff
Atropisol, 1% (mydriatic) Atropine sulfate: 0.4 mg/0.5 ml	Rectal thermometer Means for obtaining
Sterile water ampules	weight
Sterile normal saline ampules	Indwelling urinary
Calcium gluconate: 10%, 1g/ 10 ml; 97 mg (4.8 mEq)/10 ml Ca^{++}	catheter tray with collection bag Urinary dipsticks
Phenytoin: 2 ml, 50 mg/ml	
Propranolol: 40 mg tablets	
Intravenous barbiturates	

Immediate Care of Convulsions

1. If convulsions occur, turn woman onto left side to prevent aspiration of vomitus and supine hypotension syndrome.
2. Insert folded towel, plastic airway, or padded tongue blade into *side* of mouth to prevent biting of lips or tongue and to maintain airway. Do not put fingers into woman's mouth; because she may bite them involuntarily.
3. Suction food and fluid from glottis or trachea.
4. Give MgSO$_4$ (and amobarbital sodium for recurrent convulsions) as ordered (Anderson, 1987).
5. Administer oxygen by means of face mask or tent after convulsion ceases (masks and nasal catheters cause excessive stimulation). Oxygen rate may be up to 10 L/min (as opposed to 3 L/min advocated for continuous O$_2$ in chronic conditions).
6. Record time and duration of convulsions; include description.
7. Note any urinary or fecal incontinence.

Sample Nursing Care Plan

HOSPITAL MANAGEMENT OF SEVERE PREECLAMPSIA

ASSESSMENT	NURSING DIAGNOSIS (ND)/ PLAN(P)/GOAL(G)	RATIONALE/ IMPLEMENTATION	EVALUATION
Blood pressure, 160/110 or more. Proteinuria, 3+, 4+. Urinary output, scant, dark color. Weight gain, 2 kg (4 lb) in less than a week. Hematocrit increases (hemoconcentration). Generalized edema.	ND: Potential for injury: maternal and fetal, related to edema, proteinuria, hypertension. P: Decrease severity of disease to ensure a healthy mother and baby. G: Mother and fetus suffer no adverse sequelae to PIH. ND: Decreased cardiac output related to arteriolar constriction and increased peripheral resistance. ND: Altered cardiopulmonary tissue perfusion related to edema and expansion of extravascular fluid. P: Reduce edema and increase tissue perfusion. G: Normalization of intravascular volume and tissue profusion	*To monitor and minimize severity of disease and effects of edema, proteinuria, and hypertension the nurse will:* Keep woman on absolute bedrest with side rails up. Start IV and maintain rate to keep line open. Insert indwelling catheter. Have woman select people she wishes to stay with her. Limit other visitors. Maintain calm unhurried approach to care. Give rationale for care. Report on woman's progress. Assure woman that her family will be kept informed.	Woman's symptomatology of PIH regresses. Woman remains quiet. Woman's (family's) stress and anxiety kept to a minimum. Family members are kept informed.
Platelets decrease.	ND: Potential for injury: maternal and fetal, related to undetected hemoconcentration and clotting disturbances. P: Monitor for coagulopathy. G: Woman does not develop coagulopathy.	*To minimize problems with cardiac output and tissue perfusion the nurse will:* Continue surveillance of blood pressure every 1 hour or more, check for generalized edema, weight, and urinary output, hematocrit, platelets, and SGOT daily or as ordered. Report deviations immediately. Implement physician-ordered therapies.	Symptoms improve. Woman does not develop complications.
Epigastric or right upper quadrant pain. Nausea and vomiting. Headaches. Blurred vision. Hyperreflexia. Changes in level of consciousness (LOC). Seizures. Retinal detachment Blindness.	ND: Pain related to stretching of the hepatic capsule or cerebral edema. ND: Potential for injury, maternal and fetal, related to possible seizure activity or aspiration of stomach contents. ND: Sensory-perceptual alterations related to edema, proteinuria, hypertension. P: Prevent progression of	*To prevent adverse sequelae to severe PIH, the nurse will:* Control amount of external stimuli. Monitor symptoms. Assess LOC. Assess reflexes. Record findings of funduscopic examination. Report any changes. Implement physician-ordered therapy.	Seizures are prevented. Woman rests comfortably. Symptoms improve. Woman remains lucid. Eyegrounds do not change.

Sample Nursing Care Plan—Cont'd

ASSESSMENT	NURSING DIAGNOSIS (ND)/ PLAN(P)/GOAL(G)	RATIONALE/ IMPLEMENTATION	EVALUATION
	PIH; or, identify symptomatology of increasing severity, and institute appropriate therapy. G: Woman and fetus suffer no adverse sequelae to PIH.		
Presence of rales. Pulmonary edema.	ND: Impaired gas exchange related to pulmonary edema. P: Continue surveillance. G: Respiratory function remains within normal limits.	*To monitor gas exchange; the nurse will:* Listen periodically to lung sounds. Check for pulmonary edema and rales.	Breath sounds remain within normal limits.
Fetal growth retardation. Fetal distress. Late decelerations of fetal heart rate (FHR).	ND: Potential for injury: fetus, related to inadequate placental perfusion. P: Facilitate placental perfusion. G: FHR remains stable; fetus born healthy.	*To increase placental perfusion; the nurse will:* Prevent supine hypotensive syndrome: place woman on left side; when on back, raise headrest and place a wedge under right hip.	Woman remains on side. FHR remains stable.
Levels of creatinine and urea increase. Oliguria (<100 ml/4 hr). Increased proteinuria. Generalized edema. Sudden weight gain.	ND: Altered patterns of urinary elimination related to decreased renal perfusion and GFR. P: Continue surveillance. G: Urinary elimination remains within normal limits. Diuresis occurs. Proteinuria decreases/stops.	*To check urinary elimination; the nurse will:* Check urinary output every hour. Report output of <100 ml/4 hr. Keep accurate intake and output records. Check urine for protein every 4 hours. Send blood specimen to laboratory for measurement of creatinine; check results against previous tests.	Urinary elimination remains within normal limits. Diuresis occurs. Proteinuria decreases. Creatinine remains within normal limits.
Administration of MgSO$_4$	ND: Potential for injury: maternal and fetal, related to MgSO$_4$ side effects/toxicity. P: Minimize or prevent side effects/toxicity. G: Side effects/toxicity do not occur.	*To administer MgSO$_4$, the nurse will:* Follow hospital protocol (see also specific nursing care plan): Check hospital's procedure manual. Check blood levels of MgSO$_4$ periodically. Observe for toxicity. Assess reflexes and LOC periodically. Keep calcium gluconate on hand.	Further complications from MgSO$_4$ administration do not occur.
Woman (couple) anxious. Fearful of injury to fetus.	ND: Anxiety related to sudden change in condition. P: Relieve anxiety. G: Woman's (family's) anxiety is minimized.	*To monitor coping mechanisms; the nurse will:* Assess affect, restlessness, anxiety. Assess response to support person.	Woman feels free to express concerns. Support person does not make woman more anxious.

Continued.

Sample Nursing Care Plan—Cont'd

ASSESSMENT	NURSING DIAGNOSIS (ND)/ PLAN(P)/GOAL(G)	RATIONALE/ IMPLEMENTATION	EVALUATION
	ND: Ineffective individual and family coping related to stress of disease process. P: Give support and information. G: Woman (family) develop increased coping skills.	Observe for adverse behavior. Keep woman (couple) informed of progress.	
Preterm labor.	ND: Potential for injury: fetus, related to preterm birth. P: Monitor for labor; if labor occurs, minimize injury. G: Woman's pregnancy and labor result in a healthy mother and baby.	*To monitor for labor; the nurse will:* Observe woman for progress of labor. Assess for complications of labor. Prepare for delivery. Prepare woman (couple) for delivery by answering questions, supplying information and reinforcing information given to her by the physician.	Preterm labor does not occur; or, labor progresses normally. Healthy mother and baby result.

MATERNAL INFECTIONS

Pregnancy confers no immunity against infection, and both the mother and the fetus must be considered when the pregnant woman carries an infection. Sexually transmitted diseases and other infections are responsible for significant morbidity, substantial financial costs, and immeasurable suffering as a result of the disease process and its sequelae. The nurse must be knowledgeable about the various types of infections, their implications for the mother and fetus, and techniques for management. The nurse can help the woman prevent or treat infections successfully.

Acquired Immune Deficiency Syndrome (AIDS)*

I. Risk factors for developing AIDS
  A. Heterosexual, homosexual, or bisexual intercourse with person who is positive for human immunodeficiency virus (HIV)
  B. Sharing needles during intravenous drug use
  C. Multiple sexual partners, prostitution, unprotected intercourse

  D. Transfusion of blood or blood products with HIV-positive blood
  E. HIV-positive mother; transference to fetus in utero
II. Infection with HIV (all stages are infectious, and all tests positive for the antibody in 2 weeks to 6 months)
  A. Infection occurs through
    1. Infected blood or blood products
    2. Sexual intercourse (anal, vaginal, or oral)
    3. Transplacental (mother to baby)
  B. Symptoms of AIDS-related complex (ARC)
    1. Malaise
    2. Night sweats
    3. Fever
    4. Swollen lymph glands
    5. Diarrhea
    6. Weight loss (wasting syndrome—"Slim's disease")
  C. Symptoms of AIDS
    1. Pneumocystis carinii pneumonia (PCP)
    2. Kaposi's sarcoma (KS)
    3. Cancers
    4. Fungal infections
    5. Opportunistic infections
    6. Central nervous system damage
    7. Viral infections
  D. Death

*This information was current at the time of publication. Because of the dynamic nature of this disease and ongoing research, nurses are encouraged to verify data with current sources.

III. Common opportunistic infections observed with AIDS or HIV infection
   A. Fungal
      1. Histoplasmosis—disseminated
      2. Candidiasis—oral (thrush), esophagus, intestinal, vaginal
      3. Cryptococcosis—disseminated or meningitis
      4. Aspergillosis–disseminated, pulmonary, and central nervous system
   B. Parasitic
      1. Pneumocystis carinni pneumonia
      2. Toxoplasmosis—neurologic or disseminated
      3. Cryptosporidiosis—enterocolitis
   C. Viral
      1. Herpes simplex—mucocutaneous, mouth, pulmonary, gastrointestinal
      2. Cytomegalovirus (CMV)—retinas, lungs, liver
   D. Bacterial
      1. Tuberculosis—pulmonaryor disseminated
      2. *Mycobacterium avium-intracellulare*—disseminated
      3. Group B streptosepticemia
IV. Tumors associated with AIDS
   A. Kaposi's sarcoma—skin, mucous membranes, gastrointestinal tract, lungs
   B. Burkitt's lymphoma—lymph system
   C. Non-Hodgkin's lymphoma of B cell or unknown immunologic phenotype
   D. Squamous cell carcinoma—rectum, anorectum, mouth

Tests Used for the Diagnosis of HIV Infection*

The diagnosis of HIV infection† is established by isolating either the HIV or the presence of the IgG antibody to HIV by means of the following:
   1. Enzyme-linked immunosorbent assay (ELISA)
      a. Most commonly performed
      b. Commercially available, economical
      c. Sensitivity, specificity of approximately 98%
      d. Should be performed on at least two separate occasions to prevent false-negative results
   2. Western blot test
      a. Performed to confirm ELISA
      b. More expensive than ELISA
      c. More specific than ELISA
      d. Confirms presence of antibody to specific HIV antigens
These tests do not differentiate passively transferred maternal IgG antibody to HIV from that actively produced by the infant. It is therefore recommended that an HIV-positive infant be retested between the ages of 15 to 18 months, when the infant's humoral immunity is well activated.

Persons at risk for developing HIV infection may be negative at time of testing; however, research shows that it may take up to 6 months to develop antibodies. Therefore it is advisable to retest 3 to 6 months after exposure.

SEXUALLY TRANSMITTED DISEASE (STD)

Historically Defined Venereal Diseases

Syphilis: acquired, congenital (annual worldwide incidence is estimated at 50 million people, with 40,000 in the United States)
Gonorrhea (annual worldwide incidence is estimated at 250 million people, with 3 million in the United States)
Chancroid
Lymphogranuloma venereum (*Chlamydia trachomatis,* L-1, L-2, L-3)
Granuloma inguinale

Newly Defined STDs

Hepatitis B (serum hepatitis)
Herpes genitalis
Balanoposthitis; balanitis
Proctitis
Human papillomavirus: condylomata acuminata
Genital candidiasis
Gardnerella vaginalis
Chlamydial infection (serovars D through K)
Acquired immune deficiency syndrome (AIDS)

Enteric Diseases That May Be Sexually Transmitted

Salmonellosis
Amebiasis
Typhoid
Giardiasis
Shigellosis

Diseases Spread by Body Contact But Not Necessarily by Coitus

Pediculosis
Molluscum contagiosum
Scabies

---

*This information was current at the time of publication. Because of the dynamic nature of this disease and ongoing research, nurses are encouraged to verify data with current sources.
†The HIV-antibody test is *not* diagnostic for AIDS.

Table 6-13 *Maternal Infection: TORCH*

Infection	Maternal Effects	Fetal or Neonatal Effects	Counseling: Prevention, Identification, and Management
Toxoplasmosis (protozoa)	Acute infection: similar to influenza; lymphadenopathy	With maternal acute infection: parasitemia Less likely to occur with maternal chronic infection Abortion likely with acute infection early in pregnancy	Avoid eating raw meat and exposure to litter used by infected cats; if cats in house, have toxoplasma titer checked If titer is rising during early pregnancy, abortion may be given to the mother as an option
Other Hepatitis A (infectious hepatitis) (virus)	Abortion—cause of liver failure during pregnancy Fever, malaise, nausea, and abdominal discomfort	Exposure during first trimester; fetal anomalies; fetal or neonatal hepatitis; premature birth; intrauterine fetal death	Usually spread by droplet or hand contact especially by culinary workers; γ-globulin can be given as prophylaxis for hepatitis A
Hepatitis B (serum hepatitis) (virus)	May be transmitted sexually Symptomatology variable: fever, rash, arthralgia, depressed appetite, dyspepsia, abdominal pain, generalized aching, malaise, weakness, jaundice, tender and enlarged liver	Infection occurs during birth Maternal vaccination during pregnancy should present no risk for fetus; however, data are not available.	Generally passed by contaminated needles, syringes, or blood transfusions; can also be transmitted orally or by coitus, however, but incubation period is longer; hepatitis B immune globulin can be given prophylactically after exposure Hepatitis B vaccine recommended for populations at risk; vaccine consists of series of 3 IM doses Populations at risk: women from Asia, Pacific islands, Haiti, sub-Africa, Alaska (women of Eskimo descent); other women at risk include health care providers
Rubella (3-day German measles, virus)	Rash, fever, mild symptoms; suboccipital lymph nodes may be swollen; some photophobia Occasionally arthritis or encephalitis Abortion	Incidence of congenital anomalies; first month, 50%; second month, 25%, third month, 10%, fourth month, 4% Exposure during first 2 months: malformations of heart, eyes, ears, or brain, abnormal dermatoglyphics Exposure after fourth month: systemic infection, hepatosplenomegaly, intrauterine growth retardation, rash At 15-20 years of age, may experience deterioration of intellect and development or develop epilepsy	Vaccination of pregnant women contraindicated, **pregnancy should be prevented for 2 months after vaccination**; hemagglutinin-inhibition-antigen-negative parturients can be safely vaccinated after delivery
Cytomegalovirus (CMV) (a herpes virus)	Respiratory or sexually transmitted asymptomatic illness or mononucleosis-like syndrome; may have cervical discharge	Fetal or neonatal death or severe, generalized disease—hemolytic anemia and jaundice; hydrocephaly or microcephaly; pneumonitis; hepatosplenomegaly	Virus may be reactivated and cause disease in utero or during delivery in subsequent pregnancies; fetal infection may occur during passage through infected birth canal; disease is commonly progressive through infancy and childhood
Herpes genitalis (herpex simplex virus; HSV I!)	See Table 6-14		

Table 6-14 *Guidelines for Delivery of Women with Herpes genitalis*

Maternal Condition	Risk of Transmission	Mode of Delivery	Postpartum Placement	
			Mother	Newborn
Virologic or cytologic studies are negative 1 week before delivery	Low	Vaginal	Private room	Nursery permissible
Cervical lesion present *or* culture is positive *and* membranes intact or ruptured less than 4 hours before	Low	Abdominal (cesarean)	Private room	Room-in with mother
Cervical lesion present or culture is positive and membranes ruptured more than 4 hours before	High (regardless of mode of delivery)	Vaginal	Private room	Room-in with mother

Table 6-15 *Other Infections of the Vulva and Vagina*

Clinical Situation	Clinical Symptoms and Gross Findings	Nursing Actions and Management
Vulvar dermatitis	Pain; pruritus; formication*; ulceration; exudation	
Eczema	Moist dermatitis	Remove antigen or irritant
Psoriasis	Red, slightly elevated flat lesions (in body folds)	Dermatologist; topical steroid
Viral infections		
Herpes genitalis	See Table 6-14	See "Maternal Infections," pp. 208-214
Herpes zoster (shingles)	Burning, pain along sensory nerves	Analgesic, bedrest, compresses (Burow's solution of aluminum acetate)
Warts (verruca vulgaris or plana)	On skin or mucosa	May not respond to treatment, surgery, cryotherapy
Condylomata acuminata	Chronic vaginal discharge, pruritus, or dyspareunia	
Other infections		
Impetigo—hemolytic *Staphylococcus aureus* or streptococcus	Pruritus, formication, vesicles, and bullae	Isolate; topical antibiotic
Furunculosis—staphylococcus	Perifollicular abscesses, pain	Incision and drainage (I and D); isolate; systemic antibiotics
Erysipelas—β-hemolytic streptococcus	Red, raised, confluent induration; pain, fever, burning, aching, chronic exudative sores	Isolate; systemic antibiotics; hot, wet compresses (Burow's solution of aluminum acetate)
Tuberculosis—*Mycobacterium tuberculosis*		Systemic antituberculosis chemotherapy with vitamin B_6 replacement

*Abnormal skin sensation

Sample Nursing Care Plan

MATERNAL INFECTION

ASSESSMENT	NURSING DIAGNOSIS (ND)/ PLAN (P)/GOAL (G)	RATIONALE/ IMPLEMENTATION	EVALUATION
Prenatal: Assess for general malaise, fever, rashes, gland engorgement, etc. History of UTIs, vaginal infections. Assess whether the woman has any specific risk factors for infection (population, geographic). Physical assessment: 1. Fever. 2. General affect. 3. Signs and symptoms of infection. Laboratory tests: 1. Urinalysis. 2. Blood tests (Hgb, Hct, antibody titers, syphillis, AIDS, diabetes). 3. Cultures: gonorrhea, etc.	ND: Potential for injury related to infection (maternal and fetal). ND: Altered patterns of urinary elimination related to UTI. P: Monitor closely; intervene per physician's orders; provide information; and be available for discussion of concerns and questions. G: Woman will obtain prompt treatment for signs and symptoms of infection. G: Woman will follow treatment regime.	*To identify, treat, and prevent potential spread of infection, the nurse will:* Note and evaluate any complaints suggestive of infection. Note woman's infection and treatment history. Implement universal precautions to protect self and others from spread of infection. Obtain necessary lab work. Assist physician and support woman and family during tests and when test results are explained. Explain necessity of taking all antibiotic tablets as ordered. Viral infections are treated symptomatically. Suggest comfort measures that will help to relieve discomfort. All OTC preparations must be approved by a physician.	Infection is prevented or treated promptly with no or minimum sequelae to mother or infant.
Assess woman's knowledge about infection, its signs and symptoms, treatment, and potential sequelae.	ND: Knowledge deficit related to infection, its treatment, and possible sequelae. ND: Altered family processes related to interruption of sexual relations. ND: Body image disturbance, situational low self-esteem, altered role performance, and personal identity disturbance related to contagious infection. ND: Anxiety related to spread of infection. ND: Fear related to possible fetal sequelae. P: Provide information and encourage discussion of concerns. G: Woman will learn the signs and symptoms of infection. G: Woman will learn about her infection, its treatment, and possible sequelae. G: Woman will learn how to prevent spread of infection to others.	*To teach woman about infection, its treatment, potential sequelae, and necessary isolation precautions, the nurse will:* Review the signs and symptoms of infection. Explain general care issues: 1. Adequate hydration. 2. Rest. 2. Adherence to medication regime. 4. Control temperature with fluids, cool bath, and acetaminophen (Tylenol). 5. Well balanced diet. Reinforce physician's explanation of woman's infection, its treatment, and possible sequelae (maternal and fetal). Clarify misconceptions. Help woman formulate questions for physician. Assist woman in preparation to inform partner of infection and any necessary treatment he might need to seek. Teach woman how to pre-	Woman learns the signs and symptoms of infection. Woman learns how to treat and manage her infection. Woman learns how to prevent spread of infection to others. Woman verbalizes understanding of necessary isolation precautions taken by the health care team.

ASSESSMENT	NURSING DIAGNOSIS (ND)/ PLAN (P)/GOAL (G)	RATIONALE/ IMPLEMENTATION	EVALUATION
	G: Woman will verbalize understanding of necessary isolation precautions taken by the health care team during care.	vent spread of infection. Explain any isolation precautions necessary by the health care team to prevent spread of infection to others. Encourage verbalization of concerns and fears. Assist with counseling before proposed therapeutic abortion.	
Postnatal: Assess all prenatal and intrapartal data. Physical assessment: 1. Newborn—assess for symptomatology of infection. 2. Mother—vital signs, general affect, malaise, rash, gland enlargement; redness, tenderness, warmth, pain over a specific area. Laboratory tests: Culture of any exudate. Blood tests for infection. Urinalysis.	ND: Potential for injury related to infection. ND: Altered patterns of urinary elimination related to UTI. P: Follow prescribed management. G: Woman and infant will receive prompt treatment for infection and will experience no or minimum sequelae.	*To treat an infected mother and newborn, the nurse will:* Obtain specimens ordered for laboratory testing. Administer medications as ordered (medications for symptomatic relief or antibiotics). Ensure adequate rest and nutrition. Provide high-risk care to infant.	Infection is treated promptly with no or minimum sequelae for mother and infant.
Assess knowledge regarding infection: prevention, identification, treatment.	ND: Knowledge deficit related to infection.	*To teach about infection, its treatment, and possible sequelae, the nurse will:* Review possible sequelae from infection that she or her infant might experience. Counsel regarding breastfeeding (some infections are transmitted in breast milk). Encourage questions and clarify misconceptions. Teach woman the importance of adherence to the treatment regime and the need for follow-up. Assist woman and family with grieving if indicated.	Woman learns about prevention, identification, and management of infection.
	P: Provide information as needed; provide written instructions. G: Woman will learn how her infection is identified and managed.		
Assess need for isolation precautions for mother and infant.	ND: Potential for injury related to possible spread of infection to others. ND: Alteration in parenting related to fear of spreading infection to newborn. P: Provide information, demonstrate, and observe return demonstration. G: Woman will remain in isolation to prevent potential spread of infection.	*To prevent the spread of infection, the nurse will:* Isolate mother and infant if necessary (explain isolation to the mother). Teach mother how to prevent the spread of infection to her newborn. Encourage mother-infant interaction while reinforcing isolation guidelines.	Spread of infection is prevented. Mother interacts with child while maintaining isolation protocol.

Summary of Nursing Actions

NURSING CARE FOR MATERNAL INFECTIONS

I. Goals
   A. For the mother: freedom from infection
   B. For the fetus and newborn: freedom from infection and the adverse effects of infection on fetal development and neonatal well-being
   C. For the family: knowledge of methods to avoid infection and to treat it appropriately if it occurs.

II. Priorities
   A. Prompt identification of infection and initiation of therapy
   B. Education of the woman and her family for the prevention of infection
   C. Encouragement of self-care

III. Assessment
   A. Prenatal
      1. Interview
         a. General malaise, fever rashes, gland enlargement, etc.
         b. History of UTIs, vaginal infections
         c. Population at risk
      2. Physical examination
         a. Fever
         b. General affect
         c. Signs and symptoms of infection
      3. Laboratory tests
         a. Urinalysis
         b. Blood tests: Hgb, HCT, antibody titers, syphilis, AIDS, diabetes
         c. Cultures: gonorrhea, etc.
   B. Postnatal
      1. Record, interview
         a. Prenatal data
         b. Intrapartal data
      2. Physical examination
         a. Newborn: assessment for symptomatology of infection (see Summary of Nursing Actions, "Neonatal Infection," pp. 286-287)
         b. Mother: vital signs, general affect, malaise, rash, gland enlargement; redness, tenderness, warmth, pain over a specific area
      3. Laboratory tests
         a. Cultures of any exudate
         b. Blood tests for infection
         c. Urinalysis

IV. Potential nursing diagnoses
   A. Knowledge deficit
   B. Potential for injury
   C. Noncompliance (specify)
   D. Altered family processes
   E. Sexual dysfunction
   F. Altered sexuality patterns
   G. Spiritual distress
   H. Body image disturbance
   I. Self esteem disturbance: situational low self esteem
   J. Anxiety
   K. Fear
   L. Altered patterns of urinary elimination
   M. Altered health maintenance
   N. Potential altered parenting
   O. Potential activity intolerance
   P. Pain
   Q. Potential impaired home maintenance management
   R. Impaired tissue integrity
   S. Potential impaired skin integrity

V. Plan/implementation
   A. Prenatal
      1. Viral infections are treated symptomatically.
      2. Prophylactic antibiotic therapy may be instituted to prevent secondary infection.
      3. If woman is to be treated at home, assist her and family in planning how she will implement prescribed care.
      4. Assist physician and support woman and family during tests and when hearing results.
      5. Assist with counseling before proposed therapeutic abortion.
      6. If genital lesions are found (herpesvirus type 2), prepare woman for elective cesarean delivery.
      7. Isolation techniques (institute and prepare woman for this situation).
      8. Reinforce physician's explanations of cause, management, possible outcomes.
      9. General care:
         a. Adequate hydration.
         b. Rest
         c. Adherence to medication regimen (if an oral antibiotics, woman may prevent gastrointestinal upset by taking Lactinex or eating yogurt between doses).
         d. Temperature should be kept down with acetaminophen (Tylenol), fluids, cool sponge baths.
   B. Postnatal
      1. Provide nursing-medical care for high-risk infant
      2. Isolate infant and mother if indicated.
      3. Assist woman and family with grieving if indicated.
      4. Ensure bedrest and proper diet.
      5. Answer questions regarding infection, cause, management, expected prognosis.

VI. Evaluation
   A. Infection is prevented.
   B. Infection is treated promptly with no or minimum sequelae for mother and infant.
   C. Parent or parents learn about prevention, identification, and management of infection.

MATERNAL HEMORRHAGIC DISORDERS

Hemorrhagic disorders in pregnancy are medical emergencies that require expert teamwork on the part of the physician and nurse. The nurse must be alert to symptoms of hemorrhage and shock and be knowledgeable about laboratory tests and blood replacement. Nursing care includes prompt attention to physical symptoms, competent technical skill, and supportive care for the woman and her family.

Causes of Hemorrhage

The most common causes of excessive bleeding early in pregnancy are abortion and ectopic pregnancy. Later in pregnancy, premature separation of the placenta or placenta previa may be the cause of hemorrhage. The nurse must be alert to the signs and symptoms of these problems and be prepared to intervene quickly should they arise.

Table 6-16   *Assessing Abortion*

Type of Abortion	Amount of Bleeding	Uterine Cramping	Passage of Tissue	Tissue in Vagina	Internal Cervical Os	Size of Uterus
Threatened	Slight	Mild	No	No	Closed	Agrees with length of pregnancy
Inevitable	Moderate	Moderate	No	No	Open	Agrees with length of pregnancy
Incomplete	Heavy	Severe	Yes	Possible	Open with tissue in cervix	Smaller than expected for length of pregnancy
Complete	Slight	Mild	Yes	Possible	Closed	Smaller than expected for length of pregnancy
Septic	Varies; usually malodorous; fever present	Varies; fever present	Varies; fever present	Varies; fever present	Usually open; fever present	Any of the above with tenderness
Missed	Slight	No	No	No	Closed	Smaller than expected for length of pregnancy

From Gordon RT: Emergencies in obstetrics and gynecology. In Warner CG, editor: Emergency care: assessment and intervention, ed 3, St Louis, 1983, The CV Mosby Co.

Table 6-17   *Types of Spontaneous Abortion and Usual Management*

Type of Abortion	Management
Threatened	Bedrest, sedation, and avoidance of stress and orgasm are recommended. Further treatment will depend on client's course.
Inevitable and incomplete	Prompt termination of pregnancy is accomplished usually by dilation and curettage (D & C).
Complete	No further intervention may be needed if uterine contractions are adequate to prevent hemorrhage and if there is no infection.
Septic	Immediate termination of pregnancy by method appropriate to duration of pregnancy. Cervical cultures and sensitivity (C & S) studies are done and broad-spectrum antibiotic therapy (e.g., ampicillin) is started. Treatment for septic shock is initiated if necessary.
Missed	If spontaneous evacuation of the uterus does not occur within 1 month, however, pregnancy is terminated by method appropriate to duration of pregnancy. Blood clotting factors are monitored until uterus is empty. Disseminated intravascular coagulation (DIC) and incoagulability of blood with uncontrolled hemorrhage may develop in cases of fetal death after twelfth week if products of conception are retained for longer than 5 weeks.

Table 6-18 *Differential Diagnosis of Ectopic Pregnancy*

	Ectopic Pregnancy	Appendicitis	Salpingitis	Ruptured Corpus Luteum Cyst	Uterine Abortion
Pain	Unilateral cramps and tenderness before rupture	Epigastric, periumbilical, then right lower quadrant pain; tenderness localizing at McBurney's point; rebound tenderness	Usually in both lower quadrants with or without rebound	Unilateral, becoming general with progressive bleeding	Midline cramps
Nausea and vomiting	Occasionally before, frequently after rupture	Usual; precedes shift of pain to right lower quadrant	Infrequent	Rare	Almost never
Menstruation	Some aberration; missed period, spotting	Unrelated to menses	Hypermenorrhea or metrorrhagia or both	Period delayed, then bleeding, often with pain	Amenorrhea, then spotting, then brisk bleeding
Temperature and pulse	37.2°-37.8° C (99°-100° F); pulse variable; normal before, rapid after rupture	37.2°-37.8° C (99°-100° F); pulse rapid: 99-100	37.2°-40° C (99°-104° F); pulse elevated in proportion to fever	Not over 37.2° C (99° F); pulse normal unless blood loss marked, then rapid	To 37.2° C (99° F) if spontaneous; to 40° C (104° F) if induced (infected)
Pelvic examination	Unilateral tenderness, especially on movement of cervix; crepitant mass on one side or in cul-de-sac	No masses; rectal tenderness high on right side	Bilateral tenderness on movement of cervix; masses only when pyosalpinx or hydrosalpinx present	Tenderness over affected ovary; no masses	Cervix slightly patulous; uterus slightly enlarged, irregularly softened; tender with infection
Laboratory findings	WBC to 15,000/μl; RBC strikingly low if blood loss large; sedimentation rate slightly elevated	WBC: 10,000-18,000/μl (rarely normal); RBC normal; sedimentation rate slightly elevated	WBC: 15,000-30,000/μl; RBC normal; sedimentation rate markedly elevated	WBC normal to 10,000/μl; RBC normal; sedimentation rate normal	WBC: 15,000/μl if spontaneous; to 30,000/μl if induced (infection); RBC normal; sedimentation rate slightly to moderately elevated

Reproduced, with permission, from Benson RC, editor: Current obstetric and gynecologic diagnosis and treatment, ed 5, copyright 1984 by Lange Medical Publications, Los Altos, Calif.

Table 6-19 *Summary of Findings: Abruptio Placentae and Placenta Previa*

| | Abruptio Placentae | | | |
	Marginal Separation	Moderate Separation	Severe Separation* (More Than 66%)	Placenta Previa
Bleeding: external, vaginal	Minimal	Absent to moderate	Absent to moderate	Minimal to severe and life-threatening
Color of blood	Dark red	Dark red	Dark red	Bright red
Shock	Absent	Common	Very common; often sudden	Occasional
Coagulopathy	Rare	Occasional	Common	Rare
Uterine tonicity	Normal	Increased—may be localized to one region or diffuse over uterus; uterus fails to relax between contractions	Tetanic, persistent uterine contraction; boardlike uterus	Normal
Tenderness (pain)	Usually absent; if present, is localized	Increased—usually diffuse over uterus	Agonizing, unremitting uterine pain	Absent
Ultrasonographic findings				
Location of placenta	Normal—upper uterine segment	Normal—upper uterine segment	Normal—upper uterine segment	Abnormal—lower uterine segment
Station of presenting part	Variable to engaged	Variable to engaged	Variable to engaged	High—not engaged
Fetal position	Usual distribution†	Usual distribution	Usual distribution	Commonly transverse, breech, or oblique
Concurrent hypertensive state	Usual distribution	Commonly present	Commonly present	Usual distribution

*Onset is usually abrupt; fetus usually dies.
†Usual distribution refers to the usual variations or incidence seen when there is no concurrent problem.

Sequelae of Hemorrhagic Disorders

Women who develop bleeding disorders during pregnancy are at risk for coagulapathy. Therefore, blood clotting problems must be assessed and diagnosed early. If disseminated intravascular coagulation (DIC) develops or the woman goes into shock, immediate interventions are necessary.

Table 6-20 *Blood Clotting Factors*

Factor	Synonyms
I	Fibrinogen
II	Prothrombin
III	Platelet factor 3, thromboplastin
IV	Calcium
V	Labile factor, proaccelerin, AC globulin (ACG)
VI	Synonymous terms no longer used
VII	Serum prothrombin conversion accelerator (SPCA), proconvertin, autoprothrombin
VIII	Antihemotrophic factor (AHF), antihemophilic globulin
IX	Plasma thromboplastin component (PTC), Christmas factor, autoprothrombin II
X	Stuart-Prower factor, Stuart factor, Prower factor
XI	Plasma thromboplastin antecedent (PTA)
XII	Hagemen factor
XIII	Fibrin (protein) stabilizing factor

Table 6-21   *Coagulation Tests*

Test	Comments
Activated partial thromboplastin time (PTT; measures intrinsic system): 25-36 sec	Screening test of choice: very sensitive, relatively easy to perform, inexpensive. All coagulation factors except proconvertin are measured.
One-stage prothrombin time (PT; Quick test; measures extrinsic system): 9.5-11.3 sec	Test for proconvertin (VII), proaccelerin (V), Stuart-Prower factor (X), prothrombin (II), and fibrinogen deficiencies. Unfortunately, it does not measure factors necessary for earlier stages of coagulation.
Thrombin time (plasma): 10-15 sec	Test measures conversion of fibrinogen to fibrin and depends on concentration of fibrinogen or inhibitors such as fibrin split-products, antithrombins, and heparin.
Platelet count: 130,000-370,000/mm³	**Most reliable index for DIC.**
Specific factor assays (e.g., plasma fibrinogen): 195-365 mg/dl	Each of coagulation factors can be assessed by indirect clotting method using natural or synthetic factor-deficient substrates and compared with activity of normal plasma (100%). However, fibrinogen is only factor that can be measured directly by chemical method.
Bleeding time Template: 2-8 min Ivy: 1-7 min Duke: 1-3 min	Finger or earlobe puncture 5 mm deep and 2 mm wide (Bard-Parker blade no. 11) is made after antiseptic preparation of skin. Note time of puncture; touch bleeding point gently with sterile filter paper to absorb blood every 30 sec until bleeding stops.

Disseminated Intravascular Coagulation

I. Predisposing factors
   A. Abruptio placentae
   B. Intrauterine fetal death syndrome
   C. Amniotic fluid embolism
   D. Preeclampsia-eclampsia
   E. Hemorrhagic shock
   F. Saline abortion
   G. Hydatidiform mole
   H. Ruptured uterus
   I. Sepsis
   J. Tumultuous or hypertonic labor
   K. Difficult delivery
   L. Oxytocin (Pitocin) induction

II. Physical findings
   A. Spontaneous bleeding from gums or nose
   B. Excessive bleeding from site of slight trauma (i.e., venipuncture)
   C. Sudden tachycardia, diaphoresis, or restlessness with anxiety
   D. Sequelae: acute renal failure, pituitary insufficiency (Sheehan's syndrome)

III. Treatment
   A. Remove causative factor
      1. Delivery of dead fetus
      2. Treatment of infection, eclampsia
      3. Removal of hydatidiform mole
      4. Removal by cesarean delivery of fetus, abruptio placenta, or placenta previa
   B. Establish support mechanisms
      1. Woman's right hip elevated to prevent hypotensive syndrome.
      2. Oxygen administered by tight-fitting mask at 10 to 12 L/min.
      3. Parenteral therapy begun (e.g., Ringer's lactated solution).
      4. CVP monitoring begun with attempt to maintain CVP within normal limits: 6 to 12 cm H_2O.
   C. Treat condition
      1. Administer whole blood as needed at rate sufficient to maintain hematocrit (HCT) at 30% and urinary output at 30 to 60 ml/hr.
      2. Administer blood components as needed.
         One unit of platelets raises adult level by 5000.
         One unit of cryoprecipitate (fibrinogen and factor VIII) replaces depleted coagulation factors. Cryoprecipitate is more effective in restoring normal coagulation than lyophilized fibrinogen. In addition, it has the advantage of minimizing transmission of serum hepatitis (about 20% of people who receive fibrinogen acquire homologous serum hepatitis), *or*
         Two units of fresh frozen plasma replace coagulation factors and fibrinogen. The frozen plasma is thawed in the laboratory. It should be administered within 15 to 20 minutes, since the factors disintegrate as the plasma warms.
      3. Heparin may be ordered.* This is administered by constant infusion pump at 12.5 U/kg/hr to arrest coagulation and fibrinolysis.
      4. Diagnosis and treatment of sequelae; minor or major hemorrhagic diathesis, acute renal failure, pituitary insufficiency (Sheehan's syndrome), compromised newborn (usually not affected, except indirectly through hypoxia).

---

*Paradoxically, cautious intravenous heparin administration may stop the abdominal clotting and check bleeding. Heparin should be administered only after appropriate investigative studies, however, and usually in consultation with a hematologist.

Table 6-22   *Replacement Clotting Factors*

Infusate and Factors	Need	Risk	Expected Outcome
Fresh-frozen plasma; clotting factors	Depleted clotting factors	Hepatitis B	Increase fibrinogen to 10 mg/dl per unit infused
Cryoprecipitate; I,V,VII,XIII	Fibrinogen concentration below 50 mg/dl; a level of 50,000/mm^3 should be sought	Hepatitis	Increase fibrinogen 2 to 5 mg/dl, to 10 mg/dl per unit infused
Platelet concentrate; platelets	<20,000/mm^3	Rhesus isoimmunization in Rh negative women	Increase platelet count 7500/μl per unit infused

Table 6-23   *Symptoms of Shock*

	Mild	Moderate	Severe	Irreversible
Respirations	Rapid, deep	Rapid, becoming shallow	Rapid, shallow, may be irregular	Irregular, or barely perceptible
Pulse	Rapid, tone normal	Rapid, tone may be normal but is becoming weaker	Very rapid, easily collapsible, may be irregular	Irregular apical pulse
Blood pressure	Normal or hypertensive	60-90 mm Hg systolic	Below 60 mm Hg systolic	None palpable
Skin	Cool and pale	Cool, pale, moist, knees cyanotic	Cold, clammy, cyanosis of lips and fingernails	Cold, clammy, cyanotic
Urinary output	No change	Decreasing to 10-22 ml/hr (adult)	Oliguric (less than 10 ml) to anuric	Anuric
Level of consciousness (LOC)	Alert, oriented, diffuse anxiety	Oriented, mental cloudiness or increasing restlessness	Lethargic, reacts to noxious stimuli, comatose	Does not respond to noxious stimuli
CVP	May be normal (6-12 cm H$_2$O)	3 cm H$_2$O	0-3 cm H$_2$O	

Modified from Royce JA: Nurs Clin North Am **8**:377, 1973; and Wagner MM, Clinical Nursing Specialist, University of Iowa Hospitals and Clinics.

Hemoglobin and Hematocrit Below Acceptable Level for Trimester

	Hgb	Hct
First trimester	≤11 g/dl	≤37%
Second trimester	≤10.5 g/dl	≤35%
Third trimester	≤10 g/dl	≤33%
Nonpregnant	≤12 g/dl	≤37%

HAZARDS OF SHOCK THERAPY

HAZARD	NURSING ACTION
Fluid overload: moist respirations, stridor, or dyspnea	Alert physician, decrease the drip rate
Shock lung: tachypnea, dyspnea, anxiety, a rise in blood pressure, cyanosis, and harsh loud breaths	Alert physician, maintain ventilator between 50 and 70 mm Hg
Oxygen toxicity: muscular twitching about the face, followed by convulsions resembling grand mal seizures.	Alert physician; take convulsion precautions

Sample Nursing Care Plan

HEMORRHAGIC DISORDERS OF PREGNANCY

ASSESSMENT	NURSING DIAGNOSIS (ND)/ PLAN (P)/GOAL (G)	RATIONALE/ IMPLEMENTATION	EVALUATION
Vital signs and blood pressure. Affect/LOC (agitated, anxious, uncomfortable, dull). Tenderness (uterine, abdominal, cervical, perineal). Integument (color, warmth, moisture, turgor). Time in child-bearing cycle: Prenatal: duration since LMP. Postnatal: duration since delivery. Events preceding symptoms (falls, vaginal examination, coitus, childbirth). Previous obstetric history: past, current. Amount of bleeding, presence and size of clots. Associated discomfort: amount and location (uterine, referred pain, bladder). Passage of tissue. Blood: Rh and blood group, type and crossmatch as necessary; Hgb, Hct; CBC: WBC, platelets. Urine: Pregnancy test if woman suspected of being in early pregnancy; UTI; chest x-ray study if extrapelvic infection is suspected or if surgery is anticipated.	ND: Decreased cardiac output related to hemorrhage. ND: Fluid volume deficit related to hemorrhage. ND: Impaired gas exchange related to hemorrhage or its therapy. ND: Altered cardiopulmonary tissue perfusion related to hemorrhage. ND: Fluid volume excess related to blood or fluid replacement. ND: Potential for injury related to infection or excessive volume loss. ND: Pain. P: Monitor closely, or provide information, and be available to discuss concerns. G: The client will remain physiologically safe as indicated by: a. Vital signs stabilized within normal limits b. Hemodynamic stability c. Absence of infection d. Absence of pain	*To identify hemorrhage and treat appropriately, the nurse will:* Report and record findings promptly. Monitor vital signs, blood pressure, LOC, CVP, integument. Save all peripads, linens soaked with blood, clots, and tissue. Start IV infusion using large bore catheter in the event blood transfusion is needed. Hang appropriate blood product. Administer medications as ordered, (analgesics, oxytocics, antibiotics). Obtain specimen collection, (blood, urine, culture). Insert retention urine catheter. Provide preoperative and postoperative care as needed, including medications, oxygen; keep woman and family informed. Give Rh₀ (D) immune globulin, if indicated (Chapter 40).	Woman's blood loss is minimized. Vitals signs are stablized within normal limits. Complications of blood, fluid, and electrolyte replacement are averted. Fluid and electrolyte balance is maintained. Woman's reproductive capability is maintained. Surgical intervention is successful with no adverse sequelae. Comfort is maximized. Client remains free from infection. Fetus/newborn suffers no sequelae related to maternal condition.
Assess woman's learning needs in regard to hemorrhage, its management, and complications.	ND: Knowledge deficit related to identification of and care during a hemorrhagic disorder. P: Provide information and be available to discuss concerns and questions. G: Woman will be instructed about her condition and its management. G: Woman will learn the danger signals of hemorrhage.	*To teach the woman about hemorrhage, its management and complications, the nurse will:* Carefully explain known causes, management, and expected outcomes. Assist in identifying questions for the physician. Teach woman about danger signs and symptoms (bleeding, fever, cramping, pain) and whom to call should they occur. Counsel regarding antibiotic	Woman and family verbalize understanding of the condition and its management. Woman identifies danger signals and whom to notify.

Sample Nursing Care Plan—cont'd

ASSESSMENT	NURSING DIAGNOSIS (ND)/ PLAN (P)/GOAL (G)	RATIONALE/ IMPLEMENTATION	EVALUATION
	G: Woman will learn the signs and symptoms of infection.	therapy. Counsel regarding nutrition to prevent anemia. Provide information regarding contraceptives as appropriate. Refer to social services (home health care, home service, etc.).	
Assess for previous experience with loss and positive coping mechanisms utilized. Assess support system. Assess current emotional status of woman. Identify spiritual needs for clergy to be present as support or to baptize fetus or newborn.	ND: Anxiety related to actual or potential loss. ND: Body image disturbance, personal identity disturbance, situational low self-esteem, altered role performance. ND: Ineffective individual or family coping related to loss and grief. ND: Powerlessness related to loss or grief. ND: Spiritual distress related to loss or guilt. P: Provide information and be available to discuss concerns and questions. G: Woman and family will accept a loss in a positive manner. G: Guilt or blame will be averted. G: Self-concept will not be disturbed. G: Spiritual distress will be averted. G: Sense of power will be retained (participates in own care).	*To help woman and family with the experience of loss and initiate the grieving process, the nurse will:* Explain procedures, sensations, expected outcomes; answer questions. Involve family in planning and care. Encourage verbalization of concerns and feelings. Assist woman and family with emotional reactions. Implement care of woman and family experiencing perinatal loss. Explain the grief process. Give couples the opportunity to see fetus or inform them of sex. Baptize products of conception or newborn, or summon clergy if requested.	Woman verbalizes understanding of condition and its management. Woman identifies support system. Woman initiates grief process.
Disseminated intravascular coagulation (DIC) Predisposing factors: Retained dead fetus. Infection. PIH. Abruptio placenta. Amniotic fluid embolism. Signs: Spontaneous bleeding (e.g., from gums, nose). Excessive bleeding from site of slight trauma. Reduced laboratory values for platelets, fibrinogen, proaccelerin, antihemophilic factor, and prothrombin. Ecchymoses (sudden tachycardia, diapho-	ND: Anxiety, fear, pain, ineffective individual coping related to signs and symptoms of DIC. ND: Knowledge deficit related to DIC, its causes and management. ND: Fluid volume deficit or excess related to DIC or its management. ND: Altered (cardiopulmonary) tissue perfusion and injury related to DIC. P: Continuous assessment for risk factors and symptomatology and rapid identification and initiation of therapy. G: For the mother: prompt identification and ap-	*To implement therapy the nurse will:* Assist physician with treatment or removal of predisposing factors: a. Deliver dead fetus. b. Treat existing infection or PIH. c. Deliver fetus and abrupted placenta. Establish management of hemorrhagic shock or bacteremic shock. Replace clotting factors. Assist with treatment of sequelae.	The woman survives the disease with minimum or no damage to body organs or systems. The woman's blood-clotting mechanism returns to normal. The woman and her family understand the disease process and its management. The newborn survives with no adverse sequelae.

Continued.

Sample Nursing Care Plan—cont'd

ASSESSMENT	NURSING DIAGNOSIS (ND)/ PLAN (P)/GOAL (G)	RATIONALE/ IMPLEMENTATION	EVALUATION
...resis, or restlessness with anxiety). Occurrence of sequelae: Acute renal failure. Pituitary insufficiency (Sheehan's syndrome).	...propriate therapy to prevent serious sequelae to hemorrhage or its therapy. G: For the fetus or newborn: prevention of hypoxia. G: For the family: a healthy mother and newborn.		

Summary of Nursing Actions

GENERAL NURSING CARE OF PREGNANCY-RELATED HEMORRHAGE

I. Goals
  A. For the mother: a physiologically and emotionally safe experience
  B. For the lost embryo: baptism, as necesary
  C. For the viable fetus: a safe passage from intrauterine to extrauterine existence as close to term gestation as possible
  D. For the family: successful coping with the experience

II. Priorities
  A. Identify hemorrhage and treat appropriately.
    1. Replace blood, blood products, fluids, and electrolytes immediately.
    2. Monitor therapy carefully to prevent complications such as fluid overload, shock lung.
    3. Correct the underlying problem.
  B. Manage discomfort:
    1. Administer analgesics per physician's orders.
    2. Keep woman informed regarding her condition and its management.
  C. Provide emotional support:
    1. Implement care for individuals experiencing loss.
    2. Keep woman and family informed.
    3. Summon clergy or other support persons per woman's or family's request.

III. Assessment
  A. Interview
    1. Time in childbearing cycle:
      a. Prenatal: duration since LMP.
      b. Postnatal: duration since delivery
    2. Events preceding symptomatology, e.g., falls, vaginal examination, coitus; childbirth
    3. Previous obstetric history: past, current
    4. Amount of bleeding, presence and size of clots

  5. Associated discomfort: amount and location, e.g., uterine, referred pain, bladder
  6. Passage of tissue
  B. Physical examination
    1. Vital signs and blood pressures
    2. Affect/LOC, e.g., anxious, agitated, uncomfortable, dull
    3. Tenderness, e.g., uterine, abdominal, cervical, perineal
    4. Integument, e.g., color, warmth, moisture, turgor
  C. Laboratory tests
    1. Blood
      a. Rh and blood group; type and cross match as necessary
      b. Hgb, HCT
      c. CBC: WBC, platelets
    2. Urine
      a. Pregnancy test, e.g., if woman is suspected of being in early pregnancy
      b. UTI
    3. Chest x-ray; if extrapelvic infection is suspected, or if surgery is anticipated

IV. Potential nursing diagnoses
  A. Potential for infection
  B. Anxiety
  C. Fear
  D. Decreased cardiac output
  E. Pain
  F. Ineffective individual coping
  G. Ineffective family coping: compromised
  H. Potential fluid volume deficit
  I. Potential for injury
  J. Anticipatory grieving
  K. Knowledge deficit
  L. Powerlessness

Summary of Nursing Action—cont'd

M. Impaired gas exchange
N. Spiritual distress
O. Altered tissue perfusion (specify)
P. Potential altered home maintenance management
Q. Self esteem disturbance: situational low self esteem
R. Altered role performance
S. Personal identity disturbance

V. Plan/implementation
A. Technician
   1. Report and record findings promptly.
   2. Save all peripads, linens soaked with blood, clots, and tissue.
   3. Obtain specimen collection, e.g., blood, urine, culture.
   4. Administer medications, as ordered, e.g., analgesics, oxytocics, antibiotics.
   5. Start IV infusion using large-bore needle in the event blood transfusion is needed.
   6. Monitor vital signs, blood pressure, length of contractions, central venous pressure, LOC, CVP, integument.
   7. Insert retention urinary catheter.
   8. Provide pre- and postoperative care as needed.
   9. Hang appropriate blood product.
B. Support person
   1. Implement care for woman and family experiencing loss.
   2. If possible, give couples opportunity to see fetus or inform them of sex.
   3. Explain procedure, sensations, expected outcomes; answer questions.
   4. Assist woman and family with emotional reactions.
   5. Involve family in planning and care.
   6. Baptize products of conception or newborn, or summon clergy.
C. Teacher/counselor/advocate
   1. Carefully explain known causes, management, and expected outcomes.
   2. Counsel regarding antibiotic therapy.
   3. Assist with identifying questions for the physician.
   4. Refer for social services, e.g., home health care, homemaker service, etc.
   5. Counsel regarding nutrition to prevent anemia.
   6. Teach woman about danger signs and symptoms (bleeding, fever, cramping, pain) and whom to call should they occur.
   7. Provide information regarding contraceptives as appropriate.

VI. Evaluation
A. Condition is identified promptly, and appropriate therapy is instituted.
B. Blood loss is minimized.
   1. Vital signs and blood pressure remain within normal limits.
   2. DIC does not occur.
   3. Complications of blood, fluid, and electrolyte replacement are averted.
   4. Fluid-electrolyte balance is maintained.
   5. Woman's reproductive capability is maintained.
   6. Surgical intervention is successful with no adverse sequelae.
   7. Comfort is maximized.
C. Woman and family come to terms with loss in a positive manner.
   1. Guilt or blame is averted.
   2. Self-concept is not disturbed.
   3. Spiritual distress is averted.
   4. Sense of power is retained, e.g., participates in own care.
D. Woman and family verbalize understanding of the condition and its management.
E. Knowledge needs are met.

ENDOCRINE AND METABOLIC DISORDERS

Maternal endocrine and metabolic disorders have immediate and long-term consequences for the mother and her fetus or newborn. Nurses can play a major role in the management of these problems. A primary component of nursing care is client teaching. The woman who becomes an active participant in her own care has the most potential for preventing or minimizing the adverse effects of the disorder and improving the prognosis for herself and her offspring.

Diabetes Mellitus

Diabetes mellitus is a complication in about 1% to 2% of pregnant women. Improved methods for maintaining glucose levels within the normal range have improved fetal prognoses, and risk management has allowed more women to carry their pregnancies in term. The nurse must have a sound knowledge base regarding various classifications of the condition and laboratory tests and their implications. It is vital to educate the woman and her family if management is to be successful.

Classification. Following is the 1979 classification of diabetes mellitus issued by the National Diabetes Data Group.

type I diabetes mellitus Formerly called juvenile-onset diabetes or insulin-dependent diabetes; onset in people 40 years or *younger;* etiology: genetic, immunologic, viral. Prone to ketosis.

type II diabetes mellitus Formerly called maturity-onset diabetes or non-insulin-dependent diabetes; occurs in all ages, but more usual in the older, overweight person; etiology: primarily genetic. Resistant to ketosis. In pregnancy, insulin is required to control maternal plasma glucose levels (Hollingsworth, 1985).

type III diabetes mellitus Formerly called gestational diabetes; intolerance to glucose with onset during pregnancy with return to normal tolerance after delivery.

type IV diabetes mellitus Formerly called secondary diabetes; refers to abnormalities in glucose tolerance following pancreatic disease, endocrine disorders (Cushing's syndrome), drug ingestion (oral contraceptives), cirrhosis, and the like.

hyperglycemia Blood levels of glucose that exceed normal values.

White's 1978 classification of pregnant diabetic women considers age at onset, duration, and vascular or renal changes, if any (Table 6-24). Although even mild forms of diabetes pose a threat to mother and infant, the incidence of perinatal death increases with the presence and degree of vascular or renal pathologic changes (classes D, E, and F).

Table 6-24 *Classification of Diabetes During Pregnancy (Priscilla White)*

Class	Characteristics	Implications
Glucose intolerance of pregnancy	Erroneously known as gestational diabetes. Abnormal glucose tolerance during pregnancy; postprandial hyperglycemia during pregnancy.	Diagnosis before 30 weeks' gestation important to prevent macrosomia. Treat with diet adequate in calories to prevent maternal weight loss. Goal is postprandial blood glucose <130 mg/dl at 1 hour, or <105 mg/dl at 2 hours. If insulin is necessary, manage as in classes B, C, and D.
A	Chemical diabetes diagnosed before pregnancy; managed by diet alone: any age at onset.	Management as for glucose intolerance of pregnancy.
B	Insulin treatment used before pregnancy; onset at age 20 or older; duration <10 years.	Some endogenous insulin secretion may persist. Fetal and neonatal risks same as in classes C and D, as is management.
C	Onset at age 10-20, or duration 10-20 years.	Insulin-deficient diabetes of juvenile onset.
D	Onset before age 10, or duration >20 years, or chronic hypertension (not preeclampsia), or background retinopathy (tiny hemorrhages).	Fetal macrosomia or intrauterine growth retardation possible. Retinal microaneurysms, dot hemorrhages, and exudates may progress during pregnancy, then regress after delivery.
F	Diabetic nephropathy with proteinuria.	Anemia and hypertension common; proteinuria increases in third trimester, declines after delivery. Fetal intrauterine growth retardation common; perinatal survival about 85% under optimum conditions; bedrest necessary.
H	Coronary artery disease.	Serious maternal risk.
R	Proliferative retinopathy.	Neovascularization, with risk of vitreous hemorrhage or retinal detachment; laser photocoagulation useful; abortion usually not necessary. With active process of neovascularization, prevent bearing-down efforts.

From Benson RC, editor: Current obstetric and gynecologic diagnosis and treatment, ed 5, Los Altos, Calif, 1984, Lange Medical Publications.

3-Hour Glucose Tolerance Test

After a 100 g glucose load the 3-hour GTT is abnormal if 2 or more of the following values are found:

	Plasma (mg/dl)	Venous Whole Blood (mg/dl)	Plasma (Glucose Oxidase) (mg/dl)
Fasting	≥ 105	≥ 90	≥ 95
1 hour	≥ 190	≥ 165	≥ 180
2 hours	≥ 165	≥ 145	≥ 155
3 hours	≥ 145	≥ 125	≥ 140

Table 6-25   *Blood Tests for Diabetes Mellitus in Pregnancy*

Test	Instructions	Technique	Findings	Precautions
Fasting blood sugar (FBS): measures amount of glucose in blood when woman is fasting	No food for 12 hr before test, e.g., 8 PM to 8 AM; water is only fluid allowed	Blood drawn by venipuncture and sent to laboratory	Normal: 80-120 mg/dl serum Abnormal: ≥140 mg/dl on 2 occasions, diagnostic of diabetes mellitus	None
Postprandial blood sugar: measures blood sugar following meal	None	Woman eats meal containing 100 g of carbohydrate; blood drawn by venipuncture 2 hr after meal and sent to laboratory	Normal: 80-120 mg/dl serum	None
Oral glucose tolerance test (GTT): measures woman's response to measured dose of glucose	No food for 12 hr before test or during test, but may have water; no smoking, tea, coffee, during test (alter body's response to carbohydrate); minimize activity (alters glucose metabolism); minimize stress (epinephrine and cortisone raise glucose levels by promoting gluconeogenesis)	Weigh woman, obtain fasting blood and urine specimens; administer 100 g of glucose orally in lemon juice; collect blood samples at 1, 2, and 3 hr; mark each specimen with time obtained and send to laboratory	See values, in box above Abnormal fasting: elevated or two other values lie outside normal range	Caution woman she may experience dizziness, sweating, weakness, nausea, vomiting, or diarrhea during second and third hour Diuretics and glucocorticoids may distort findings; do not use if fasting blood sugar (FBS) over 200 mg/dl
Intravenous (IV) glucose tolerance test: preferred test in pregnancy since absorption of glucose from intestinal tract is variable and may result in distorted findings in oral GTT	Same as oral GTT	Weigh woman; obtain fasting blood and urine specimens: administer 50 ml of 50% glucose in distilled water IV over a 4 min period and serial blood specimens obtained until 2 hr is reached, labeled as to time obtained, and sent to laboratory	Plasma glucose level Normal fasting: <100 mg/dl 2 hr: level not higher than fasting level	Caution woman she may experience facial flushing and dizziness as glucose is being administered Other precautions: same as for GTT
Tolbutamide response test not used since tolbutamide may have teratogenic effect on fetus				

Table 6-26 *Differentiation of Hypoglycemia, Ketoacidosis, and Hyperglycemic Hyperosmolar Nonketotic Coma (HHNK)*

	Hypoglycemia (Insulin Reaction)	Ketoacidosis (Diabetic Coma)	HHNK
Causes	Too much insulin Not enough food (delayed or missed meals) Excessive exercise or work Indigestion, diarrhea, vomiting	Too little insulin Too much or wrong kind of food Infection, injuries, illness Insufficient exercise	Abnormally high glucose levels without ketoacidosis in mild or suspected diabetic—pancreatic disorders that lower production of insulin Complication of extensive burns, excess steroids (i.e., with steroid therapy), acute stress, TPN,† hemodialysis, peritoneal dialysis
Onset	Sudden (regular insulin) Gradual (modified insulin or oral agents)	Slow (days)	Rapid if woman dehydrated

Symptomatology	Hunger
	Sweating
	Nervousness
	Weakness
	Fatigue
	Blurred or double vision
	Dizziness
	Headache (especially with NPH insulin* or PZI)
	Pallor, clammy skin
	Shallow respirations
	Normal pulse
	Laboratory values
	  Urine: negative for sugar and acetone
	  Blood glucose: 60 mg/dl or less
		Thirst
		Nausea or vomiting
		Abdominal pain
		Constipation
		Drowsiness
		Dim vision
		Increased urination
		Headache
		Flushed, dry skin
		Rapid breathing
		Weak, rapid pulse
		Acetone (fruity) breath odor
		Laboratory values
		  Urine: positive for sugar and acetone
		  Blood glucose: 250 mg/dl
			Polyuria
			Thirst (intracellular dehydration)
			Hypovolemia
			Blood serum levels
			  FBS: 600-3000 mg/dl
			  Acetone level: normal or slightly elevated
			Dry skin
			Coma, death

Nursing actions	Notify physician Give low-fat milk If orange juice is given for a fast supply of sugar, follow it later with milk Obtain blood and urine specimens for laboratory testing	Notify physician Keep woman flat in bed and warm Record intake and output Check and record vital signs	Administer insulin in line with blood glucose levels Monitor IV therapy (sodium and water deficits corrected without extreme shift of fluid into intracellular compartment with no reduction of hyperosmolarity of blood) Monitor woman for dehydration; record intake and output Check and record vital signs Notify physician of changes in symptomatology

Modified from form used at Santa Clara Valley Medical Center, San Jose, Calif.
*NPH: neutral protamine Hagedorn; PZI: protamine zinc insulin
†TPN (total parenteral nutrition) replaces the term *hyperalimentation*.

Guidelines for Client Teaching

DIABETES

ASSESSMENT

1. Pregnant woman of >25 years old.
2. Obese prepregnant and pregnant weight.
3. Glycosuria.
4. One hour blood sugar >190 mg/dl.
5. Large fetus.
6. Hydramnios.

NURSING DIAGNOSES

Knowledge deficit related to gestational diabetes.

Altered nutrition: more than body requirements related to obesity.

Altered nutrition: less than body requirements related to dysfunctional carbohydrate metabolism.

Potential for injury: mother and fetus, related to dysfunctional carbohydrate metabolism.

Potential self-care deficit related to procedures necessary to maintain euglycemia.

Fluid volume excess related to fluid retention and vascular changes.

GOALS

Short-term

Woman will learn about gestational diabetes.

Woman (couple) will learn how to test blood sugar with fingerstick.

Woman (couple) will learn how to assess glycosuria with chemstrip.

Woman (couple) will learn basics of diet management.

Woman (couple) will learn insulin administration.

Intermediate

Woman will learn to maintain euglycemia.

Woman will maintain proper nutrition and exercise.

Long-term

Woman will have a healthy baby with minimal or no problems postpartum.

REFERENCES AND TEACHING AIDS

Pamphlets from insulin manufacturers (i.e., Lilly, SKF).

Pamphlets from chemstrip and blood sugar testing apparatus manufacturers.

A-V materials on diabetes.

Chemstrips for urine.

Insulin needle, sterile water, alcohol sponges, orange or grapefruit.

Chart showing injection sites.

CONTENT/RATIONALE	TEACHING ACTIONS
To inform woman (couple) about diabetes: Discuss pathophysiology of diabetes with woman and support person.	Using a chart or A-V materials, show couple (woman) where insulin is manufactured in the body. Discuss what insulin does in carbohydrate metabolism. Show how diabetes changes this regulatory mechanism and how it effects the mother and the fetus.
Explain how the glucose gets into the urine from the bloodstream.	Demonstrate how to test a sample of woman's urine with a chemstrip. Ask for a return demonstration and observe the accuracy with which she interprets the results. Show woman how to record the results.
To discuss self-assessment: Discuss how to do the fingerstick and test it for glucose. Allow for woman to be ready to learn (demonstrate understanding and caring).	Demonstrate how to test blood for glucose level. If woman is shy about sticking her own finger, ask the support person to do a return demonstration on the woman. Show how to read the results and where to record it. If the woman is on a sliding scale of insulin, show woman (couple) how to read the scale and interpret how much insulin she should have at that time.
To teach self-administration of insulin: Explain the use of the equipment for the procedure by using the exact equipment the woman will use at home. This avoids confusion and gives the woman (couple) hands-on experience. Stress importance of accuracy. Stress importance of using correct syringe with correct insulin. Teach and stress importance of rotating sites. Current bottle of insulin can be used at room temperature, unused bottle to be kept refrigerated.	Show woman (couple) the procedure for drawing up the insulin, reading the syringe, and administering the insulin. For practice injections, use the fruit. When it comes time for the real injection, ask the woman (couple) to give a return demonstration to you while you supervise. The first injection is usually the most difficult. Nurse may have to help the woman (support person) pierce the skin.

Continued.

Guidelines for Client Teaching—cont'd

CONTENT/RATIONALE	TEACHING ACTIONS
To avoid complications through self-care:	Review adverse effects of ketoacidosis.
Review signs and symptoms of ketoacidosis. Point out that illness, especially infection, vomiting, diarrhea may precipitate ketoacidosis.	
Stress importance of continuing urine and blood testing during sick days and staying in constant contact with the physician.	Review relationship between available glucose and insulin needs.
Explain causes and dangers of hypoglycemia to woman (couple).	Review causes and dangers of hypoglycemia to woman (couple).
Describe care and treatment and prevention of hypoglycemia. List foods to take during an insulin reaction, discuss amount to take. Discuss what to do in case of insulin coma. Support person must understand what to do (Glucagon injection).	Stress importance of carrying fast-acting sugar and consuming extra carbohydrate before exercise. Stress importance of bedtime snack.
	Stress relationship between diet and exercise. Give Medic-Alert information.
Explain importance of carrying identification pointing out woman is a diabetic.	Teach role diet plays in disease management. Provide printed material for woman to take home for future reference.
Discuss diet management. Have registered dietitian (RD) see woman/couple. Reinforce information given by him/her.	
Discuss increased susceptibility to infection, eye problems, neurologic changes.	Discuss with woman importance of good skin and foot care. Stress importance of wearing proper fitting shoes, discourage extremes of temperature.
Explain role of exercise in helping to balance insulin and blood glucose.	Stress that exercise enhances use of glucose and decreases need for insulin. Talk about the exercises and activities that she is to do regularly.
Discuss exercise and activities that have been prescribed for her by the physician.	
Explain the importance of contacting her physician before any long-term travel. Review dangers of not being prepared for complications.	Stress the importance of not doing any unnecessary long-term travel. Stress importance of carrying insulin, syringes, fast-acting sugar. Wear ID bracelet and carry an exchange list for dietary needs.
Stress the need for follow-up care during this time.	Give woman (couple) appointment for next time. Write down numbers of importance for the woman (couple) and give them to her to take with her.
	Allow time for questions.

EVALUATION Woman (couple) is receptive to information presented. Competence is evident in return demonstrations and questions. Woman and fetus complete pregnancy with no adverse sequelae to diabetes mellitus.

Sample Nursing Care Plan

DIABETES MELLITUS

ASSESSMENT	NURSING DIAGNOSIS (ND)/ PLAN (P)/GOAL (G)	RATIONALE/ IMPLEMENTATION	EVALUATION
How long has woman had diabetes mellitus? Has woman administered insulin? Knowledge about diabetes. Knowledge about care needed during pregnancy to prevent sequelae for the mother and fetus. Assess feelings about diabetes.	ND: Knowledge deficit related to diabetes mellitus, its management, and potential effects on the pregnant woman and fetus. ND: Ineffective individual coping related to woman's responsibility in managing her diabetes mellitus during pregnancy. P: Provide information, be available for discussion, demonstrate, and observe return demonstration. G: Woman will learn about diabetes mellitus, its management, and potential sequelae during pregnancy. G: Woman will demonstrate technique of home monitoring tests and verbalize understanding of the results she should report. G: Woman will verbalize her concerns and feelings about her disease and its possible sequelae.	*To teach woman about diabetes mellitus, its management, and effects on pregnancy, the nurse will:* Review pathophysiology of the disease. Encourage verbalization of concerns and feelings. Assist woman in formulating questions for the physician. Clarify misconceptions. Teach home monitoring tests, demonstrate techniques, interpretation, and recording of results. (Urine test should be controlled at +1 sugar to avoid hypoglycemia, which is extremely dangerous to the fetus). Review the effects of diabetes on the pregnant woman and fetus (especially the uncontrolled diabetes sequelae). Teach (written and oral) the danger signs of diabetes and whom to notify. Stress importance of weekly prenatal visits during second half of pregnancy. Refer woman to community diabetic support group.	Woman verbalizes understanding of instruction. Woman accurately demonstrates how to perform home monitoring tests. Woman verbalizes her concerns and feelings about her disease and its possible sequelae, without undue anxiety. Woman keeps all scheduled appointments. Woman notifies caregiver if danger signs appear. Woman joins and participates in community diabetic support group.
Assess verbal and nonverbal actions regarding diabetes and pregnancy. Assess woman's support system. Note previous successful coping mechanisms.	ND: Anxiety, fear, ineffective individual coping, dysfunctional grieving, powerlessness, body image disturbance, self-esteem disturbance, altered role performance, personal identity disturbance, spiritual distress, altered family processes related to diabetes and its potential sequelae on the pregnant woman and fetus. P: Establish a therapeutic relationship, provide information, be available for discussion, and assist with problem solving.	*To assist woman in verbalizing concerns and adjusting to the strict management of her disease, the nurse will:* Provide private area for conversation. Discuss issues in an unhurried manner. Provide consistency in caregivers. Encourage verbalization of concerns and feelings. Answer questions honestly. Assist woman in formulating questions for physician. Clarify misconceptions. Offer woman choices when possible. Compliment woman on suc-	Woman verbalizes her concerns and feelings. Woman participates in her plan of care. Woman identifies her support system. Woman identifies previous successful coping mechanisms.

Continued.

Sample Nursing Care Plan—cont'd

ASSESSMENT	NURSING DIAGNOSIS (ND)/ PLAN (P)/GOAL (G)	RATIONALE/ IMPLEMENTATION	EVALUATION
	G: Woman will verbalize concerns and feelings regarding diabetes and its potential sequelae on the pregnant woman and fetus. G: Woman will identify her support system. G: Woman will identify previous successful coping mechanisms.	cessful learning, problem solving, and coping. Identify previous successful learning, problem solving, and coping. Identify with woman her support system. Involve significant others in plan of care. Refer to community diabetes support group. Refer to psychologist, clergy, social worker, etc.	
Assess knowledge regarding insulin and its administration.	ND: Knowledge deficit related to insulin effects and its administration. ND: Potential for injury related to improper insulin administration. P: Provide information and time for discussion, demonstration, and observation of return demonstration. G: Woman will learn the purpose and effects of insulin in the body. G: Woman will administer insulin to herself correctly.	*To teach woman about insulin, its effects on the body, and proper administration, the nurse will:* Explain insulin's effect in the body. Review peak action of insulin and signs of hypoglycemia. Stress importance of administration of correct dose with correct syringe. Demonstrate correct withdrawal and administration of insulin. Explain importance of site rotation and identify the sites that can be used. Teach proper techniques of insulin storage. Monitor woman's self-administration of insulin until techniques are learned and understood. Explain why insulin needs will be higher during the third trimester.	Woman learns the purpose and effect of insulin. Woman administers her own insulin properly. Woman understands changing insulin needs during pregnancy.
Assess knowledge of hyperglycemia.	ND: Knowledge deficit related to hyper- or hypoglycemia. ND: Potential for injury related to hyper- or hypoglycemia to the pregnant woman and fetus. P: Provide information to woman conducive to discussion for woman and other family members. G: Woman will verbalize the signs and symptoms of hyper- or hypoglycemia. G: Woman will seek medical attention when dan-	*To teach woman about hyperglycemia, the nurse will:* Explain that illness, infection, vomiting, and diarrhea can precipitate ketoacidosis. Encourage woman to call physician when illness occurs and continue to administer insulin. Teach danger signs of ketoacidosis.	Woman learns the signs and symptoms of hyperglycemia. Woman verbalizes danger signs and whom to notify if they occur. Woman notifies caregiver promptly if danger signs appear. Woman experiences no episodes of hyperglycemia.

Sample Nursing Care Plan—cont'd

ASSESSMENT	NURSING DIAGNOSIS (ND)/ PLAN (P)/GOAL (G)	RATIONALE/ IMPLEMENTATION	EVALUATION
	ger signs and symptoms occur. G: Woman will use preventive measures to avoid hyper- and hypoglycemia.		
Assess knowledge of hypoglycemia, its signs and symptoms, and its treatment. Assess knowledge of preventive measures for hypoglycemia.		*To teach woman about hypoglycemia, the nurse will:* Teach signs and symptoms of hypoglycemia. Review causes and dangers of insulin reaction. Stress importance of carrying fast-acting sugar when traveling and of having milk on hand at home. Review relationship of exercise and diet. Explain importance of seeking medical attention for hypoglycemia because of its dangerous effects on self and fetus. Give Medic-Alert information and encourage woman to wear bracelet or necklace. Review the signs of hypo- and hyperglycemia with significant others and who to notify when danger signs occur.	Woman verbalizes signs and symptoms of hypoglycemia. Woman carries supply of fast-acting sugar and verbalizes having milk on hand at home. Woman wears Medic-Alert bracelet at all times. Woman experiences no episodes of hypoglycemia. Family verbalizes knowledge of signs of hypoglycemia and its treatment.
Review knowledge of diabetic diet. Assess cultural and financial influences on food served. Who prepares the meals? Who buys the food? Woman's likes/dislikes.	ND: Knowledge deficit related to the diabetic diet and its importance to a woman with diabetes during pregnancy. ND: Altered nutrition: less or more than body requirements, related to diabetes and pregnancy. P: Provide information and climate conducive to discussion. G: Woman will learn about the diabetic diet and verbalize the importance of adhering to its protocol during pregnancy.	*To teach the woman about diabetes diet management during pregnancy, the nurse will:* Consider cultural and financial implications when planning teaching. Ascertain type of diet woman is to follow at home. Refer to registered dietitian (RD). Explain importance of a balanced diet. Encourage woman to design sample menus. Stress importance to maintain or achieve appropriate weight and pattern of weight gain during pregnancy.	Woman verbalizes understanding of instruction. Woman gains weight according to protocol for the pregnant woman with diabetes. Woman implements diet prescribed by and developed with caregiver.
Intranatal: Perform assessments for normal laboring woman. Assess for hypoglycemia.	ND: Potential for injury related to hypoglycemia. ND: Potential for injury related to preeclampsia.	*To monitor woman and fetus for signs of labor complications the nurse will:*	Woman is monitored and treated promptly for preeclampsia and hypoglycemia.

Continued.

Sample Nursing Care Plan—cont'd

ASSESSMENT	NURSING DIAGNOSIS (ND)/ PLAN (P)/GOAL (G)	RATIONALE/ IMPLEMENTATION	EVALUATION
Assess for signs of pre-eclampsia. Assess fetal monitor strip. Assess anxiety level. Assess for excessive uterine size associated with hydramnios and fetal macrosomia. Assess for dyspnea and supine hypotension related to excessive uterine size.	ND: Anxiety related to labor. ND: Altered (cardiopulmonary) tissue perfusion related to supine hypotension. P: Monitor maternal-fetal well-being, prevent supine hypotension, and identify and treat complications promptly. G: Woman will be monitored closely and treated for signs of hypoglycemia, preeclampsia, and supine hypotension. G: Fetus will be monitored closely for signs of distress.	Monitor vital signs, especially blood pressure, frequently. Monitor and report signs and symptoms of pre-eclampsia and hypoglycemia. Evaluate and record labor pattern. Continuously monitor fetal heart rate (FHR) and report fetal distress. Monitor IV fluids of 10% dextrose in water and insulin as ordered; titrate infusion to frequent blood glucose determinations to maintain euglycemia. Monitor the administration of oxytocin for induction as ordered. Provide supportive labor nursing, which is especially important to prevent hypoglycemia secondary to anxiety. Prepare for induction or cesarean delivery (fetal distress, fetopelvic disproportion, lack of labor progression). Alert pediatrician and nursery personnel.	Supine hypotension is avoided. Euglycemia is maintained. Woman remains free of anxiety. Woman experiences no adverse sequelae to fluid therapy and oxytocin induction or augmentation of labor. Fetus remains free from distress as indicated by FHR.
Postnatal: Perform normal postpartum assessment. Note frequent blood and urine glucose levels. Note signs and symptoms of hypo- or hyperglycemia. Assess signs and symptoms of hemorrhage and infection.	ND: Potential for injury related to fluctuating blood glucose levels after delivery. ND: Potential for injury related to complications of involution (hemorrhage, infection), or postpartum appearance of preeclampsia. P: Monitor woman's progress, provide information, and be available for discussion. G: Woman's blood glucose level will be monitored closely for initial 24-48 hours postdelivery and remain within normal limits. G: Woman will progress through normal involution without complication.	*To monitor and treat womans' fluctuating glucose levels, the nurse will:* Perform frequent fractional urine tests. Obtain blood for glucose level as ordered. Monitor foods and fluids taken. Evaluate for signs and symptoms of hypo- or hyperglycemia. Adjust insulin intake according to protocol ordered. Explain the need to triple caloric intake and decrease insulin by one-half to successfully produce breast milk. If mother develops acetonuria, discard her breast milk until resolved. Explain that hypoglycemia decreases milk production.	Woman's blood glucose stabilizes within normal limits; woman experiences minimum or no sequelae from hypo- or hyperglycemia. Woman remains free of hemorrhage, infection, or preeclampsia. Woman verbalizes understanding of instruction.

Sample Nursing Care Plan—cont'd

ASSESSMENT	NURSING DIAGNOSIS (ND)/ PLAN (P)/GOAL (G)	RATIONALE/ IMPLEMENTATION	EVALUATION
		Counsel woman to eat every meal on time even if it means others must wait. *To monitor involution, the nurse will:* See postpartum sample care *To monitor involution, the nurse will:* See postpartum sample care plan, pp. 179-183.	Woman progresses through involution without complication.

Summary of Nursing Actions

DIABETES MELLITUS

I. Goals
  A. For the mother: the woman and pregnancy suffer no adverse sequelae to diabetes mellitus
  B. For the fetus or newborn: the fetus or newborn suffers no adverse sequelae to diabetes mellitus
  C. For the family: the family copes with the complication successfully and learns ways to prevent progression of the disease. If the fetus or newborn is lost, the family copes successfully with the loss.
II. Priorities
  A. The woman and family become active participants in self-care.
  B. Gestational diabetes mellitus is identified and treatment begun promptly.
  C. Euglycemia is maintained.
III. Assessment
  A. Antepartum period
    1. Interview/record
      a. Existence of insulin-dependent diabetes mellitus
      b. Presence of factors suggesting pregnancy at risk for gestational diabetes mellitus
      c. Knowledge of disease and its management
      d. Woman's and family's response to disease and its management
      e. Woman's and family's need for referral to social services (housekeeping aid, financial assistance, peer support group)
      f. Success with home monitoring and management of the condition
    2. Physical examination
      a. Symptomatology of diabetes mellitus and its sequelae
      b. Diabetic complications, e.g., hypoglycemia, hyperglycemia, ketosis, ketoacidosis, glycosuria (Table 6-33)
      c. Obstetric conditions complicating diabetes, e.g., nausea or vomiting, PIH

      d. Associated conditions complicating pregnancy, e.g., infection
      e. Fetal well-being: fundal height, nonstress test ([NST, see guide for interpretation of NST, p. 196], fetal activity determination [FAD]), and contraction stress test (CST, see guide for interpretation of CST, p. 195)
    3. Laboratory tests
      a. Blood tests (Table 6-32)
      b. Urine tests for diabetic status, urinary traction infections (UTIs), fetal well-being (estriols)
  B. Intranatal period
    1. Observe woman for hypoglycemia: palpitation, tachycardia, hunger, weakness, sweating, tremor, pallor.
    2. Observe woman for preeclampsia.
    3. Monitor urine for amount and presence of protein and glucose.
    4. Monitor intravenous infusions: insulin, oxytocin.
    5. Culture urine following clean-catch collection for asymptomatic urinary tract infection.
    6. Monitor labor.
      a. Monitor induction: maternal/fetal responses.
      b. Use electronic fetal monitor if available.
      c. Assess amount and character of amniotic fluid.
  C. Postnatal period
    1. During first 24 to 48 hours after delivery insulin requirements fluctuate rapidly. Termination of pregnancy reverses gestation-induced endocrine changes: high serum blood glucose level, elevated levels of human growth hormone (HGH) and its potentiator, human placental lactogen (HPL).
      a. Do frequent fractional urine tests.
      b. Monitor foods and fluids taken.
      c. Assess woman for clinical manifestations of high or low serum glucose levels.
    2. Monitor vital signs, amount of bleeding, uterine

Continued.

Summary of Nursing Actions—cont'd

contractility, output, and so on as per usual post-delivery routine.

3. Assess woman's and family's reaction to experience, especially if fetal-neonatal death occurs or infant is malformed or at risk.

IV. Potential nursing diagnoses
 A. Anxiety
 B. Fear
 C. Ineffective family coping: compromised
 D. Ineffective individual coping
 E. Anticipatory grieving
 F. Altered family process
 G. Altered health maintenance
 H. Potential for injury
 I. Knowledge deficit
 J. Noncompliance (specify)
 K. Altered nutrition: more or less than body requirements
 L. Powerlessness
 M. Feeding self care deficit
 N. Body image disturbance
 O. Toileting self care deficit
 P. Dressing/grooming self care deficit
 Q. Bathing/hygiene self care deficit
 R. Personal identity disturbance
 S. Self esteem disturbance: situational low self esteem
 T. Spiritual distress
 U. Impaired home maintenance management

V. Plan/implementation
 A. Antepartum period
  1. Ascertain level of understanding and knowledge of client and family and receptiveness to teaching.
  2. Assess feelings about diabetes.
  3. Discuss pathophysiology with client or significant other.
  4. Check with physician about S/A method client will do at home.
  5. Teach, demonstrate techniques, interpret results (second voiding), and record results.
  6. Supervise client or significant other.
  7. Clinitest tablets—emphasize the following:
   a. Pass-through phase: 20 ml (4 tsp)—orange→muddy brown→orange.
   b. Wait 15 sec before shaking for final reading.
   c. Do not touch tablets.
   d. Store tablets in cool, dark place.
  8. Ketodiastix—emphasize the following:
   a. Read acetone after 15 sec
   b. Read sugar after 30 sec
  9. Determine correct injection technique (check angle used).
   a. □ 45-degree angle
   b. □ 90-degree angle
  10. Teach strict aseptic technique for withdrawal and administration of insulin.
  11. Stress importance of giving and drawing up accurate dose.
  12. Stress importance of using correct syringe with correct insulin.

  13. Have client or significant other practice drawing up with normal saline and giving injection to an orange for a day.
  14. Teach importance of rotation and sites available.
  15. Woman to give own injection with RN supervision remainder of hospital stay.
  16. Use U100 insulin unless ordered otherwise.
  17. Stress that current bottle of insulin being used can be stored at room temperature; unused bottle in refrigerator.
  18. Point out that illness, especially infection, vomiting and diarrhea, may precipitate ketoacidosis.
  19. Review causes and dangers of insulin reaction with client or significant other
   a. See Table 6-26, "Differentiation of Hypoglycemia, Ketoacidosis, and Hyperglycemic Hyperosmolar Nonketotic Coma (HHNK)"
   b. See Guidelines for Client Teaching, "Diabetes," pp. 227-228

 B. Prenatal period
  1. First half of pregnancy
   a. Elicit woman's and family's cooperation in management of diabetes and pregnancy; make sure she keeps appointments and follows up on missed appointments, performs daily urine tests and/or blood glucose determinations accurately, maintains strict dietary control, gets adequate rest and exercise, and receives early treatment for infection and symptoms of insulin shock (reaction).
   b. Reinforce need for keeping the urine test at 1 + sugar level (to be assured of mild hyperglycemia and therefore of a control over hypoglycemia and hyperinsulinemia, which are very dangerous to the embryo and fetus). (Urine should be freshly voided.)
   c. If complications develop, refer woman to physician.
  2. Second half of pregnancy
   a. Encourage visits every week to supervise management.
   b. Keep woman and family informed; reinforce physician's explanations (e.g., that insulin needs are usually higher during the third trimester).
   c. Maintenance: NPH until delivery.
   d. Fractional urine specimens tested four times daily as necessary. Woman's diet may need adjustment for rapid growth needs of fetus. Prepare for tests (Table 6-25).
   e. Observe the woman closely during teaching sessions to see how well she is dealing with what is being taught. Encourage woman's and family's expression of feelings regarding self and infant.
   f. If the woman is hospitalized, provide care as appropriate for hospitalization (e.g., NST). Provide diversional activities for woman if appropriate.

Summary of Nursing Actions—cont'd

C. Intranatal period
1. The physician and nurse keep woman and family informed of treatment and fetal status.
2. Do not allow woman to consume anything by mouth. Monitor intravenous fluids per order for the following:
   a. For induction (with oxytocin [Pitocin]).
   b. 10% dextrose in water and insulin to meet woman's caloric and insulin needs for work of labor.
3. Provide supportive labor nursing, which is especially important to prevent hypoglycemia and acidosis from anxiety.
4. Prepare for induction or cesarean birth (e.g., in case of fetal distress, fetopelvic disproportion, or lack of response to induction).
5. Alert pediatrician and nursery personnel.

D. Postnatal period
1. Adjust insulin intake (usually regular insulin) according to protocol ordered. Woman may need no insulin for first 24 hours to 48 hours. Progress to NPH according to physician's orders. Allow woman to take over insulin injections when she desires.
2. Provide postdelivery nursing care (after vaginal or cesarean birth) according to routine.
3. Provide supportive care for woman and family after fetal/neonatal death or if neonate is malformed or at risk.
4. Keep woman and family informed of her status and infant's condition.
5. Give instructions on breast-feeding:
   a. Caloric intake and insulin requirements will need adjusting; for example, women requiring large doses of insulin may need to triple caloric intake and decrease insulin by one half because of antidiabetogenic action (free glucose is used in production of lactose).
   b. If mother develops acetonuria, discontinue breast-feeding (pump breasts and discard milk) and contact physician for supervision.
   c. If mother becomes hypoglycemic from lack of food or anxiety or other reason, her epinephrine level increases, which decreases her milk supply and inhibits the letdown reflex.
6. Counsel woman regarding personal care: she *must* eat on time even if it means that others must wait; it will take more energy to add care of the new baby to her previous routine.
7. Couple may request genetic counseling. Infant will not necessarily acquire the disease.
8. Counsel couple on contraception, sterilization, and planning for future pregnancies.

VI. Evaluation
A. Antepartum period
1. Ability to cope with diagnosis—verbalizes reactions and comprehension
2. Verbalizes knowledge of normal and altered use of insulin and glucose in body.

3. Verbalizes reasons for testing and significance of results
4. Demonstrates accurate testing of urine ac and hs or as ordered (second voiding)
5. Records results and interprets each test; follows urine testing schedule without being reminded (keep at bedside)
6. Demonstrates correct care of equipment
7. Demonstrates correct withdrawal and administration of insulin to self
8. Verbalizes importance to site rotation and identifies sites used
9. Verbalizes proper techniques of insulin storage
10. Woman gives own injection daily with RN supervision
11. Explains signs and symptoms, describes care and treatment of hypoglycemia, hyperglycemia, and ketoacidosis (Table 6-33)
12. Carries diabetic identification

B. Prenatal period
1. The woman and family understand the disease process and are informed about and willing to participate actively in its management.
2. Adverse effects of associated problems (i.e., changes in glucose tolerance, alterations in insulin metabolism, and use and increased tendency to ketosis) have a minimal effect on the mother and fetus.
3. The woman suffers no sequelae of diabetes (e.g., nephropathy, retinopathy) or worsening of preexisting complications.
4. The woman suffers no related complications during pregnancy: hyperemesis gravidarum, preeclampsia-eclampsia, hydramnios.
5. Through home monitoring of blood glucose and management of diet, exercise, and insulin, the woman maintains euglycemia.
6. Verbalizes importance of consultation with a physician before travel and obtaining necessary supplies.
7. Verbalizes reason for carrying insulin on self.
8. Discusses realistically exercise and activity to be maintained and reason for regular exercise.

C. Intranatal period
1. Woman suffers no related complications during labor, e.g., vena cava hypotensive syndrome, dystocia, energy/insulin imbalance.
2. Parent-newborn attachment occurs; or if newborn exhibits a disorder or dies, the grieving process is initiated.

D. Postnatal period
1. Woman suffers no related complications during the early postpartum period, e.g., wide variations in blood glucose, PIH, hemorrhage (especially after delivery of large baby or polyhydramnios).
2. Parent-child attachment occurs; or if newborn exhibits a disorder or dies, the grieving process is initiated.

Hyperemesis Gravidarum

Hyperemesis gravidarum is excessive vomiting during pregnancy, and it can lead to dehydration and starvation. In about 1 of every 1000 pregnant women, severe intractable emesis requires hospitalization. The definitive cause of hyperemesis during pregnancy is still unknown and is subject to debate. Some theorize that it is psychologic and caused by the unstable woman's reaction to pregnancy; others describe it as a hormonal problem, since it surfaces in unusual pregnancy conditions such as multiple gestation, hydatidiform mole, or an elevated T_4.

Regardless of the cause, nurses play an important role in the care of women suffering from this disorder. The following sample nursing care plan and summary of nursing actions provide a basis for management of the woman with hyperemesis gravidarum.

Sample Nursing Care Plan

HYPEREMIS GRAVIDARUM

ASSESSMENT	NURSING DIAGNOSIS (ND)/ PLAN (P)/GOAL (G)	RATIONALE/ IMPLEMENTATION	EVALUATION
Assess for signs and symptoms: Excessive vomiting. Dehydration: rapid weight loss, poor skin turgor. Metabolic acidosis: headache, mental dullness, hyperpneic leading to disorientation, stupor, coma, and death. Starvation: hypoproteinemia and hypovitaminosis.	ND: Potential fluid volume deficit and impaired gas exchange related to vomiting and metabolic acidosis. ND: Altered nutrition: less than body requirements related to nausea and vomiting. P: Maintain constant vigilence for excessive vomiting. G: Woman's vomiting episodes are eliminated, fluid and electrolyte balance returns, and adequate nutrition is assured.	*To support women's physiologic processes, the nurse will:* Assist physician or initiate intravenous fluid therapy per physician's order. Give antiemetics as ordered. Maintain woman NPO as ordered. Support woman's nutritional needs through TPN, addition of nutrients (vitamins, etc.) into peripheral or central lines. Keep room clean and fresh with adequate ventilation. When oral foods/fluids are allowed, provide small amounts of attractively served foods to fit her preferences.	Hyperemesis gravidarum abates and does not recur. Fluid/electrolyte balance is restored. Adequate nutrition is reestablished.
Assess woman's affect, emotional state, and support system.	ND: Potential ineffective family or individual coping related to age, life-style, pregnancy, hyperemesis, or other disturbance. P: Assist with identification of etiologic factor(s) and with therapeutic management to meet her emotional/psychologic needs. G: Etiologic factor(s) is (are) identified and appropriate therapy initiated.	*To support woman's emotional/psychologic processes, the nurse will:* Provide safe, confidential, private space for identifying and discussing concerns. Mobilize support group/ person of her choice. Maintain 'no visitor' policy or monitor her visitors, prn. Keep woman and family informed of maternal and fetal status.	Woman is able to identify and discuss her concerns and begin to problem-solve solutions. Support system is mobilized, it is determined whether etiologic factors had an emotional or psychologic basis. Woman states she felt comfortable with and part of the team.

Sample Nursing Care Plan—Cont'd

ASSESSMENT	NURSING DIAGNOSIS (ND)/ PLAN (P)/GOAL (G)	RATIONALE/ IMPLEMENTATION	EVALUATION
Assess for etiologic factors.	ND: Potential fluid volume deficit and impaired gas exchange related to persistence of etiologic factors. P: Assess collaboratively with appropriate team members (e.g. endocrinologist). G: Etiologic factor(s) is (are) identified and managed so that hyperemesis does not recur.	*To assist with assessment the nurse will:* Follow-through with collection of specimens and prescribed therapies. Carefully document woman's responses.	Etiologic factor(s) is (are) identified, appropriate therapy is instituted, and hyperemesis does not recur.
Assess knowledge and understanding of the disorder.	NP: Knowledge deficit related to condition, its cause, and management. P: Meet woman's knowledge needs. G: Woman states she understands condition.	*To meet woman's knowledge needs, the nurse will:* Provide content in amount and manner to meet individual woman's needs. Provide sufficient time for discussion, repetition, etc.	Woman states content accurately, and, after discharge, reports early signs/symptoms of recurrence immediately.
Assess for severe (rare) complications of jaundice, hemorrhage, fetal distress.	ND: Potential for injury related to severe complications. P: Maintain careful surveillance; report signs, symptoms immediately. G: Woman and fetus suffer no adverse sequelae.	*To prevent progression of severe complications, the nurse will:* Remain vigilant for complications. Report findings immediately and initiate therapy as ordered.	Woman and fetus suffer no adverse sequelae related to hyperemesis gravidarum or its management.

Summary of Nursing Actions

HYPEREMESIS GRAVIDARUM

1. Goals
   A. For the mother: a physiologically safe and psychologically satisfying pregnancy
   B. For the fetus: a physiologically safe intrauterine environment
   C. For the family: effective family coping with the condition
II. Priorities
   A. Prevention of dehydration and starvation
   B. Support of family coping
III. Assessment
   A. Amount of vomiting
   B. Dietary progress and daily weight, fluid intake, and urinary output
   C. Woman's affect and response to home environment and pregnancy
   D. Fetal heart rate and growth of fetus
   E. Jaundice (a rare occurrence)
   F. Abnormal bleeding, for example, from mucosal surfaces (a rare occurrence)
   G. Intravenous line for infiltration, etc.
IV. Potential nursing diagnoses
   A. Anxiety
   B. Fear
   C. Ineffective individual coping
   D. Ineffective family coping: compromised
   E. Altered family processes
   F. Potential fluid volume deficit
   G. Knowledge deficit
   H. Altered nutrition: less than body requirements
   I. Powerlessness
   J. Body image disturbance
   K. Self esteem disturbance: situational low self esteem
   L. Altered pole performance
   M. Parental role conflict
   N. Personal identity disturbance
   O. Pain
   P. Altered health maintenance
   Q. Impaired home maintenance management

V. Plan/implementation
   A. Management of hyperemesis gravidarum includes hospitalization in a pleasant, well-ventilated room.
   B. Parenteral fluids, electrolytes, sedatives, and vitamins will be required.
      1. For the first 48 hours parenteral fluids are used to maintain hydration and restore fluid and electrolyte balance.
      2. Cautious resumption of a dry diet in six small feedings with clear liquids an hour after meals generally is acceptable.
   C. Accept woman's behavior in gentle, nonjudgmental manner.
   D. Encourage woman to discuss her feelings, emphasizing her complete recovery. Keep conversational topics pleasant.
   E. Keep family informed as to progress. (Family may feel anger or hurt at being excluded from visiting, as well as contempt for wife and mother.)
   F. Maintain excellent daily hygiene.
   G. If additional psychotherapy is indicated, the physician will give woman referrals.
   H. Report and record fetal heart rate abnormalities, maternal jaundice, and bleeding from mucosal surfaces.
   I. Change intravenous tubing per hospital protocol to prevent infection. Reinsert intravenous line at another site if infiltration or venous thrombosis occurs.
VI. Evaluation
   A. Severe vomiting episodes are resolved; fluid and electrolyte homeostasis is achieved, and weight gain occurs.
   B. No adverse sequelae, maternal or fetal, develop as a result of condition.
   C. If medical treatment is unsuccessful, surgical intervention to terminate pregnancy is undertaken.
   D. Woman comes to terms with self, pregnancy, and life situation.

LABOR AND DELIVERY AT RISK

Complications during birth can result in both physical and emotional sequelae. Prolonged and difficult labor is physically debilitating at best. If remedial measures are not instituted promptly and expertly, the mother and fetus may sustain injury or die. Many complications can be diagnosed before labor begins, and preparation can limit their effects. Others are sudden, and the safety of the mother and infant depend on the judgement of health care personnel.

Dystocia and Prolonged Labor

Dystocia is as difficult birth as opposed to easy (normal) birth, or eutocia. Dystocia results from differences in the normal relationships between any of the five essential factors of labor. This section presents the various types of conditions that cause dystocia.

Prolonged labor is usually defined as active labor that continues more than 20 hours. The nurse should carefully monitor patterns of labor and report deviations to the physician or midwife.

Nursing care is similar for both of these problems. Uterine contractions may be augmented either by an amniotomy or by the administration of oxytocics; or cesarean delivery may be determined to be the best course of action. Nursing actions for both of these strategies are presented.

Table 6-27   *Pelvic Dystocia*

Factor	Inlet Contracture	Midpelvic Contracture	Outlet Contracture
Description	Diagonal conjugate less than 11.5 cm	Sum of interischial spinous and posterior sagittal diameters of midpelvis 13.5 cm or less Interischial spinous diameter less than 9 cm	Interischial spinous diameter 8 cm or less Outlet contraction alone, without midplane contraction, rare
Change in pattern of labor	Rupture of membranes, early, spontaneous Dilation of cervix slows or ceases Descent does not occur	Descent arrested (transverse arrest of the fetal head); fetal head cannot undergo internal rotation and descend Contractions decrease in frequency and intensity Dilation of cervix slows	Descent arrested
Potential maternal effects	Intrauterine infection Rupture of abnormally thinned lower segment of uterus Pathologic retraction ring develops Formation of fistulas Psychologic trauma from difficult delivery	Rupture of uterus Exhaustion Psychologic trauma from difficult delivery	Extensive perineal lacerations Exhaustion
Potential fetal effects	Fetal asphyxia Fetal and neonatal death Excessive molding of fetal head Prolapse of cord	Fetal asphyxia Fetal death Excessive molding of head	Fetal asphyxia Fetal death
Medical management	Cesarean delivery if safe vaginal delivery not possible	Cesarean delivery if fetal head cannot pass obstruction Forceps delivery if fetal head passes obstruction (head descends, perineum bulges, vertex is visible) Vacuum extractor when cervix fully dilated	Extensive mediolateral episiotomy

LABOR PATTERNS IN NORMAL AND PROLONGED LABOR

Normal Labor

1. Dilation: continues
   a. Latent phase: <4 cm and low slope
   b. Active phase: >5 cm or high slope
   c. Deceleration phase: ≥9 cm
2. Descent: active at ≥9 cm dilation
3. Normal labor progresses rapidly; multiparas faster than nulliparas

Prolonged Labor Patterns	Nulliparas	Multiparas
1. Prolonged latent phase	>20 hr	>14 hr
2. Protracted active-phase dilation	<1.2 cm/hr	<1.5 cm/hr
3. Secondary arrest: no change for	≥2 hr	≥2 hr
4. Prolonged deceleration phase	>3 hr	>1 hr
5. Protracted descent	<1 cm/hr	<2 cm/hr
6. Arrest of descent	≥1 hr	≥½ hr

Table 6-28   *Dysfunctional Labor: Primary and Secondary Powers*

Factor	Hypotonic Uterine Dysfunction	Hypertonic Uterine Dysfunction	Inadequate Voluntary Expulsive Forces
Description	Cause may be contracture and fetal malposition, overextension of uterus (twins), or unknown (primary powers)	Usually occurs before 4 cm dilation; cause not yet known, may be related to fear and tension (primary powers)	Involves abdominal and levator ani muscles Occurs in second stage of labor; cause may be related to conduction anesthesia, heavy analgesia, paralysis, or intense pain with contractions (secondary powers)
Change in pattern of progress	Contractions decrease in frequency and intensity Uterus easily indentable even at peak of contraction Uterus relaxed between contractions (normal)	Pain out of proportion to intensity of contraction Pain out of proportion to effectiveness of contraction in effacing and dilating the cervix Contractions increase in frequency Contractions uncoordinated Uterus is contracted between contractions (basal hypertonus), cannot be indented.	No voluntary urge to push or bear down
Potential maternal effects	Infection Exhaustion Psychologic trauma	Loss of control related to intensity of pain and lack of progress Exhaustion	Spontaneous vaginal delivery prevented
Potential fetal effects	Fetal infection Fetal and neonatal death	Fetal asphyxia with meconium aspiration	Fetal asphyxia
Medical management	Oxytocic stimulation of labor Prostaglandin stimulation of labor	Analgesic (morphine, meperidine) if membranes not ruptured or fetopelvic disproportion not present Relief of pain permits mother to rest; when she awakens, normal uterine activity may begin	Coach mother in bearing down with contractions Analgesia to counteract pain Cesarean delivery only if fetal distress

Table 6-29   *Dystocia of Fetal Origin*

Factor	Fetopelvic Disproportion	Malposition	Malpresentation: Breech
Description	Fetal macrosomia with normal or small pelvis Fetal anomaly	Persistent occiput posterior position (OP) Leopold's manuevers reveal small parts against abdominal wall Abdominal contours differ Vaginal examination: the cervix may need to be fully dilated before examiner can feel direction of suture lines in relation to fontanels	Related to prematurity; most infants assume a longitudinal lie with vertex presenting at term Related to multiple fetuses, hydramnios, oligohydramnios, fetal or maternal anomalies Breech presentations revealed by abdominal and vaginal examinations, x-ray films, and sonography Breech presentation occurs in four types
Change in pattern of progress	Engagement does not occur Descent does not occur Uterus unusual size or contour Membranes rupture early Cervical dilation slows Contractions decrease in frequency and intensity	Contractions are diminished in frequency and intensity Backache is accentuated Cervical dilation slows Descent is delayed Second stage of labor may be prolonged	Heart sounds loudest slightly above the umbilicus Labor not unduly prolonged Spontaneous complete expulsion seldom successfully accomplished Aftercoming head does not have time to mold during descent and therefore expulsion may be prevented
Potential maternal effects	Infection Development of pathologic ring Rupture of uterus Vaginal fistulas	Exhaustion Increased sensitivity to pain Extension of episiotomy Psychologic trauma from prolonged labor	Morbidity and mortality increased as result of operative delivery including cesarean delivery
Potential fetal effects	Infection Prolapse of cord Excessive molding of the head; may result in intracranial hemorrhage	Fetal asphyxia	Prematurity Congenital anomalies Birth trauma, asphyxia from cord compression, or placental separation during birth Fetal death Infant has little molding of the head
Medical management	Cesarean delivery if vaginal delivery poses a potential threat to mother or fetus	Conservative approach followed as most of fetuses (70%) in OP position: • Rotate spontaneously to an anterior position and deliver spontaneously • May deliver in the face-to-pubes position if posterior position persists Mediolateral episiotomy done to permit manual or forceps rotation Low forceps delivery of vertex may be needed Cesarean delivery if head does not engage, rotation cannot be accomplished, or face-to-pubes delivery not possible	External version may be attempted after 34 weeks' gestation Extra sterile towels and **Piper forceps** are added to delivery table for mechanism of labor Cesarean delivery is commonly used in nulliparas and in multiparas with fetuses estimated to be larger than 3360 g (7¼ lb) if labor is ineffective or when hazardous complications arise

Procedure 6-2

INDUCTION OF LABOR

DEFINITION

An obstetric procedure in which labor is started or augmented artificially by means of amniotomy or administration of oxytocics.

PURPOSE

To initiate or augment the uterine contractions of labor.

EQUIPMENT

Oxytocin (Pitocin)* or synthetic oxytocin (Syntocinon); container of 1000 ml 5% dextrose in water or normal sterile saline for oxytocin solution; container of 1000 ml 5% dextrose in water or normal sterile saline for piggyback set-up (maintenance IV); infusion pump (IVAC) or standard pump (Harvard); amnihook or Allis clamp (for AROM); bedpan or fracture pan.

NURSING ACTIONS	RATIONALE
Fetal stress: fetal bradycardia, tachycardia, or heart irregularity (oxytocin is stopped and 5% dextrose in water is infused).	
Wash hands before and after touching woman and equipment. Glove.	To prevent nosocomial infection and to implement universal precautions.
Apply fetal and maternal electronic monitor before beginning induction.	To obtain constant, accurate recording of FHR and contractions.
	To obtain baseline information.
Explain technique, rationale, and reactions to expect:	To promote cooperation of woman and family.
IV fluid route and rate: what "piggyback" is for.	To lessen anxiety over technique.
Reasons for use: induce labor, improve labor.	To assure woman and family of careful monitoring.
	To prepare woman and family for chances of success.
Discuss:	To prepare woman for sensations. Preparation dispels fear of the unknown.
Reactions to expect—nature of contractions: Intensity of contraction increases more rapidly, holds the peak longer, and ends more quickly. The contractions will begin to come regularly and more often.	
Monitoring to expect:	
Maternal: blood pressure, pulse, uterine contractions, uterine tone.	To reassure woman of continued care.
Fetal: heart rate, activity	
Success to expect: reaffirm physician's explanation that if inertia is not overcome in 8 hours or less (using 5 U of oxytocin), the chance of success is minimal.	To help woman orient herself in time; to know an end point.
Position woman in left lateral position.	To maximize placental perfusion and oxygenation of fetus.
Prepare solutions and administer according to prescribed orders with pump delivery system:	To promote safety, a piggyback setup is used; this permits the induction solution to be stopped while the vein remains open with the second solution.
Set up infusion pump and solution.	
Flag solution containing oxytocin (Pitocin) with a red label.	
Connect piggyback solution to IV line.	
Begin induction with 1 mU/min (Appendix B).	To ensure that the least amount of medication necessary is used for a favorable outcome.
Increase dose arithmetically by 2 mU increments (e.g., 1,3, and 5 mU/min at 15 min intervals) (Appendix A).	To determine minimum amount of medication necessary for success.

*If the pregnancy is complicated by diabetes mellitus, higher doses of oxytocin are usually needed.

INDICATIONS FOR CESAREAN DELIVERY AND MATERNAL AND FETAL EFFECTS

INDICATIONS FOR CESAREAN DELIVERY	EFFECTS OF CESAREAN DELIVERY	TYPE OF UTERINE INCISIONS
Maternal	**Maternal**	**Classic Cesarean Incision**

1. Fetopelvic disproportion
2. Previous cesarean delivery
3. Breech presentation
4. Medical complications (e.g., PIH)
5. Placental abnormalities (i.e., placenta previa, premature separation of the placenta)
6. Infections (e.g., herpesvirus, type 2)
7. Trauma to the pelvis
	1. Mortality (1:1000) from
	  a. Anesthesia
	  b. Severe sepsis
	  c. Thromboembolic episodes
	2. Morbidity higher than with vaginal delivery because of:
	  a. Infection
	  b. Injury to the urinary tract
		Incision is vertical through skin and vertical through contractile portion of uterus. It is used when rapid delivery is necessary, in shoulder presentation, and in placenta previa when the placenta is implanted on the anterior wall. Classic cesarean delivery is useful when general anesthesia is unavailable, since this operation can be carried out with local infiltration anesthesia. The potential for rupture of the scar (1% to 2%) with a subsequent pregnancy and the frequent occurrence of small bowel adhesions to the anterior suture line have limited the use of this type of cesarean delivery.

Fetal	**Fetal**	**Lower Segment Cesarean Incision**

1. Fetal hypoxia
2. Prolapse of cord
3. Breech presentations
4. Malpresentations (e.g., shoulder)
5. Fetal anomalies (e.g., hydrocephalus)
	1. Mortality has declined where cesarean delivery is used in conjunction with improved perinatal care
	2. Morbidity
	  a. Birth trauma is reduced
	  b. Reduced morbidity in breech deliveries, transverse lie of the fetus, and placenta previa
		Lower segment cesarean delivery is possible by means of a vertical incision or a transverse incision. The transverse incision is the preferred method. It "(1) results in less blood loss, (2) is easier to repair, (3) is located at a site least likely to rupture with extrusion of the fetus into the abdominal cavity during a subsequent pregnancy, and (4) does not promote adherence of bowel or omentum to the incisional line" (Pritchard, McDonald, and Gant, 1985).

Table 6-30 *Bishop's Scale*

	Score*			
	0	1	2	3
Dilation (cm)	0	1-2	3-4	5-6
Effacement (%)	0-30	40-50	60-70	80
Station (cm)	−3	−2	−1	+1
Cervical consistency	Firm	Medium	Soft	
Fetal position	Posterior	Midline	Anterior	

*Parous woman can be induced at score of 5; nulliparous woman, at score of 7.

The *preparation* of the woman for cesarean birth is the same for either elective or emergency surgery. The obstetrician discusses the need for the cesarean delivery and the prognosis for mother and infant with the woman and her family. The anesthesiologist assesses the woman's cardiopulmonary system and presents the options for anesthesia. Informed consent is obtained for the procedures. Procedure 6-3 contains the nursing care necessary in preparation for surgery.

Procedure 6-3

CESAREAN DELIVERY: PREPARATION

DEFINITION

Delivery of the fetus by an abdominal and uterine incision.

PURPOSE

To complete the preparation for surgery as competently and quickly as possible.

To provide emotional support through a caring attitude, calm manner, and technical competence.

To decrease client anxiety by reassurance.

EQUIPMENT

Skin preparation kit (for shaving); retention (Foley) catheter kit; IV infusions (as ordered); medications (as ordered).

NURSING ACTIONS	RATIONALE
Wash hands before and after touching woman and equipment. Glove, prn.	To prevent nosocomial infection and to implement universal precautions.
Explain procedures to be carried out.	To keep the family informed, decrease anxiety, and elicit cooperation.
Complete preoperative preparation of abdomen. The abdomen is shaved beginning at the level of the xiphoid process and extending to the flank on both sides and down to the pubic area.	To minimize potential for infection.
Insert a retention catheter (Foley). It is attached to a continuous drainage system. Care must be taken that catheter is placed properly within the bladder and is draining adequately.	To ensure the bladder remains empty during the operation.
Administer preoperative medications as ordered:	
Analgesia.	To promote relaxation before surgery.
Atropine.	To minimize amount of secretions in bronchial tree.
Antacid.	To prevent irritative pneumonia if aspiration of gastric juice from stomach occurs.
If spinal or epidural anesthesia is used, an antacid may be the only medication administered.	
Begin IV infusion. 1000 ml Ringer's lactate solution, or 5% dextrose in water or saline.	To maintain hydration.
	To have a line open for administration of blood, medications, etc. if needed.
Send specimens to laboratory for analysis.	To replace blood loss during surgery or postpartum if excessive.
Send blood for typing and cross-matching. Two units of matched blood are kept in reserve for 48 hours after surgery.	
Send urine for routine analysis.	To establish baseline data.
Send blood for CBC and chemistry.	To establish baseline data.
Take and record vital signs, blood pressure, FHR.	To establish baseline data.
Complete preoperative care including removal of dentures, contact lenses, rings, and fingernail polish. Valuables are given to support person or put into safekeeping.	To protect client.
Ready the woman's chart for use in surgery and to see whether permission forms for care of the mother and infant are signed. If the woman has received an analgesic or anesthetic, the responsible adult accompanying the woman signs the necessary forms.	To provide data base for future comparison.
	To provide data base for implementation of the next steps in the nursing process.
	To promote collaboration with other members of the health care team.
Provide as much information as possible to the woman and her family while carrying out the necessary care.	To relieve apprehension and promote understanding

Guidelines for Client Teaching

PREPARATION FOR CESAREAN DELIVERY

ASSESSMENT
1. Woman in third trimester of pregnancy.
2. Woman to be prepared for possible cesarean delivery.
3. Woman to have repeat cesarean delivery.

NURSING DIAGNOSES
Knowledge deficit related to cesarean delivery.
Knowledge deficit related to testing for fetal well-being and fetal lung maturity.
Anxiety and fear related to possible or actual cesarean delivery.
Self-esteem disturbance related to unsatisfied planned birth experience.
Potential altered parenting.
Personal identity disturbance related to loss of control over decisions and powerlessness.

GOALS
Short-term
Woman (couple) will learn that a cesarean delivery can be a positive birth experience.
Woman (couple) will learn the reasons for the cesarean delivery.

Intermediate
Woman (couple) will learn the rationale for prenatal testing and how the results determine cesarean delivery.
Woman (couple) will learn rationale for testing for fetal lung maturity.
Woman (couple) will learn about medications and forms of anesthesia given for cesarean deliveries.

Long-term
Woman (couple) will take a tour of the operating room/delivery room.
Woman (couple) verbalizes feelings about cesarean delivery.
Woman (couple) will learn immediate preoperative preparation for cesarean delivery.
Woman (couple) understands breast-feeding is still an option.
Woman understands that pain relief will be provided.

REFERENCES AND TEACHING AIDS
Books and pamphlets describing cesarean delivery in a positive way.
Discussion and lecture, use of slides, charts, illustrations.
Films or videos depicting a cesarean birth.
Tour of the hospital's labor and delivery suite, including the operative area and recovery area.
Discussions with parents who have experienced cesarean delivery.

CONTENT/RATIONALE	TEACHING ACTIONS
To meet information needs regarding cesarean delivery and rationale:	
Explain the anatomy and physiology pertaining to cesarean delivery and how it differs from a vaginal delivery.	Use charts, diagrams, audio-visual aids to show difference between a vaginal and cesarean delivery.
Discuss prenatal testing and how it illustrates fetal well-being.	Use diagrams or audio-visual aids if possible; discuss parents' questions and concerns.
Nonstress test (NST); used as a screening test, looking for accelerations of FHR in conjunction with fetal movement. Reactive test shows at least 2 FHR accelerations >15 beats per minute above the baseline and lasting 15 seconds or more in conjunction with fetal movements in a 10-minute period. Nonreactive test does not fulfill the above criteria and is an indication for further evaluation.	Discuss rationale behind each test. Explain where these tests are done and by whom. Discuss questions and concerns.
Contraction Stress Test (aka oxytocin stress test, stress test). This test evaluates fetal response to labor contractions (i.e., can the fetus withstand the stress of normal labor?)	
Negative test shows no late decelerations of FHR during 3 contractions over a 10-minute period.	
Positive test—late decelerations are observed during this time; shows fetoplacental unit cannot withstand the stress of normal labor. There are terms of classification in between. For this test, intravenous oxytocin may be administered or the woman may be asked to provide nipple stimulation to produce natural oxytocin in the body.	Indicate that interpretations of this test will be explained by the physician at the time the test is taken.

Continued.

Guidelines for Client Teaching—cont'd

CONTENT/RATIONALE	TEACHING ACTIONS
Ultrasonography, either done alone or in cojunction with amniocentesis, provides information on approximate gestational age and maturity of the fetus.	Explain what ultrasound testing is and what information it provides the physician. Show a picture of the machine, a diagram of how it works, and a picture of a fetus from an ultrasound done previously.
Biophysial profile, a combination of ultrasonography, NST, fetal movement, and placental grading, tells the physician how the maternal-fetal-placental unit is working.	Explain the parameters of this test and what the significance of the test shows.
Amniocentesis (Procedure 6-1) may be done to provide information on fetal lung maturity by way of L/S ratio, phosphatidylglycerol (P/G) ratio, or Foam Stabilizing Index (FSI).	Explain what information this test provides.
Discuss the types of medications the woman may be given to mature the fetal lungs if a cesarean delivery is necessary	Review what the physician's instructions were at this point. Clarify any questions.
To provide anticipatory guidance for pre- and postoperative care:	
Discuss types of anesthesia that are used for cesarean delivery.	Show a diagram or picture of a woman receiving an epidural or spinal.
Explain the difference between epidural and spinal anesthesia. If continuous morphine or fentanyl is used in your institution, explain what this is.	
Explain preoperative preparation and postoperative assessment that will be implemented.	Explain shaving the abdomen, insertion of an indwelling urinary catheter, starting intravenous infusion.
	Discuss what will be done in the recovery area after the operation.
	Reassure woman, if she is up to it, and her newborn is well, she may hold the baby at this time.
Discuss alternate positions for breast-feeding so that the incision is not interfered with.	Reassure her that she may still breast-feed.
Arrange for a tour of the labor and delivery area, include the operating and recovery areas.	Take woman (couple) on a tour. Point out important sights, sounds, and smells at that time. Leave time for questions.

EVALUATION Couple verbalizes understanding of information presented, they ask appropriate questions. Woman (couple) sees cesarean delivery as a positive, alternate method of childbirth, and it is a satisfying experience for them.

Preterm Labor

Preterm labor, a problem experienced by many women, is frightening for the woman and family and dangerous for the immature fetus. If recognized early, preterm labor can be stopped or controlled until the fetus' lungs and organs are mature enough to withstand extrauterine life.

Nurses play an important role as client educator. If the woman recognizes the signs and symptoms of preterm labor, she can seek assistance. The following pages contain material to help the practitioner educate clients about preterm labor, as well as guidelines for the care of a woman receiving ritodrine hydrochloride to delay delivery.

Guidelines for Client Teaching

PRETERM LABOR: HOME MANAGEMENT

ASSESSMENT

Gravida 2 carrying twins, 30 weeks' gestation.

First baby born at 34 weeks' gestation.

Preterm labor has been diagnosed and treated; woman is now ready for discharge with medication; or,

Preterm labor is to be treated at home.

NURSING DIAGNOSES

Knowledge deficit related to management of preterm labor.

Potential for injury: maternal and fetal, related to recurrence of preterm labor and delivery.

Anxiety, mild to moderate, related to possible recurrence of preterm labor and delivery.

GOALS

Short-term

Gravida learns home management after preterm labor episode.

Intermediate

Gravida implements home management.

Long-term

Gravida carries pregnancy to or near term and gives birth to healthy mature twins.

REFERENCES AND TEACHING AIDS

Printed materials available through drug companies, hospitals, and clinics.

CONTENT/RATIONALE	TEACHING ACTIONS
To understand preterm labor, its causes, signs, and symptoms:	
Review guidelines for client teaching: preterm labor recognition.	Implement teaching actions as required from guidelines.
To foster understanding and self care:	
Bedrest	
Bedrest is intended to keep the pressure of the fetus off the cervix and to enhance uterine perfusion. Kneeling or sitting in bed does not keep the fetus from pressing on the cervix. Physical rest is facilitated by peace of mind. Someone other than the mother must assume care of older children, cooking, and cleaning. Many women are allowed out of bed only for use of the bathroom.	Develop care plan mutually with woman/couple/family. Mobilize assistance for home management. Advise woman to lie on her left side with her head flat or raised on a small pillow.
Medications	
If the woman is being maintained at home on an *oral* dose of tocolytic medication (ritodrine hydrochloride or terbutaline), woman must know rationale, side effects, and danger signs.	Medications are reviewed and the woman is given written instructions regarding care. Inform woman about the action and side effects of the drug. Instruct her how to take her pulse and report any rate greater than 120 beats per min to her physician, how to report symptoms, including palpitations, tremors, agitation, and nervousness.
Some over-the-counter drugs may cause deleterious effects. Oral administration may be better tolerated when taken with food. Sedation is often ordered to facilitate relaxation and rest.	Caution her not to use ritodrine with any over-the-counter drugs unless her physician approves. Advise and give written instructions (for herself and her family) regarding the medication. This includes the prescription for sedation, dosage, times for administration, and side effects.
Avoidance of activities that could stimulate labor:	
Sexual stimulation is contraindicated because (1) prostaglandins in semen can stimulate labor in a susceptible woman and (2) touching the cervix or pressure against the posterior wall of the vagina may stimulate Ferguson's reflex (the increase in myometrial contractility that follows mechanical stretching or touching of the cervix). Nipple stimulation may induce oxytocin production that can cause recurrence of uterine activity.	Encourage discussion of this sensitive topic.
To identify hazards and intervene in a timely manner:	
Review danger signs of preterm labor.	Review verbally and provide written instructions regarding:

Continued.

Guidelines for Client Teaching—cont'd

CONTENT/RATIONALE	TEACHING ACTIONS
Review danger of infection if membranes are not intact.	a. What to do and whom to notify in case of onset of labor or rupture of membranes. b. Maintaining personal hygiene if membranes have ruptured earlier. c. Assessing for signs of infection (e.g., odor of vaginal discharge, increase in body temperature).
To assist with home maintenance: Social service consultation may be helpful if the woman has to be transported into a center from an outlying area. Living arrangements, meals, transportation, and financial assistance may be needed for some families.	Refer to appropriate agency after discussion and mutual planning with family.

EVALUATION The nurse can be reasonably assured that teaching was effective if the goals for care are achieved. The woman and her family are able to implement self-care so that preterm labor is stopped, there are no adverse sequelae to medication, and positive family processes are maintained. The woman delivers healthy infants at or near term.

DANGER SIGNS

Ritodrine Toxicity

1. Central nervous system: severe nervousness or anxiety, tremulousness, headache, restlessness.
2. Respirations: dyspnea, hyperventilation.
3. Cardiovascular system: severe palpitations or cardiac irregularities, chest pain; pulmonary edema.
4. Gastrointestinal: severe nausea or vomiting, epigastric distress, diarrhea.

Terbutaline Toxicity

1. Central nervous system: severe dizziness, drowsiness, headache, nervousness, restlessness; clouded sensorium.
2. Blood pressure: severe hypertension.
3. Heart rate: continuous palpitations.
4. Musculoskeletal: severe muscle cramps and weakness.
5. Gastrointestinal: continuous nausea and vomiting.

Procedure 6-4

NURSING CARE OF A WOMAN RECEIVING RITODRINE HYDROCHLORIDE

DEFINITION

The use of a β-sympathomimetic agent to stop the uterus from contracting, thereby stopping preterm labor.

PURPOSE

Suppression of preterm labor.

EQUIPMENT

Intravenous infusion equipment, sphygmomanometer, stethoscope, equipment for cardiopulmonary arrest, fetal monitoring equipment.

HAZARDOUS SYMPTOMS

See danger signs: ritodrine hydrochloride, p. 248.

NURSING ACTIONS	RATIONALE
Identify client and check physician's orders.	To provide the right therapy for the right person.
Wash hands before and after touching client or equipment. Glove, prn.	To prevent nosocomial infection and to implement universal precautions.
Assess maternal vital signs and FHR.	To obtain baseline data.
Monitor vital signs and blood pressure every 15 minutes until stable and then follow hospital protocol. *Maternal pulse should not exceed 140 beats per minute for more than 10 minutes.* Note regularity and quality.	To detect complications: cardiac arrhythmias are adverse effects of β-adrenergic therapy, pulmonary edema, and fluid overload.
Prepare mother for use of cardiac monitor.	
Note breath sounds when counting respiratory rate.	
Monitor FHR: *should not exceed 180 beats per minute.* Intermittent evaluation should continue during oral therapy also.	
Observe for any untoward symptoms.	
Ask woman to report symptoms.	To elicit subjective symptoms.
Send blood samples to laboratory for analysis of levels of glucose, potassium, and hematocrit.	To assess for hypokalemia and acidosis.
	As glucose moves into cells, potassium shifts from the extracellular space.
Maintain absolute bedrest during intravenous infusion.	To minimize stress and reduce pressure on cervix.
Prevent hypotension; keep woman in left-lateral position or place wedge under right hip if in supine position.	To maintain placental perfusion.
Apply antiembolism stockings.	To prevent pooling of blood in lower extremities.
Do not use under knees. Encourage passive leg exercises.	
Maintain adequate hydration, 2000 to 3000 ml daily.	To maintain cardiac output.
Prevent overhydration:	
Measure intake and output.	To detect overhydration.
Weigh daily.	
Prevent undue stress:	
Prepare woman for potential side effects (i.e., agitation, palpitations, nervousness, tremors, tachycardia).	To promote relaxation through anticipatory guidance.
Instruct woman to report symptoms.	To elicit subjective symptoms.
Treat for complications:	
Hold medication. If intravenous, keep line open with plain solution.	To minimize effects of medication.
Notify physician and prepare antidote as ordered.	To initiate immediate therapy.
Maintain woman in high Fowler's position.	To minimize effects of possible pulmonary edema.
Administer oxygen.	To maintain sufficient oxygenation.
Initiate CPR for arrest if necessary.	To maintain oxygenation and body functions.

MEDICAL, SURGICAL, AND PSYCHOSOCIAL CONDITIONS COMPLICATING PREGNANCY

Preexisting medical disorders, surgical procedures, emotional problems, and substance abuse all can have a serious impact on the pregnant woman and her fetus. A thorough understanding of each problem is required, and the maternity nurse must have a general knowledge of medical-surgical nursing and mental health nursing. A detailed discussion on the impact of these numerous conditions is beyond the scope of this manual. This section therefore includes general information on four problems: cardiovascular disorders, sickle cell disease, general surgery, and substance abuse.

DANGER SIGNS

Cardiac Decompensation
Cardiac Decomposition

Gravida: Subjective Symptoms

1. Increasing fatigue or difficulty breathing or both with her usual activities
2. Feeling of smothering
3. Need to cough frequently
4. Rapid pulse; feeling that her heart is "racing"
5. Swelling of feet, legs, fingers (rings do not fit anymore), or face

Nurse: Objective Signs

1. Irregular rapid pulse ($\geq$100 beats per minute)
2. Progressive, generalized edema
3. Rales at base of lungs
4. Orthopnea; increasing dyspnea
5. Rapid respirations ($\geq$25 per minute)
6. Frequent cough
7. Increasing fatigue

Sample Nursing Care Plan

HEART DISEASE AND CHILDBEARING

ASSESSMENT	NURSING DIAGNOSIS (ND)/ PLAN (P)/GOAL (G)	RATIONALE/ IMPLEMENTATION	EVALUATION
Prenatal care: Assess for factors that increase stress on the heart (anemia, infection, household activities). Assess for signs of cardiac decompensation: generalized edema, rales at the base of lungs, pulse irregularity. Patterns of weight gain. Vital signs. Edema. Discomforts of pregnancy. Urinalysis (protein, blood acetone, glucose). Blood work (Hgb, Hct, WBC, platelets). Check for side effects and interactions of medications. Assess dietary patterns.	ND: Altered tissue perfusion related to hypotensive syndrome. ND: Increased cardiac output related to pregnancy. ND: Impaired home maintenance management related to mother's restricted household activities or confinement to bed. P: Provide information, be available for discussion, and continuing ongoing surveillance for maternal well-being. Home visit may be considered. Explore community resources for home assistance. G: Woman will maintain adequate perfusion as exhibited by stable blood pressure, clear lung fields, no edema,	*To closely monitor a woman with heart disease for decompensation, the nurse will:* Reinforce physician's explanation for need of close medical supervision. Schedule weekly appointments and evaluate problems pertaining to missed appointments. Review symptoms of cardiac decompensation. Monitor weight and dietary patterns. Monitor vital sign patterns. Note and report edema ("Are your shoes getting tight?") Obtain urine and blood specimens, and evaluate and report results. Monitor for side effects and interactions of medications. Encourage adequate rest.	Woman remains free from cardiac decompensation. Woman attends weekly health care appointments. Woman obtains adequate rest and avoids restricted activities. The home situation is controlled with assistance provided as necessary. Woman self-administers heparin as ordered by a physician.

Sample Nursing Care Plan—cont'd

ASSESSMENT	NURSING DIAGNOSIS (ND)/ PLAN (P)/GOAL (G)	RATIONALE/ IMPLEMENTATION	EVALUATION
	and regular pulse. G: Woman will attend scheduled appointments. G: Woman will avoid restricted activities and achieve adequate rest. G: Woman will self-administer heparin as ordered.	Restrict activities such as housework and shopping and refer to child care and home health agencies. Teach woman how to self-administer heparin as ordered.	
Assess client's baseline knowledge of her heart disease. Assess client's knowledge of how pregnancy will affect her heart disease.	ND: Knowledge deficit related to care required by a woman with heart disease during pregnancy. ND: Fear related to increased peripartum risk. P: Provide information, be available for discussion, and mobilize resources and support. G: Woman and family will learn how to monitor and care for her heart disease during pregnancy. G: Woman and family will learn the risks of pregnancy on her heart disease.	*To teach the heart disease client how to care for herself during pregnancy, the nurse will:* Review effects pregnancy will have on her health. Help woman formulate questions for the physician. Evaluate woman's desire to continue with the pregnancy given all the peripartum risks and review her option for termination of the pregnancy. Teach symptoms of cardiac decompensation (verbal and written). Review restricted activities and need for rest. Teach nutrition and the need for a high iron, high protein, and adequate caloric diet to gain about (10.8 kg) 24 lb during pregnancy. Tell woman to avoid foods high in Vitamin K if she is receiving heparin therapy. Teach woman regarding danger of infection, its signs, and symptoms. Review information pertaining to management of labor and the early postdelivery period.	Woman and family verbalizes an understanding of the risks of pregnancy on woman's health. Woman learns how to care for herself during pregnancy and knows whom to contact should danger signs present. Woman and familily utilize community resources and support. Woman and family follow prescribed diet and treatment regimen.
Intrapartum care: Routine assessments for a laboring woman. Vital signs every 10 to 30 minutes. Alert physician to heart rate >100 or >25 respirations per minute. Assess respiratory status frequently for dyspnea, coughing, or rales at base of lungs.	ND: Increased cardiac output related to the stress of labor and delivery. ND: Altered (cardiopulmonary) tissue perfusion related to hypotension (maternal or fetal). P: Promote cardiac function, provide emotional support, and remain alert for potential complications.	*To increase perfusion by alleviating cardiac stress, the nurse will:* Promote cardiac function by: A. Alleviating anxiety. B. Placing woman in side-lying position. C. Medicating or sedating for discomfort. D. Preventing, recognizing, reporting, and treating hypotension, which may	Woman maintains adequate perfusion during labor and delivery. Fetus will remain adequately perfused in utero as demonstrated by acceptable FHR patterns.

Continued.

Sample Nursing Care Plan—cont'd

ASSESSMENT	NURSING DIAGNOSIS (ND)/ PLAN (P)/GOAL (G)	RATIONALE/ IMPLEMENTATION	EVALUATION
Note and record color and skin temperature. Assess for signs of cardiac shock. Assess for suspicious FHR deceleration patterns (Chapter 17).	G: Woman will maintain adequate perfusion, exhibited by stable blood pressure, regular pulse, warm pink extremities, and clear lung field. G: Woman will maintain adequate perfusion to the placenta as exhibited by a stable FHR during labor.	follow anesthesia. For delivery, place on left side or supine with left hip elevated. Administer medications and report signs of cardiac decompensation. Monitor contractions and FHR response.	
Watch for symptoms of emotional stress.	ND: Anxiety related to fear for infant's safety. ND: Fear of dying related to perceived inability to control stress of labor. P: Minimize or eliminate emotional stress. G: Woman will be comforted and anxiety relieved by stress reduction techniques.	*To control the client's level of stress, the nurse will:* Answer any questions of concern the client might have about labor and delivery. Help client formulate questions for the physician. Correct misconceptions. Explain upcoming procedures, feelings, or sensations she might experience. Encourage support person to provide comfort techniques (back rub, pressure to lumbar spine, etc.). Encourage support person to remain at bedside with the woman as a comfort measure. Administer medications for discomfort or sedation as ordered.	Woman reports comfort or demonstrates reduced anxiety by measures instituted.
Postdelivery care: Close assessment for cardiac decompensation. Routine postpartum assessments. Assess for signs and symptoms of infection and hemorrhage. Monitor intake/output closely.	ND: Decreased cardiac output related to fluid shifts after delivery. ND: Altered (cardiopulmonary) tissue perfusion related to rapid fluid shifts on a compromised cardiovascular system. ND: Potential for injury related to hemorrhage or infection. ND: Knowledge deficit regarding methods to reduce stress on cardiac system. P: Promote cardiac function and involution, provide emotional support, and remain alert for potential complications.	*To monitor for, and prevent, cardiac decompensation, the nurse will:* Evaluate for cardiac decompensation up to 7 days after delivery. Perform all routine postpartum care and teaching. Apply abdominal binder or tourniquets as ordered by a physician after delivery. Administer medications as ordered (oxygen, digitalization therapy, etc.) Elevate head of bed and encourage side-lying. Teach regarding stool softeners, fluids, and diet to reduce strain of bowel movements. Prevent overdistended bladder after delivery.	Woman remains free from signs and symptoms of cardiac decompensation. Woman remains free from hemorrhage and infection. Woman verbalizes understanding of instructions. Woman experiences normal involution.

Sample Nursing Care Plan—cont'd

ASSESSMENT	NURSING DIAGNOSIS (ND)/ PLAN (P)/GOAL (G)	RATIONALE/ IMPLEMENTATION	EVALUATION
	G: Woman will not demonstrate signs of cardiac decompensation after delivery.	Isolate from sources of infection. Prevent or promptly treat hemorrhage or infection. Facilitate mother-infant interactions that do not stress the mother.	
Assess woman's support system. Assess family's response to the birth and infant. Assess the need for outside resources (home care, child care).	ND: Ineffective family coping: compromised, related to added child care and household tasks. ND: Altered family processes related to assuming woman's responsibilities after delivery. ND: Self-care deficit related to need for bedrest. ND: Situational low self-esteem related to restriction placed on involvement in care of infant. P: Facilitate parent-child relationship and mutually develop a plan for care utilizing outside resources as necessary. G: Woman will rest and recuperate after delivery. G: Woman will not be stressed by child care or household activities after delivery.	*To assure that the woman has the needed rest to recuperate, the nurse will:* Identify with the client her support systems. Observe the family's response to the infant and child care activities. Examine the family's time and resources to assist the client with child care and household tasks. Notify outside resources to assist with the care of the woman, house, and child (homemaker, child care, home health care). Encourage woman to spend "quiet moments" with her child but to allow family to provide most of the child care activities. Remind woman that she can assume all child care activities once she allows her body to recuperate from childbirth.	Woman achieves the needed rest to recuperate. The mother and family accept the limitations imposed on the woman by the presence of heart disease. Woman's family or outside services assumes responsibility of children and household tasks until client recuperates. The parent-child relationship is fostered by the family.

Table 6-31　*Sickle Cell Disease: Potential Problems, Prevention, and Maintenance*

Potential Problem	Prevention and Maintenance
1. Inadequate oxygen to meet needs of labor and prevent sickling	1. a. Monitor hemoglobin level and hematocrit to maintain hemoglobin at 7 g or more and hematocrit at 20% or more b. Assist with transfusions c. Administer oxygen d. Coach for relaxation and to lessen anxiety
2. Infection resulting from anemia: urinary tract infection, pyelonephritis, pneumonia	2. a. Continue actions as under no. 1 b. Maintain adequate hydration c. Administer antibiotics, as ordered d. Maintain strict asepsis e. Encourage frequent voiding to keep bladder empty
3. Sequestration crisis caused by need for and destruction of RBCs	3. Administer folic acid supplement (15-30 mg) to decrease erythropoietic demands and reduce probability of capillary stasis
4. Crisis caused by hypoxia, hypotension, acidosis, dehydration, exertion, sudden cooling, low-grade fever	4. a. Continue actions as under no. 1 b. Avoid supine hypotension c. Maintain adequate hydration d. Maintain comfortable room temperature; use warm blankets or cool cloths as needed e. Assist with analgesia and anesthesia
5. Pseudotoxemia (hypertension, and proteinuria; *no* large weight gain); often accompanies bone pain crisis	5. a. If true PIH occurs, care is the same as for PIH b. Monitor blood pressure and urine c. Administer heparin, as ordered
6. Thrombophlebitis (from increased blood viscosity)	6. a. Monitor for positive Homans' sign b. Initiate bedrest if Homans' sign is positive or if reddened, warm areas, or a lump are found c. Maintain adequate hydration d. Administer heparin, as ordered e. Apply warm compresses f. Apply antiembolism stockings
7. Congestive heart failure	7. a. Assess pulse, respiratory rate every 15 minutes b. Auscultate for rales frequently c. Place in semirecumbent position d. Administer oxygen and medications (e.g., digitalis, antibiotics, diuretics, analgesics) e. Prevent bearing down; reassure woman about low forceps delivery under anesthesia (local or regional)
8. Pulmonary infarction (hemoptysis, cough, temperature to 38.9° C [102° F], friction rub)	8. Assess for this possible complication to facilitate early diagnosis
9. Postpartum hemorrhage (resulting from heparin therapy)	9. Administer ordered oxytocic medication

Table 6-32   *Preoperative Management of the Pregnant Woman*

	Collect Data	Psychologic Preparation	Physical Preparation	Legal Status
Physician	Aid in medical diagnosis Determine need, type, and extent of surgery Identify potential complications requiring medical intervention Obtain baseline data for future comparison	Explain need, type, and extent of surgery to woman and significant others Explain effect on fetus and pregnancy	Prescribe and carry out tests Prescribe diet, drugs Prescribe actions to ensure safety and comfort during surgery	Obtain informed, signed consent for procedure Complete physician's preoperative orders
Nurse	Identify psychologic readiness for surgery Identify knowledge of events that will occur Identify potential complications requiring nursing intervention Obtain baseline data for future comparison	Verify woman's understanding and clarify as indicated Give explanations about tests Give opportunities to express feelings and concerns Support significant others	Assist woman and physician in carrying out tests Help woman meet basic needs in preparation for surgery Assist woman in carrying out physician's orders	Ensure that identification bands are on and correct Complete preoperative checklist

Modified from Phipps WJ, Long BC, and Woods NF: Medical-surgical nursing: concepts and clinical practice, ed 3, St Louis, 1987, The CV Mosby Co.

Table 6-33   *Some Causes of Vital Sign Changes in Early Postoperative Phase*

Increase	Decrease
Temperature	
Stress reaction (low-grade fever)	Cold operating room and recovery room
Pulse rate	
Jarring during transfer Shock, hemorrhage Hypoventilation Acute gastric dilation Pain Anxiety Cardiac arrhythmias	Digitalis overdose Cardiac arrhythmias
Respiratory Rate	
Hypoventilation: poor positioning, right chest or upper abdominal dressing, obesity, gastric dilation	Drugs: anesthetics, narcotics, sedatives
Blood Pressure	
Anxiety ($\uparrow$ systolic) Pain	Jarring during transfer Severe pain Cardiac arrhythmias Shock: fluid loss, hemorrhage, acute gastric dilation

From Phipps WJ, Long BC, and Woods NF: Medical-surgical nursing: concepts and clinical practice, ed 3, St. Louis, 1987, The CV Mosby Co.

Table 6-34   *Signs and Symptoms of Alcohol and Drug Problems*

Drug	Psychologic Signs	Physiologic Signs
Alcohol		
Intoxication	Mood lability or change Impaired attention or memory Irritability Talkativeness	Slurred speech Flushed face Incoordination, unsteady gait Nystagmus
Withdrawal	Anxiety Depressed mood or irritability Maladaptive behavior	Nausea and vomiting Malaise or weakness Autonomic hyperactivity Coarse tremor of hands, tongue, eyelids Orthostatic hypotension
Opioid*		
Intoxication	Euphoria, dysphoria Psychomotor retardation Apathy Maladaptive behavior Impaired attention or memory	Pupillary constriction Drowsiness Slurred speech
Withdrawal	Insomnia	Lacrimation, rhinorrhea Pupillary dilation Piloerection; sweating

Continued.

Table 6-34—cont'd.   *Signs and Symptoms of Alcohol and Drug
                      Problems*

Drug	Psychologic Signs	Physiologic Signs
Withdrawal—cont'd		Diarrhea Yawning Mild hypertension Tachycardia Fever
Cocaine		
Intoxication	Psychomotor agitation Elation Grandiosity; talkativeness Hypervigilance Maladaptive behaviors	Tachycardia Pupillary dilation Hypertension Perspiration; chills Nausea; vomiting
Withdrawal	Depressed mood Disturbed sleep Increased dreaming	Fatigue
Phencyclidine (PCP)	Euphoria Psychomotor agitation Increased anxiety Emotional lability Grandiosity Sensation of slowed time Synesthesias Maladaptive behaviors	Vertical or horizontal nystagmus Hypertension Increased heart rate Numbness Decreased response to pain Ataxia; dysarthria

*Most commonly abused narcotics: heroin (the most potent), codeine, morphine.

ADOLESCENT PREGNANCY AND PARENTHOOD

Much has still to be done before the problem of adolescent pregnancy and its sequelae for infant, mother, family, and society in general is solved.

There is a definite societal acceptance toward allowing adolescents more freedom to make decisions and to exercise autonomy and self-determination in their relationships with health care providers and with others in the social system.

In spite of the development of many successful programs, adolescent pregnancy remains the most pressing problem in maternity and gynecologic nursing care today.

Table 6-35 *Adolescent Development and Readiness for Childbearing*

	Early Adolescence (11-14)	Middle Adolescence (15-17)	Late Adolescence (18-20)
Parent most related to conflicts	Beginning to loosen ties with her mother. Vacillates between wanting to be closer (i.e., a mother herself) and wanting to be babied (i.e., cannot conceive of herself as a mother).	Struggling to break from both parents and become autonomous.	Personal identity stronger; some emotional independence from parents; ready for outside love interest.
Quality and style of relationships with others	Strong relationships with other girls. Experiences crushes on safe (i.e., unattainable) adults.	Relationships with peers intense; parents replaced with peers; difficulty with authority figures, cannot either accept or compromise. Friends are heterosexual but self-identity needs (who am I), not intimacy needs, are uppermost. Sexual experimentation and risk taking.	Conflict with parents lessens, nurturant feelings for others emerge, wants to share love and commitment.
View of herself	Self-concept inconsistent and fluctuating; parallels rapid physical changes and capability changes. Vague sense of self as female.	Self-involvement a critical need. Ambivalence and uncertainty predominate. Senses her femininity and has a beginning awareness of responsibility for actions. Definitive commitments not yet necessary. Unresolved dependency needs preclude her wanting to accept dependency of others.	More realistic about who and what she is. Behaviors and responses more predictable. Capable of personal reflections, more in touch with her own feelings. Accepts adult body.
Defense mechanisms	Primary defense is denial, manifested by unwillingness to hear pertinent information (e.g., almost never protected by contraception during sexual experimentation).	Magical thinking and feelings of greater power pervade fantasy, mood swings experienced, any nonsuccess is a tragedy. Exaggeration of response prevents an accurate assessment of real tragedy.	Uses reality-based strategies to cope with stress. Can think through problems, uses rational thought.
Goals and interests	Is "now" oriented. The immediacy of her needs requires instant gratification. Operates by fixed rules and authority, little ability to "give and take," therefore rigid and punitive. Denial is major defense.	Goals and interest reflect growing ability to problem solve. Dependency-independency needs make her inconsistent in approach. Intensely narcissistic (self-centered). Generally unempathetic and unable to tolerate others' demands that detract from her self-focus. Impulsive, unpredictable behavior.	Goals and interests reflect longer-range view. More ready to accept responsibility for self and others. Recognizes need to develop educational or vocational skills. Approximates the adult in being able to provide warm, nurturing care for a child.

Modified from Sahler OJ: In McAnarney ER, editor: Premature adolescent pregnancy and parenthood, New York, 1983, Grune & Stratton, Inc.

KILOCALORIE REQUIREMENTS AND SAMPLE MENUS FOR PREGNANT ADOLESCENTS

Calculating Kilocalorie Requirements*   **Kilocalories**

1. Allow kilocalories for maximum daily growth needs: 123
2. Add RDA† of kilocalories for pregnancy: 300
3. Add average RDA† of kilocalories for age and growth percentile for nonpregnant female.   2100

                                                                                                              2523 total daily
4. *Underweight:* Add 500 additional kilocalories per day, 16% of which should be protein (20 g):   3023 total daily
5. *Overweight:* Use lower range of "normal" suggested values or 38 kcal/kg or 17 kcal/lb pregnancy weight.

Sample Menus

	DAY 1	DAY 2
Breakfast	Egg and ham on English muffin (fast food)	1 cup cornflakes with 1 cup milk
	1 cup milk	2 Tbsp raisins
	1 glass orange juice (6 oz; 180 ml)	1 glass orange juice (6 oz; 180 ml)
Snack	1 pkg peanut butter crackers	1 pkg nuts
	1 can apple juice (6 oz; 180 ml)	1 carton chocolate milk (8 oz; 240 ml)
Lunch	Cheeseburger on bun with lettuce and tomato	"Sub"—1 slice each ham, salami, and cheese with lettuce, tomato, onion, green pepper, 1 Tbsp dressing
	1 carton chocolate milk (8 oz; 240 ml)	1 can apple juice (6 oz; 180 ml)
	1 slice watermelon	1 cup buttered popcorn
Snack	Ice cream cone	2 cups spaghetti and meatballs
Dinner	Baked chicken leg and thigh	1 slice Italian bread
	½ cup rice	Tossed salad—lettuce, tomato, onion
	½ cup string beans	1 Tbsp dressing
	1 cup milk	1 tsp margarine
	½ cup fruit cocktail	Milkshake, vanilla
Snack	1 slice pizza	

KILOCALORIES	PROTEIN (G)	FAT (G)	CHOLESTEROL (G)	KILOCALORIES	PROTEIN (G)	FAT (G)	CHOLESTEROL (G)
2604	119	132	286	2857	115	147	248

Underweight: replace cheeseburger with extra-large hamburger deluxe; add 1 cup orange juice to evening snack   *Underweight:* add 1 carton chocolate milk to afternoon snack, extra cheese or cold cuts to lunch, 2 Tbsp dressing for salad

KILOCALORIES	PROTEIN (G)	FAT (G)	CHOLESTEROL (G)	KILOCALORIES	PROTEIN (G)	FAT (G)	CHOLESTEROL (G)
3149	133	155	334	3353	137	172	278

Overweight: replace ice cream cone with 1 can apple juice (6 oz; 180 ml)   *Overweight:* replace milkshake with 1 cup skim milk

KILOCALORIES	PROTEIN (G)	FAT (G)	CHOLESTEROL (G)	KILOCALORIES	PROTEIN (G)	FAT (G)	CHOLESTEROL (G)
2354	111	114	270	2400	112	131	196

From Frank D et al: J Calif Perinatal Assoc 3(1):21, 1981.
*These calculations are based on the maximum kilocalorie allowance for growth. The best indication of whether a pregnant female is getting sufficient kilocalories is to monitor her growth. If inadequate or excess weight gain occurs, consultation with a nutritionist is recommended.
†Recommended daily dietary allowance.

Sample Nursing Care Plan

TEENAGE PREGNANCY

ASSESSMENT	NURSING DIAGNOSIS (ND)/ PLAN (P)/GOAL (G)	RATIONALE/ IMPLEMENTATION	EVALUATION
Note previous obstetric history. Assess knowledge regarding: pregnancy, childbirth, parenthood. Cultural beliefs. Financial status. View of pregnancy. Does client want to continue with the pregnancy? Does client want to be a parent or put the child up for adoption? Assess teen's support systems, boyfriend, peers, family, outreach service, in community.	ND: Knowledge deficit related to choices regarding pregnancy, childbirth experience, and parenthood. P: Supply information about choices and community resources and support. G: Client will learn about pregnancy, childbirth, and parenthood. G: Client will learn about her choice to maintain or abort the pregnancy, keep the child, or place the child for adoption.	*To teach client about pregnancy, childbirth, and parenthood, the nurse will:* Examine own views regarding sexuality to be able to maintain nonjudgmental approach. Listen and give honest answers. Accept and expect repeated testing from the adolescent. Create a safe and stable environment that engenders trust. Evaluate which of the three stages of development the adolescent is experiencing. Teach the adolescent about pregnancy choices, childbirth, and parenthood. Utilize group teaching as a means for learning and establishing teen support. Encourage questions and verbalization of fears or concerns. Compliment teen on well-thought-out questions and reference to learned issues. Encourage support person to attend and participate in prenatal care. Refer to childbirth and parenthood class.	Client learns about her pregnancy choices, childbirth experience; and parenthood. Client makes a choice with which she is comfortable. Client is able to effectively utilize community resources or support from family or friends.
Note teen's current obligations (school, work, home). Accessibility to health care.	ND: Ineffective individual coping, related to situational crises of teen pregnancy. P: Establish a trusting relationship and ensure confidentiality. G: Client will learn the importance of early and continuous prenatal care. G: Client will keep her appointments and participate in her care.	*To encourage client to attend prenatal care, the nurse will:* Provide consistency of caregivers. Explain the need to closely monitor her pregnancy. Create safe, stable environment. Evaluate transportation needs to health care center. Schedule appointments around school or work activities.	Client attends prenatal care. Client participates in her plan of care.

Continued.

Sample Nursing Care Plan—Cont'd

ASSESSMEMT	NURSING DIAGNOSIS (ND)/ PLAN (P)/GOAL (G)	RATIONALE/ IMPLEMENTATION	EVALUATION
		Use creative forms of health care delivery to maximize services. Note maternal responses to pregnancy and the adolescent's interpretation of them. Provide obstetric, psychosocial, and outreach services in one setting, if possible. Offer teen as many choices as possible and encourage her to take an active role in her plan of care.	
How do you feel about yourself? How do you feel about pregnancy? How do you feel about becoming a mother? What are your goals for the future? Support system.	ND: Body image disturbance, situational low self-esteem, altered role performance, related to pregnancy. ND: Potential for altered growth and development related to concurrent adolescence and pregnancy. ND: Potential for social isolation from family or peers related to pregnancy. P: Help client increase problem-solving skills to plan for a future and to communicate caring and support. G: Client will discuss concerns and feelings about pregnancy. G: Client will identify her support system. G: Client will continue to develop in her stage of adolescence during her pregnancy.	*To assist the client in maintaining her self-concept, the nurse will:* Show interest in client, her thoughts and feelings. Provide private place to talk and discuss matters in an unhurried manner. Encourage verbalization. Identify support system with teen. Evaluate teen's adolescent stage to counsel and support her in achieving her developmental tasks. Compliment teen on her appearance, verbalization of feelings, and learning. Refer to outside resources, guidance counselor, tutor.	Client verbalizes her concerns and feelings about pregnancy. Client identifies her support system. Client develops in her own stage of maturity.
Assess for teen's use of: alcoholic beverages, smoking, street drugs. Ask if teen's close friends use alcohol, drugs, or tobacco products.	ND: Altered health maintenance related to substance abuse. ND: Potential for injury (maternal and fetal) related to substance abuse. ND: Potential for infection related to intravenous drug abuse. P: Provide information and be available for discussion of concerns and questions. G: Client will learn how substance abuse will af-	*To promote a pregnancy free from substance abuse, the nurse will:* Examine teen's substance abuse habit: 1. Duration of abuse. 2. Time and circumstances when substances are used. Explain the dangers of substance abuse on the pregnant woman and fetus. Utilize group teaching to promote peer support against substance abuse.	Client learns about the effects of substance abuse on pregnancy. Client avoids nonprescribed drugs, smoking, and alcoholic beverages during pregnancy.

Sample Nursing Care Plan—Cont'd

ASSESSMEMT	NURSING DIAGNOSIS (ND)/ PLAN (P)/GOAL (G)	RATIONALE/ IMPLEMENTATION	EVALUATION
	fect herself and her baby during pregnancy. G: Client will avoid non-prescribed drugs, smoking, and alcoholic beverages during pregnancy.	Examine with teen her current peer group and their influence with the use of drugs, smoking, and alcohol. Involve support person in plan to reduce, then eliminate, substance abuse. Refer teen to social services and a "quit smoking" or addiction program.	
How many meals are eaten daily? Who prepares the meals? Cultural and religious influences on food. Knowledge of the four basic food groups. Client's food likes/dislikes. Does she take vitamins? Financial status.	ND: Knowledge deficit related to nutritional needs of the mother and fetus during pregnancy. ND: Altered nutrition: less than body requirements, related to increased nutrient requirements during pregnancy and adolescence. P: Increase client's knowledge about nutrition and involve her in "taking charge" of what happens to her by mutual planning. G: Client will learn about the nutritional needs of pregnancy. G: Client will design sample meals that are balanced with the basic food groups.	*To increase the client's knowledge about nutrition during pregnancy, the nurse will:* Review the four basic food groups. Instruct on the importance of adequate nutrition during pregnancy. Examine cultural and financial considerations when planning nutrition instructions. Refer to financial support agencies for low-income cases (welfare, Women, Infants, and Children [WIC]). Mutually select foods to meet nutrition needs, personal preferences, budget requirements, and seasonal availability. Assist client in designing sample menus. Teach client how to prepare foods to ensure optimum nutritive value.	Client verbalizes understanding of instruction. Client prepares sample menus that meet the daily nutrition requirements during pregnancy.
Note baseline blood pressure and monitor at every prenatal visit. Note edema (are your shoes fitting tight?) Note proteinuria. Note fetal heart rate after 8 to 12 weeks. Note fetal activity after 16 weeks.	ND: Altered tissue perfusion related to inadequate placental perfusion secondary to PIH. ND: Potential for injury, maternal and fetal, related to PIH. P: Monitor for potential complications. G: Client will be monitored closely for signs and symptoms of pregnancy-induced hypertension (PIH). G: Client will be treated promptly if she demonstrates PIH.	Adolescents at great risk for PIH.	Client remains free from PIH or condition is identified and treated promptly so mother and fetus demonstrate no or minimum sequelae. Client experiences no complications.

Continued.

Sample Nursing Care Plan—Cont'd

ASSESSMEMT	NURSING DIAGNOSIS (ND)/ PLAN (P)/GOAL (G)	RATIONALE/ IMPLEMENTATION	EVALUATION
Has adolescent cared for a child before? Who will be assisting in child care? Support system. Knowledge of infant needs.	ND: Knowledge deficit related to infant care activities, growth patterns, and developmental needs. P: Provide information and encouragement, demonstrate, and observe reverse demonstration. G: Client will learn infant care activities, growth pattern, and developmental needs. G: Client will identify her support system for child care.	*To teach adolescent about infant care activities, growth patterns, and developmental needs, the nurse will:* Identify baseline knowledge. Begin infant care activities instruction during prenatal period. Involve support person in teaching sessions. Focus teaching toward adolescent's maturity and cognitive level. Refer client to parenthood classes. Refer to and make initial contact with social services for a future resource person if problems arise in child care.	Client learns infant care activities, growth patterns, and developmental needs. Client identifies her support system. Client's self-esteem increases with increase in skill.

References

Anderson GD: A systematic approach to eclamptic convulsion, Contemp OB/GYN 29(3):65, 1987.

Danforth DN and Scott JR, editors: Obstetrics and gynecology, ed 5, Philadelphia, 1986, JB Lippincott Co.

Hollingsworth DR: Maternal metabolism in normal pregnancy and pregnancy complicated by diabetes, Clin Obstet Gynecol 128:457, 1985

Knuppel RA and Drukker JE: High-risk pregnancy: a team approach, Philadelphia, 1986, WB Saunders Co.

Lindheimer MD and Katz AI: Current concepts: hypertension in pregnancy, N Engl J Med 313(11):675, 1985.

National Diabetes Data Group: Classification and diagnosis of diabetes mellitus and other categories of glucose intolerance, Diabetes 28:1039, 1979.

Phipps WJ, Long BC, and Woods NF: Medical-surgical nursing: concepts and clinical practice ed 3, St Louis, 1987, The CV Mosby Co.

Sibai BM: Seeking the best use for magnesium sulfate in preeclapmsia-eclampsia, Contemp OB/GYN 29(1):155, 1987.

Bibliography

Bennett EC: Sexually transmitted diseases: current approaches, NAACDG Newsletter 14(8):1, 1987.

Corbett M and Meyer JH: The adolescent and pregnancy, Boston, 1987, Blackwell Scientific Publications, Inc.

Finnegan LP: Substance abuse: implications for the newborn, Perinatolology-Neonatology July/August 1982.

Haggerty L: TORCH: a literature review and implications for practice, JOGN Nurs 14:124, Mar/Apr 1985.

Metcalf J, McAnulty JH, and Ueland K: Burwell and Metcalfe's Heart disease and pregnancy: physiology and management ed 23, Boston, 1986, Little, Brown & Co, Inc.

Pritchard J, MacDonald P, and Gant N: Williams' Obstetrics, ed 17, New York, 1985, Appleton-Century-Crofts.

Silver H et al: Addiction in pregnancy: highrisk intrapartum management and outcome, J Perinatol 793:178, 1987.

7

Complications of the Newborn

Early identification and prompt management are imperative in treating newborns with complications. A solid knowledge base, sharp assessment skills, and expert clinical technique enable the nurse to play a vital role in the care of the compromised neonate. When an infant is born with problems, the family goes through stages of shock, denial, and guilt. The nurse must be prepared for the barrage of questions and emotions that accompany these situations and provide support to the family.

GESTATIONAL AGE AND BIRTHWEIGHT

Infants born at risk for gestational age and weight problems exhibit physiologic and pathologic states related to degree of maturity. Advances in modern technology have improved the survival rate and overall health of preterm infants, but problems remain. The nurse's skills in observing and recording often form the foundation for early diagnosis and appropriate treatment. The plan of care for premature infants is based on an understanding of infant behavior.

This section provides assessment guides for physical and neuromuscular maturity as well as a summary of potential problems. Nursing care emphasizes the need for parental support in facilitating the development of a positive parent-child relationship. Information presented here will assist the nurse to identify the special needs of parents who have experienced preterm delivery.

Table 7-1   *Physical Maturity Scales*

Criterion	Findings and Assigned Scores					Infant Score*
	0	1	2	3	4	
Skin						
Edema	Edema evident over hands and feet; pitting seen over tibia	Pitting edema over tibia	No edema obvious	—	—	_____
Texture and opacity	Gelatinous, transparent; veins seen especially over abdomen	Visible, veins; thin, smooth	Few larger veins seen, especially over abdomen; medium-thick smooth skin	Veins rarely seen; some thickening superficial cracking	No vessels; parchmentlike, thick, cracking; if leathery, very cracked, and wrinkled, give score of 5	
Color	Dark red (infant is quiet for evaluation)	Pink	Pale pink	Pale; pink mainly over palms, soles, lips, and ears		
Lanugo	None	Abundant over body; long; thick	Thinning, especially over lumbosacral area	Bald areas; thinning over other areas	Mostly bald of lanugo; at least half of back bald	_____
Plantar creases	No creases seen	Faint red marks on upper half of sole	Red marks obvious over more than upper half; deeper lines over less than one third	Indentations noticeable over more than one third; lines seen over two thirds	Creases cover entire sole	_____
Breast	Nipple barely perceptible; no palpable breast tissue	Flat, smooth areola present around well-defined nipple; some breast tissue	Stippled areola but edge flat; 1-2 mm breast bud	Stippled areola with edges raised; 3-4 mm breast bud	Full areola; 5–10 mm breast bud; may have breast milk	_____
Ear form Cartilage	Pinna flat, soft, easily folded	Slight incurving of pinna; soft, easily folded; slow recoil	Well-incurved pinna; soft; ready recoil	Upper pinna well curved; formed and firm to edge; instant recoil	Thick cartilage; ear stiff	_____
Genitals Male	No testes in scrotum and no rugae over scrotum	—	Testes descending; few rugations	Testes within scrotum good rugae	Scrotum pendulous with rugae covering scrotum	_____
Female	Prominent clitoris and labia minora; labia majora do not cover labia minora	—	Labia majora and labia minora equally prominent	Labia majora appear large; labia minora, small	Labia majora completely cover clitoris and labia minora	
					TOTAL	_____

*Highest score possible = 25

Table 7-2   *Preterm Infant's Potential Problems and Their Physiologic Bases*

Potential Problem	Physiologic Bases
Initiating and maintaining respirations	Paucity of functional alveoli; incomplete aeration of lungs caused by deficient surfactant
	Smaller lumen and greater collapsibility or obstruction of respiratory passages
	Weakness of respiratory musculature
	Insufficient calcification of bony thorax
	Absent or weak gag reflex
	Immature and friable capillaries in brain and lungs
	Few functional alveoli in infants less than 28 weeks' gestational age (usually nonviable); marginal function in infants at 29-30 weeks
Maintaining body temperature	Large surface area in relation to body weight (mass)
	Absent or poor reflex control of skin capillaries (no shiver response)
	Small, inadequate muscle mass activity; absent or minimum flexion of extremities on body
	Meager insulating subcutaneous fat
	Friable capillaries and immature temperature regulating center in brain
	The smaller the infant, the more difficult it is for her or him to maintain normal body temperature
Maintaining adequate nutrition	Mechanical feeding problems
	• Absent or weak sucking and swallowing reflexes; unsynchronized
	• Absent or weak gag and cough reflexes
	• Small stomach capacity
	• Immature cardiac sphincter (stomach)
	• Lax abdominal musculature
	Absorption and assimilation problems
	• Paucity of stored nutrients: vitamins A and C; calcium, phosphorus, iron; loss of fat and fat-soluble vitamins in stool
	• Immature absorption, decreased amount of hydrochloric acid
	• Impaired metabolism (enzyme systems) or enzyme pathology
Maintaining central nervous system (CNS) function	Birth trauma: damage to immature structures
	Fragile capillaries and impaired coagulation process; prolonged prothrombin time
	Recurrent anoxic episodes
	Tendency toward hypoglycemia
Maintaining renal function	Impaired renal clearance of metabolites and drugs
	Inability to maintain acid-base, fluid, and electrolyte homeostasis
	Impaired ability to concentrate urine
	Paucity of stored nutrients from mother
Resisting infection	Paucity of stored immunoglobulins from mother
	Impaired ability to synthesize antibodies
	Thin skin and fragile capillaries near surface
	Impaired ability to muster white blood cells
Resisting hematologic problems	Increased capillary friability and permeability
	Low plasma prothrombin levels (increased tendency to bleed)
	Relatively slowed erythropoietic activity in bone marrow
	Relatively increased rate of hemolysis
	Loss of blood for laboratory specimens
Maintaining musculoskeletal integrity	Weak, underdeveloped muscles
	Immature skeletal system (bones, joints)
	Meager subcutaneous fat with its cushioning effect
Maintaining retinal integrity	Immature vascular structures in retina
	Need for oxygen therapy

Table 7-3 *Neuromuscular Maturity Scales**

Criterion	Method of Assessment	0
Posture	Position: supine Activity: quiet Assessment: extension and flexion of arms, hips, legs	Complete extension
Square swindow (wrist)†	Position: supine Method: with thumb supporting back of arm below wrist, apply gentle pressure with index and third fingers on dorsum of hand; do not rotate infant's wrist Assessment: angle formed between hypothenar eminence and forearm	Very premature (<30 weeks) 90°
Arm recoil‡	Position; supine Method; flex forearms on upper arms for 5 sec; pull on hands to full extension and release Assessment: degree of flexion	No recoil; arms remain extended 180°
Popliteal angle	Position: supine; pelvis on flat, firm surface Method: flex leg on thigh; then flex thigh on abdomen; holding knee with thumb and index finger, extend leg with index finger of other hand behind ankle Assessment: degree of angle behind knee	Complete extension; very premature 180°
Scarf sign	Position: supine Method: support head in midline with one hand; pull hand to opposite shoulder Assessment: position of elbow in relation to midline	Elbow to opposite arm like scarf around neck
Heel to ear	Position: supine, pelvis is kept flat on surface Method: pull foot up toward ear on same side; do not hold knee Assessment: distance of foot from ear and degree of extension of knee	Toes touch ear; leg completely extended (180°)

*Compare the combined scores for physical and neuromuscular maturity to the "maturity rating" scores and read estimated weeks of gestational age. Estimate of gestational
  All three measurements should fall within same approximate range, for example, all within SGA, LGA, or AGA. If one measurement is excessively large (falling into LGA
†Counterpart: ankle dorsiflexion. ‡Counterpart: leg recoil.

		Finding and Assigned Scores			Infant Score	
1	2	3	4	5	X	0
Extension of arms; slight flexion of hips, legs	Extension of arms	Slight flexion of arms; full flexion of legs	Complete flexion	—	_____	_____
Premature (30-35 weeks) 60°	Premature (30-35 weeks) 45°	Maturing (35-38 weeks) 30°	Term: hand lies flat on ventral surface of forearm 0°	—	_____	_____
—	Some recoil; sluggish response 100°-180°	Maturing (35-38 weeks) 90°-100°	Brisk recoil to complete flexion >90°	—	_____	_____
Prematue (30-35 weeks) 160°	Premature (30-35 weeks) 130°	Maturing (35-38 weeks) 110°	Maturing (35-38 weeks) 90°	Extension is resisted >90°	_____	_____
Elbow beyond midline of thorax	Elbow just beyond midline	Elbow at midline	Elbow does not reach midline	—	_____	_____
Toes almost reach face (130°)	Knees flexed (110°)	Knees flexed (90°)	Knees flexed politeal angle is less than 90°	—	_____	_____

NEUROMUSCULAR MATURITY TOTALS _____ _____

PHYSICAL MATURITY TOTALS _____ _____

(see Table 7-1).

COMBINED SCORE _____ _____

age obtained is accurate only to plus or minus 2 weeks. After gestational age is estimated, infant's length, weight, and head circumference are entered on appropriate graphs.
range) and other two fall into SGA range, growth deviation should be assessed. X, First examination; O, second examination.

Table 7-4   *Differences in Experiences of Term and Preterm Delivery*

Term Delivery	Preterm Delivery
The parents have gone through the full developmental process of a 40-week pregnancy.	The parents have not completed the psychological and emotional growth of a 40-week-gestation pregnancy.
The infant is healthy and has the physiologic, motor, and state control and social capacities common to full-term infants.	The infant is small, immature, often physically unattractive, and sick.
The parents have an enormous surge of emotion postpartum, which is derived from a combination of feelings of achievement and pride in their own success and fulfilled expectations about the intactness and healthiness of their infant.	The parents are often overwhelmed by feelings of failure, loss, fear, and sadness.
Full-term infants in the first 1 to 2 hours after birth have a period of alert time during which they open their eyes, look around, breast-feed, and generally behave like or exceed most parent's fantasies of a little baby.	The infant has none of the cute, appealing behaviors of a full-term infant. The infant is not alert, does not suck, and may be too sick to be held at all.

From Sammons W and Lewis J: Premature babies: a different beginning, St Louis, 1985, The CV Mosby Co.

Table 7-5   *Parental and Medical Milestones*

	Parental Milestones	Medical Milestones
Preterm birth of baby Preterm termination of pregnancy	Deprived of last trimester of pregnancy, a time of major adjustment during which the following are accomplished: 1. Resolution of issues of competency of parenting 2. Formulation of future hopes for the child 3. Change in couple's relationship as they approach parenthood	Hospital admission
Parents apart—different areas of hospital or different hospital Isolation Issues of fault	Reverse of caregiving role: father there first Initial time is a period of extreme disorganization 1. Loss of family and community supports 2. Long period before social interaction with baby (parents may need this) 3. Sense of distance from baby Death issue Loss of fantasy child dream	Transport Ventilator Multiple procedures Intravenous or arterial catheters
Mother discharged from hospital	Adaptation to NICU* environment 1. Initial distance—uncertain where baby is 2. Numbers and machinery 3. Parents relate to different machine: breast pump	Baby physiologically unstable
Parents together	Observers of the nurse's role with the baby Begin to understand some of what the technicalities and the numbers mean Start to use the medical jargon on the telephone Start to see other people developing a relationship with the baby Dependent on relationships with nurse and physician	Getting better Nasogastric feedings Temperature instability Beginning of nursing and staff attachment to baby
Begin caregiving: adoption of the staff role	Competition with the staff Fathers start to perceive change in focus to mother-infant relationship Start to offer show of affection for the baby Signs Attachment to head "doughnut" support Toys Clothes	Baby off of major support systems Still on monitors Weight single focus of well-being

Table 7-5, cont'd *Parental and Medical Milestones*

	Parental Milestones	Medical Milestones
Attempts to read social cues of infant	Holding the baby; difficult to get to know the baby 1. Feeding problems 2. Caregiving but little attachment 3. Still feel like it is not "our baby" 4. Energy consumption: beginning to sense how to "help" the baby 5. Conflicting messages: "okay" but monitors just to make sure	Removal of last physical barriers Out of Isolette to bassinet
Changes in visiting patterns May visit separately	Need to form their own relationship—beginning of attachment 1. Subjective: not measureable by number of phone calls, duration of visits, etc. 2. What they want to do, not what they are told to do by staff Differentiation of mother and father roles 1. Different caregiving routines 2. Different visiting times 3. Competition over who had the "magic touch" at the last visit Reassessment of competency issues, parents' and infant's 1. Breast-feeding: continuation or failure 2. Less competition over caregiving 3. Joy at increased awake time 4. Joy at increased response to inanimate stimulation	Off monitors Feeling that the baby has made it Parallel questions of whether the parents are ready
Nesting behavior	Start forming identity of child 1. Push for discharge date, sometimes inappropriately soon before an emotional base established 2. Settle lingering medical and developmental concerns: apnea etc.; necessary for security to feel comfortable going home 3. Start to use name actively—not just she or he	Nursing detachment issues
Start forming present role	Initial joy of predictable social response 1. Conflicting feelings of hope and risk 2. How do we form a relationship? Is it the same as for full-term infants? 3. Understanding child vs. understanding instructions, orders, and how to read behavior cues	
Grandparents and friends visit	Need to reestablish community and family supports	
Discharge	Final home preparations Often seem anxious—trying to adjust to facing new responsibilities Frequent questions	Medical discharge What to tell parents about high risk vs. recovery Is the premie normal?
Coming home: learning to live together	New sense of isolation—need to be self-sufficient Working out feeding and sleeping issues; new questions, uncertain answers Increased sense of competence of the parent-infant response system Predictability New feelings of crisis and doubt Medical visits or illnesses Grocery store at 6 months of age Overprotection, doubt about the premie Self-doubt	Visits to follow-up clinic

Answering questions about the future	Increasing sense of who the child is
	Independence vs. dependence issues
	New milestones:
	    Smiles
	    Laughter
	    Talking
	    Elicit attention
	    Originate social games	

Feeling like the premie has made it	Personal time Another child Vacations	

From Sammons W and Lewis J: Premature babies: a different beginning, St Louis, 1985, The CV Mosby Co.
*Neonatal intensive care unit.

NURSING CARE OF THE COMPROMISED NEWBORN

The woman, her family, and the compromised neonate are highly vulnerable. Protection of the newborn by maintenance of a warm environment, adequate oxygen, and safety is an important part of nursing care. The newborn's nutrition, fluid, and elimination needs must be monitored and met carefully.

This section provides procedures with rationales for the nursing interventions most commonly required by the compromised newborn. The nurse must keep in mind that parents need constant support. Holistic nursing care includes educating parents about the therapy their infant is receiving and helping them cope with feelings of guilt and grief.

Procedure 7-1

WEANING FROM OXYGEN THERAPY

DEFINITION

Withdrawing an infant from ventilator and extraneous oxygen dependence.

PURPOSE

To prepare infant to breathe room air. To stop ventilator use.

EQUIPMENT

Equipment already in use by infant being weaned; pulse oximeter (if available); regular bassinet, blankets, linens as needed after infant is weaned.

NURSING ACTIONS	RATIONALE
Identify client and check physician's orders.	To provide the right therapy for the right person.
Wash hands before and after touching client or equipment. Glove, prn.	To prevent nosocomial infection and to implement universal precautions.
Proceed with weaning process gradually.	To minimize the possibility of complications. The hazards of sudden cyanosis and respiratory collapse become greater with increased time that infant has received oxygen therapy.
Decrease oxygen by 10% every 30 to 60 minutes (or 2 to 4 hours) as child improves.	To minimize the possibility of reopening right-to-left shunts: foramen ovale, ductus arteriosus.
Attach infant to pulse oximeter during weaning.	To provide information on oxygen saturation of the tissues.
Monitor laboratory values simultaneously: blood pH, PaO$_2$,* partial pressure of carbon dioxide in arterial blood (PaCO$_2$), arterial hemoglobin concentration.	To provide data for modifying rate of weaning process.
Observe infant closely for the following:	To prevent adverse reactions to weaning:
Pulse.	Pulse elevation.
Respiratory effort.	Respiratory distress.
Skin color.	Cyanosis.
If symptoms occur, increase oxygen and proceed with slower weaning process.	

*Blood gas values given in Appendix C. Hospital intensive care units have protocols for care based on blood gas values.

Procedure 7-2

FEEDING NEWBORN WITH CLEFT LIP AND PALATE

DEFINITION

Congenital defects characterized by a fissure(s) in the palate and upper lip, resulting from the failure to fuse during embryonic development.

PURPOSE

To facilitate feeding when infant has difficulty creating a vacuum and sucking.

To prevent aspiration of feeding.

To prevent discomfort from increased amount of swallowed air.

EQUIPMENT

Lamb's nipple; Duckey nipple with flange to fit over defect; Brecht feeder; Rubber-tipped Asepto syringe.

NURSING ACTIONS	RATIONALE
Identify client and check physician's orders.	To provide the right therapy for the right person.
Wash hands before and after touching client or equipment. Glove, prn.	To prevent nosocomial infection and to implement universal precautions.
Prepare thickened formula as ordered, usually with dried rice cereal.	To increase gravity flow of fluid into stomach, and prevent aspiration.
Choose appropriate nipple and enlarge hole in nipple as needed.	To assist infant in creating a vacuum during sucking and to encourage development of normal sucking pattern.
	To permit passage of thickened formula.
Check infant for clear airway.	To minimize possibility of aspiration.
During feeding check infant for the following signs: aspiration—choking and cyanosis; swallowed air—abdominal distention.	To prevent abdominal distension and aspiration that can compromise respirations.
Hold infant in upright position.	To minimize possibility of aspiration and return of fluid through nose and to aid swallowing.
Interact with infant: talk and make eye contact with her or him.	To stimulate psychosocial development. If mother sees nurse doing this, it may facilitate her acceptance of the child.
Burp or bubble infant frequently.	To minimize amount of air that is swallowed when there is unnatural passage between nose and mouth. Technique increases infant's comfort and minimizes regurgitation and aspiration.
	To facilitate feeding.
When feeding with a rubber-tipped Asepto syringe, place rubber tip on top of and to side of infant's tongue.	To prevent tip of syringe from entering cleft in palate.
Offer feeding slowly.	To allow infant time to swallow.
NOTE: The child with a cleft lip only may be able to feed well with a regular or "preemie" nipple.	

Procedure 7-3

GAVAGE FEEDING

DEFINITION

A procedure in which a tube is passed through the nose or mouth into the stomach to feed an infant with weak sucking, uncoordinated sucking, and swallow or respiratory distress.

PURPOSE

To meet the nutrition and fluid needs of the infant who cannot suck.

EQUIPMENT

Sterile feeding tube: rubber or plastic, rounded tips, sizes 5 to 10, infant lengths; clearly calibrated syringe for feeding; stethoscope and sterile medication syringe without needle; sterile water for lubrication; feeding formula; medications.

NURSING ACTIONS	RATIONALE
Identify client and check physician's orders.	To provide the right therapy for the right person.
Wash hands before and after touching client or equipment. Glove, prn.	To prevent nosocomial infection and to implement universal precautions.
The infant's anatomy makes it difficult to enter the trachea. One or more of the following tests are done to determine correct stomach placement:	*To ensure paper placement of the nasal or oral tube for gavage feedings.*
Use sterile syringe to inject 0.5 ml of air through catheter into stomach, Simultaneously, listen for sound of air bubbling or "growling" in stomach with stethoscope over epigastric region.	Sound of air bubbling confirms tube placement in stomach.
The most complete procedure involves listening with stethoscope first over the epigastrium and then on each side of the anterior chest.	The sound of rushing air heard over the anterior chest should be considerably diminished intensity compared with that heard over the epigastrium.
Aspirate small amount of stomach contents.	Aspiration of stomach contents confirms proper placement of tube.
Fill tube with stomach contents, and pinch off tube; add syringe containing feeding.	This avoids allowing air into stomach with feeding.
Oral insertion: intermittent or indwelling catheter:	*To accomplish oral insertion:*
Position infant: head of mattress up one notch, folded towel under shoulders to slightly extend neck.	Opens oropharynx. Extends and straightens esophagus.
Select size 8 French feeding tube.	Is adequate size for feeding. Less apt to fold over or curl up.
Measure distance between bridge of nose, to earlobe, and then to lower end of xiphoid process. Mark distance with 5 cm (2 in) thin strip of paper tape. Fold tape over tube, leaving two long ends with which to secure tube when it is in place.	Determines length necessary to reach into stomach without folding back on itself. Facilitates anchoring tubing, if it is to be indwelling. Paper tape is usually less irritating to skin.
Lubricate tube in sterile water.	Prevents trauma and infection.
Pass tube along base of tongue, advancing it into esophagus as infant swallows.	Offers less risk of vagal stimulation or of accidental entry into trachea. Stimulates esophageal peristalsis and opens cardiac sphincter.
Test placement of tube.	Avoids introduction of formula, vitamins, and medicines into trachea or esophagus.
Aspirate and measure any residual feeding in stomach. If 1 ml or less, subtract same amount from this feeding. If more than 1 ml, physician may wish to have this feeding skipped.	Avoids overfeeding. Excessive fluid in stomach suggests intestinal obstruction.
Slowly pour warmed formula into syringe barrel and allow it to flow by gravity into stomach. Hold reservoir 15 to 20 cm (6 to 8 in) above infant's head. If gravity flow is too rapid, lower syringe, or insert plunger into syringe, and inject *slowly*. Feeding time should approximate that of nipple feedings (20 minutes or about 1 ml/min.)	Rapid entry of formula into stomach causes rapid rebound response with regurgitation, thus increasing danger of aspiration or abdominal distension, which compromises respiratory effort.
Do not allow level of formula to go below neck of syringe.	Prevents entry of air into stomach to minimize risks of regurgitation and distension.

Procedure 7-3, cont'd

NURSING ACTIONS	RATIONALE
Observe infant's response.	Prevents respiratory distress. Assists gastrointestinal functioning.
Follow formula with specified amount of sterile water.	Gets all formula into stomach and clears tubing of formula.
Pinch tubing (or clamp it off) and withdraw it rapidly.	Prevents entry of air into stomach. Creates vacuum to hold fluid in tubing to prevent dripping it into trachea on withdrawal.
Burp or bubble infant. With left hand, support infant's head and shoulders. Raise to a sitting position and lean infant onto right hand. Right hand supports infant's chest with palm and infant's jaw with thumb and forefinger. Gently rub back with left hand.	Increases comfort. Prevents regurgitation.
Position on right side with small rolled drape or towel.	Facilitates stomach emptying.
Record the following:	Provides basis for evaluation and readjustment of feeding regimen. Facilitates communication among personnel.
Amount of residual gastric aspirate	
Type and amount of feeding, medicine	
Time of feeding	
Infant response: fatigue, peaceful sleep, abdominal distension, respiratory distress, type and amount of vomiting or regurgitation; heart and respiratory rate	
Nasal route: intermittent or indwelling catheter:	*To accomplish nasal insertion:*
Position as for oral route.	Opens oropharynx. Extends and straightens esophagus.
Select size 3½ to 5 French feeding tube.	Is adequate size for feeding and small enough to allow breathing space around it, since neonates are obligate nose breathers.
If indwelling, change every 2 or 3 days (48 to 72 hours) or more frequently if otitis is present, alternating sides of nares.	Prevents infection, irritation; excess mucus, ulceration, bleeding
Observe infant for respiratory distress.	If tube causes distress, remove it. Infants are obligate nose breathers. Use oral route.
May be preferred route for indwelling tube for continuous drip feeding.	Very small preterm infant often better tolerates feeding by continuous drip, stomach is not overloaded.
Measure distance from bridge of nose to earlobe, and then to xiphoid process (just beyond tip of sternum). Mark spot with 5 cm (2 in) thin strip of paper tape, and overlap tube, leaving ends free	Provides adequate length to reach stomach without curling. Facilitates anchoring of tubing. Decreases risk of skin irritation from tape.
Lubricate with sterile water.	Prevents tissue trauma.
Insert tube, holding it horizontally until it reaches back of nares; then lift tubing slightly and continue to advance. Allow infant to swallow tube while it is being advanced.	Accommodates to bend in back of nares and minimizes direct tissue damage. Stimulates peristalsis and opens cardiac sphincter.
Continue as for oral route.	Same as for oral route.
Nursing care after feedings:	*To provide supportive care after feedings:*
Burp infant gently after feedings.	Promotes comfort and prevents vomiting.
Turn infant's head or position the infant on right side after feeding and burping.	Protects against aspiration of stomach contents if vomiting occurs. Allows release of air from baby's stomach.
Postpone postural drainage and percussion for a minimum of 1 hour after feeding.	Promotes retention of feeding.
Avoid feeding the infant within an hour before a laboratory test for blood glucose.	Promotes accurate reading in laboratory tests.

Procedure 7-4

MONITORING PARENTERAL FLUID ADMINISTRATION

DEFINITION

Administration of fluids and nutrients to an infant by a route other than the alimentary canal, usually by intravenous route, either peripheral vein or umbilical artery.

PURPOSE

To meet the newborn infant's fluid needs.

EQUIPMENT

1. Supplies to start or maintain intravenous therapy by way of a peripheral vein, venous cutdown, or umbilical catheter.
2. Supplies to prevent accidental overhydration:
   a. Bottles containing 250 ml of infusion fluid.
   b. Administration sets with enclosed reservoirs and minidropper.
   c. Infusion pump with automatic alarm to signal an empty fluid chamber.
   d. Medicine cup (paper) or other appliance to protect insertion site if using scalp vein.

NURSING ACTIONS	RATIONALE
Identify client and check physician's orders.	To provide the right therapy for the right person.
Wash hands before and after touching client and/or equipment. Glove, prn.	To prevent nosocomial infection and to implement universal precautions.
Prepare equipment.	To avoid searching for missing articles after procedure has begun.
Restrain infant.	To provide for infant's safety and increased ease of starting parenteral fluids.
Provide pacifier to infant if appropriate.	To provide comfort for the infant who can handle a pacifier.
Continue care of intravenous infusion. Regulate rate of flow.	*To provide for adequate infusion.*
Infusion pump: check setting; double-check by counting drops per minute every hour, and note amount infused every 4 hours.	Ensures a more accurate and constant flow rate. Double-checks for equipment malfunction.
Reposition extremity or infant's head.	Ensures proper body alignment and prevents breakdown of skin. Protects infusion site.
Do not make up deficiency or excess by changing rate of flow without consulting physician.	Fluid may *overload* infant's system. An infant who has received more than prescribed amount for period must be assessed for overhydration and cardiac decompensation.
Check infusion site every hour.	*To prevent trauma to tissues. Ensures adequate hydration. Possible complications:*
Check for tissue infiltration (swelling).	Infection
Check for tissue trauma: color, temperature.	Thrombophlebitis.
If needle is in extremity, compare and contrast with other extremity.	Tissue and vein trauma.

Procedure 7-4, cont'd

NURSING ACTIONS	RATIONALE
If needle is in scalp vein, check head and face for symmetry of contour and movement.	Needle out of vein with injection of fluid into surrounding tissues and possible tissue breakdown.
Evaluate infant's hydration every hour.	*To determine adequate rate of flow.*
Urinary output: collect or weigh diapers.	Assesses amount of urine excreted.
Specific gravity of urine.	Assists in assessing appropriate solute or fluid infant needs and kidney function.
Weight: infant may be weighed every 8, 12, or 24 hours (same scale, naked, before feeding).	Weight gain or loss greater than 2% of body weight within a 24-hour period is cause for concern.
Urine: check for glucose every 8 to 24 hours.	Presence of excess glucose in the urine would indicate an excessive glucose load in the intravenous fluid.
Other: tissue turgor; fever; sunken fontanels; soft, sunken eyeballs; or behavior changes may be present.	Assesses state of hydration.
Record the following:	*To provide complete data.*
Type of fluid being used.	Evaluates treatment.
Amount of fluid absorbed every hour and amount scheduled to have been absorbed.	Meets infant's changing needs.
Amount of fluid in bottle or fluid chamber.	Identifies possible cause of any existing or new problem.
Flow rate.	Provides base line for continuation at present rate or change in rate.
Infant's condition.	Indicates infant's response to this regimen and readiness for progression.
Change intravenous tubing and bottle every 24 hours.	To decrease possibility of infection.
Irrigate intravenously.	*To maintain patency of system.*
Three-way stopcock may be used to connect tubing to needle.	Facilitates flushing needle while decreasing chance of contamination and loss of blood during procedure.
Without three-way stopcock, clamp intravenous tubing and disconnect at junction with needle. Keep tubing end sterile. Attach syringe containing 1 to 3 ml of normal saline solution or heparinized saline solution to needle.	Clears out small occluding clots; prevents formation of clots.
Slowly inject fluid into vein. Disconnect syringe and reconnect to intravenous tubing. Unclamp intravenous tubing and regulate flow of infusion.	Prevent trauma to vein or dislodging the needle.
Never flush a clogged needle.	To avoid pushing blood clot through infant's circulation.
After intravenous fluid is discontinued:	*To ensure adequate nutrition and hydration.*
Observe infant for hypoglycemia for 24 hours.	Hypoglycemia often is seen after discontinuation of parenteral therapy.
Observe infant for adequacy of nutrition and hydration.	Assesses infant's ability to take and utilize nutrients and fluids by mouth or gavage.
Continue to assess infant for thrombophlebitis at previous insertion site and sloughing.	Begins definitive treatment and prevents tissue damage.

Procedure 7-5

TOTAL PARENTERAL NUTRITION (TPN)

DEFINITION

The administration of a nutritionally adequate hypertonic solution consisting of glucose, protein hydrolysates, minerals, and vitamins through an indwelling catheter in the superior vena cava or umbilical artery.

PURPOSE

To provide continuous nutrition at a prescribed rate for extended periods of time.

EQUIPMENT

Equipment for starting intravenous infusion or cut-down; silastic catheter of appropriate size; millipore intravenous filter; constant infusion pump; TPN solution (infusion fluid); pacifier and mobiles; restraints as necessary.

NURSING ACTIONS	RATIONALE
Identify client and check physician's orders.	To provide the right therapy for the right person.
Wash hands before and after touching client or equipment. Glove, prn.	To prevent nosocomial infection and to implement universal precautions.
Gather equipment as necessary.	To be efficient and save time.
Procedure may be done in operating room. Nursing actions are the same as those for care of an infant receiving intravenous therapy, except for the following notable additions:	To maintain strict aseptic technique.
Avoid using the catheter for purposes other than the infusion solution (e.g., not to be used for blood or medications).	To maintain patency; avoid mixing incompatible fluids.
Avoid making up excess or deficit by altering the drip rate without consulting the physician.	To avoid fluid overload or deficit.
Order prescribed mixture from pharmacy. Do not tamper with mixed solution. Do not add to mixture.	To ensure accuracy of amounts and prevent microbial contamination and admixture problems.
Check on rate of flow.	To avoid overfeeding or underfeeding.
Check pump setting.	To avoid using malfunctioning equipment.
Check amount given from calibrated, enclosed reservoir every 2 to 4 hours.	
Change bottle, tubing and Millipore filter every 24 hours.	To decrease risk of microbial contamination.
Change dressing around catheter.	To prevent infection, and allow observation of needle insertion site.
Monitor infant's weight daily, at same time, on same scale, before feeding.	To provide index of response to this form of therapy.
Provide pacifier, mobiles, infant stimulation pictures.	To provide sucking satisfaction and visual stimulation.
Observe infant for complications associated with TPN.	To facilitate prompt identification and treatment of problems:
	Sepsis.
Catheter and its insertion: local skin infection septicemia, blood vessel thrombosis, obstruction or dislodgment of catheter, cardiac symptoms such as dysarrhythmia. *Candida* septicemia is common.	
Infusion solution—type and amount: glucosuria, dehydration, acidosis, amino acid imbalance.	Metabolic complications.

NEWBORN OF DIABETIC PREGNANCY

Wide fluctuations of blood glucose above and below the normal range adversely affect embryonic and fetal development. It is therefore critical to monitor carefully the pregnant woman with known diabetes. Unforunately, gestational diabetes is diagnosed after the crucial period of organogenesis.

Infants born to diabetic mothers require special care. The nurse needs to be knowledgeable about the problems that these neonates commonly develop and the appropriate interventions.

Table 7-6   *Timetable: Monitoring Pregnancy Complicated with Diabetes Mellitus*

Assessment	Gestational Age
Out of hospital	
α-Fetoprotein	10 weeks
Hb$_{Alc}$ (glycosylated hemoglobin)	Weekly
Ultrasound	18 and 28 weeks for fetal growth
Serial urine or serum estriols	Weekly starting at 32 weeks
Nonstress test	Weekly starting at 34 weeks
Amniocentesis (lecithin/sphingomyelin ratio, phosphatidyl-glycerol)	36 weeks
Repeat amniocentesis for evaluation of lung maturity	If previous test showed immaturity
Hospitalization	
Protracted nausea and vomiting	Anytime for control of condition; at 36 weeks if good glucose/insulin control has not been achieved or if other risk develops
Infection (e.g., urinary tract infection)	
Inadequate diabetic control	

Sample Nursing Care Plan

COMPLICATIONS OF INFANTS OF DIABETIC MOTHERS

ASSESSMENT	NURSING DIAGNOSIS (ND)/ PLAN (P)/GOAL (G)	RATIONALE/ IMPLEMENTATION	EVALUATION
Review prenatal records, especially noting: maternal glucose control, ultrasound results for growth, nonstress test results, amniocentesis (L/S ratio, phosphatidyl-glycerol). Assess infant frequently within the first hours of life for (in order of incidence). Respiratory distress, and congenital anomalies or disorders. Birth trauma (cephalhematoma, paralysis of the facial nerve, fracture of the clavical). Meconium aspiration (amniotic fluid is stained, or if skin, nails, or cord is stained). Gestational age, weight (LGA, appropriate for	ND: Altered breathing pattern related to lung immaturity as manifested by respiratory distress. ND: Altered breathing pattern related to secretions or meconium in airway after birth. P: Monitor continuously and modify plan of care as data emerge. G: Infant will maintain an open airway and show no signs of respiratory distress.	*To ensure maintenance of an open airway, the nurse will:* Note maternal history, especially presence of phosphatidyl-glycerol (if obtained). Have oxygen and resuscitative equipment available. Note and report signs of respiratory distress. Monitor breath sounds every 15 minutes for 6 hours. Position newborn on side, with head slightly lower and neck slightly extended. Suction neonate's mouth and nose as necessary and report meconium-stained secretions. Report and evaluate any birth trauma or congenital	Infant maintains an open airway and respiratory distress is prevented or treated quickly. Infant suffers no birth trauma; or, trauma is promptly identified and treated with no adverse sequelae. Infant's gestational age is correctly determined and

Continued.

Sample Nursing Care Plan—cont'd

ASSESSMENT	NURSING DIAGNOSIS (ND)/ PLAN (P)/GOAL (G)	RATIONALE/ IMPLEMENTATION	EVALUATION
gestational age [AGA], SGA), and degree of maturity (Tables 7-1, 7-2).		anomaly that might interfere with adequate ventilation. Treat infant as premature, regardless of weight, until gestational age and respiratory maturity are established.	appropriate care is initiated.
Assess tests for hypoglycemia: Dextrostix, Clinistix. 30 min of age. 1 ½ hr of age. 4 hr of age. 9 hr of age. 12 hr of age. 24 hr of age. Then once daily for 8 days. Evaluate serum blood glucose levels compared with Dextrostix value. Assess for signs of hypoglycemia: Feeding difficulty, hunger. Apnea. Irregular respiratory effort. Cyanosis. Weak, high-pitched cry. Jitteriness, twitching, eye rolling, seizures. Lethargy.	ND: Potential for injury related to hypoglycemia. ND: Altered nutrition: less than body requirements, related to hypoglycemia. P: Monitor closely and follow agency's protocols for care. G: Infant will maintain acceptable blood glucose levels and remain free from signs of hypoglycemia.	*To evaluate for hypoglycemia and prevent its occurrence, the nurse will:* Perform blood glucose test according to schedule. Obtain blood glucose test by laboratory once daily to compare with Dextrostix or if Dextrostix value <30 mg/dl during the first 72 hours of life or <45 mg/dl after first 3 days of life in the full term infant or <20 mg/dl in the preterm infant. Observe and report signs of hypoglycemia. If suck and swallow reflex is intact, feed the infant according to hospital protocol. Feedings should be in small frequent amounts beginning at 1 hour of age. Administer intravenous fluids as ordered if infant unable to feed. Report blood glucose <30 mg/dl; physician may administer 10% glucose in water intravenously.	Newborn suffers no hypoglycemic episodes. Newborn suffers no brain damage from hypoglycemia.
Assess blood levels for hypocalcemia (50% incidence with infants of insulin-dependent mothers). Assess signs of hypocalcemia within first 48 hours (edema, apnea, intermittent cyanosis, and abdominal distension). After 48 hours the classic symptoms of tetany may be noticed.	ND: Potential for injury related to hypocalcemia. P: Monitor closely and follow agency's protocols for care. G: Newborn will maintain acceptable blood calcium levels.	*To monitor calcium levels and treat hypocalcemia, the nurse will:* Obtain blood for serum calcium laboratory test once daily as ordered. Observe and report signs of hypocalcemia. Obtain intravenous access for calcium gluconate 10% solution as ordered (no scalp vein sites). Monitor calcium gluconate infusion. If heart rate < 100 beats/minute, discontinue infusion and notify physician. Apply firm pressure to intravenous site when catheter	Newborn suffers no episodes of hypocalcemia. Newborn has no episodes of tetany.

Sample Nursing Care Plan—cont'd

ASSESSMENT	NURSING DIAGNOSIS (ND)/ PLAN (P)/GOAL (G)	RATIONALE/ IMPLEMENTATION	EVALUATION
		is removed from vein to prevent seepage of the calcium gluconate into surrounding tissues. Reduce environmental stimuli. Observe for and take precautions against seizures.	
Assess for polycythemia between 6 and 24 hr of life (if present).		*To assess for polycythemia the nurse will:* Obtain blood for complete blood cell count (CBC) and report results.	
If polycythemia is present, closely monitor for hyperbilirubinemia.		See Summary of Nursing Actions, "Hyperbilirubinemia," p. 306.	
Assess for congenital anomalies or disorders (4% increased risk). Birth trauma (cephalhematoma, paralysis of the facial nerves, fracture of the clavical). Assess parent-newborn interactions. Assess educational needs for child care.	ND: Knowledge deficit related to care of an IDM. ND: Anxiety, fear, grieving, powerlessness, situational low self-esteem, spiritual distress, ineffective individual or family coping, altered family processes—related to having, and caring for a child with a birth defect. P: Monitor closely and institute appropriate care; be available to parents for discussion of questions; demonstrate care and observe return demonstration. G: Parents will verbalize understanding of the explained congenital anomalies or birth trauma and their effects or complications to the child's well being. G: Parents will verbalize feelings and concerns regarding their infant.	*To aid parents in adjusting to and caring for a child with an anomaly or transient birth injury, the nurse will:* Note and report congenital anomalies or birth trauma. Weigh newborn soon after delivery, then daily. Measure head and chest circumference. Explain all procedures to parents. Explain congenital anomalies or birth trauma and their effects on child. Answer questions and correct misconceptions. Encourage open communication. Demonstrate child care activities. Observe parent-infant interactions. Schedule appointments for lab studies and follow-up physical examination. Refer to outside resources (child care, homemaker, clergy, home health).	Parents verbalize understanding of instructions. Parents express feelings and concerns about their infant. If child has an anomaly or dies, parents experience appropriate grief response. Parents learn how to care for their child.

Summary of Nursing Actions

INFANT OF DIABETIC MOTHER (IDM)

I. Goals
- A. For the mother: a physically safe and emotionally satisfying pregnancy and delivery
- B. For the fetus and newborn: a healthy intrauterine environment and transition to extrauterine existence
- C. For the family: an understanding of diabetes mellitus and willing compliance with management. If newborn exhibits a disorder or dies, the grieving process is initiated.

II. Priorities
- A. Maintenance of euglycemia throughout pregnancy
- B. Safe delivery of a live infant
- C. Prevention of or early identification and treatment of neonatal hypoglycemia and other conditions associated with maternal diabetes
- D. Initiation of a positive family-newborn attachment

III. Assessment
- A. Review prenatal records.
- B. Assess the newborn frequently for the following associated clinical problems (in order of probable appearance):
  1. Respiratory distress and ventilatory adequacy
  2. Congenital anomalies or disorders (incidence is 6% compared to 2% in all deliveries)
  3. Birth trauma (e.g., cephalhematoma, paralysis of the facial nerve, fracture of the clavicle
  4. Meconium aspiration (if amniotic fluid was stained or if skin, nails, or cord is stained with meconium)
  5. Gestational age and degree of maturity (LGA, AGA, SGA)
  6. Hypoglycemia (within the first 3 hours)
  7. Polycythemia (by 6 hours of age)
  8. Hypocalcemia (within 24 to 36 hours)
  9. Hyperbilirubinemia (on day 2 or 3)
- C. Weigh newborn soon after birth, then daily. Measure head and chest circumference.
- D. Assess parent-newborn interaction.

IV. Potential nursing diagnoses
- A. Infant
  1. Impaired gas exchange
  2. Ineffective airway clearance
  3. Ineffective breathing pattern
  4. Altered nutrition: less or more than body requirements
  5. Ineffective thermoregulation
  6. Potential for injury
  7. Potential for aspiration
  8. Potential altered growth and development
  9. Potential ineffective breast-feeding
  10. Potential for infection
- B. Parents
  1. Anxiety
  2. Fear
  3. Ineffective individual coping
  4. Ineffective family coping: compromised
  5. Altered family processes
  6. Anticipatory grieving
  7. Knowledge deficit
  8. Noncompliance (specify)
  9. Altered nutrition: less or more than body requirements
  10. Powerlessness
  11. Personal identity disturbance
  12. Self esteem disturbance: situational low self esteem
  13. Body image disturbance
  14. Altered role performance
  15. Potential altered parenting
  16. Spiritual distress
  17. Potential sleep pattern disturbance
  18. Potential impaired adjustment

V. Plan/implementation
- A. At birth
  1. Maintain equipment and ensure adequate oxygen and other supplies for resuscitative measures.
  2. Assist with resuscitation as necessary.
  3. Protect newborn against loss of body heat by drying, wrapping in warmed blankets, and positioning under a heat source.
  4. Reinforce explanations to parents by physician.
  5. Provide emotional support to parents.
- B. Subsequent care
  1. Position newborn on the side, with head slightly elevated and neck slightly extended.
  2. Report and record signs of respiratory distress.
  3. Treat as if infant is premature, regardless of weight, until gestational age and respiratory maturity are established.
     - a. Place in incubator that has been set between 32° and 36° C (90° and 97° F) (depending on infant's maturity, size).
     - b. Attach thermistor probe or take axillary temperature every 15 minutes until stabilized and then hourly. Temperature should stabilize at 36.5° C (97.6° F).
     - c. Check respiratory rate every 15 minutes for 6 hours; place newborn on respiratory monitor if respirations are irregular.
     - d. Have oxygen and resuscitative equipment available.
  4. Feed as necessary (glucose, calcium). Monitor parenteral fluid therapy.
  5. Carry out orders for decreasing bilirubin levels.
  6. Promptly report and record any signs of anomalies, dysfunction, or disorder.
  7. Keep parents informed. Nurse is available to parents for their questions (e.g., explain that infant's condition is reflection of maternal condition rather than infant diabetes), discussion of feelings, and so on.

VI. Evaluation
- A. The newborn's airway remains patent, and respiratory distress is prevented or treated quickly.
- B. The newborn does not experience cold stress, and the newborn's temperature stabilizes within 8 to 10 hours after birth.

Summary of Nursing Actions—cont'd

C. The newborn experiences no hypoglycemia episodes (below 30 mg/dl), and blood glucose levels stabilize in the physiologic range (approximately between 45 and 130 mg/dl).

D. The newborn experiences no hypocalcemic episodes.

E. Bilirubin levels are maintained below toxic levels.

F. Fluid and electrolyte balance is maintained.

G. A positive relationship is established between parent and newborn.

H. Parents understand the care provided to the newborn.

I. Discharge planning is adequate:
1. Parents feel ready to provide care to the newborn.
2. Public health referral is made, if appropriate.
3. Referral to other community resources is made, if appropriate.
4. Parents stage motivation to carry out follow-up care.

SUMMARY OF NURSING CARE OF INFANT WITH HYPOCALCEMIA, HYPOGLYCEMIA, OR SEPSIS

GOALS	RESPONSIBILITIES
Recognize early signs of pathophysiologic state	Assess each system for signs and symptoms suggestive of each condition; correlate findings with general impression of progress of infant (feeding, weight gain, response to stimuli, and sleeping patterns).
Prevent or decrease potential side effects of medical intervention	
Hypocalcemia	Administer calcium gluconate slowly; if heart rate falls below 100 beats per min, stop infusion.
	Prevent extravasation of calcium gluconate into tissues:
	Avoid scalp vein.
	Ensure placement of needle before administering drug.
	Tape needle securely at site of insertion.
	Apply pressure to puncture site after removal of needle.
	Counsel mother regarding infant feeding (breast-feeding or appropriate formulas).
Hypoglycemia	Begin oral feeding as soon as possible after birth.
	Administer glucose infusion carefully; avoid overloading the system by speeding up intravenous administration.
	Observe for signs of hyperglycemia (acidosis) and possible need for insulin.
	Decrease intravenous administration of glucose slowly to prevent hypoglycemia from physiologic hyperinsulinemia.
Sepsis	Observe for side effects of antibiotics.
	Regulate infusion carefully to allow for antibiotic to be administered within 1 hour.
	Use piggyback setup if main intravenous solution has added drugs.
Monitor environment to decrease factors that will complicate recovery from each condition	Maintain thermoregulation, hydration, and oxygenation of infant.
	Monitor vital signs and correlate with infant's progress.
Hypocalcemia	Reduce environmental stimuli.
	Organize care to ensure minimum handling of infant.
	Discuss with parents reasons for minimum holding.
	Institute seizure precautions.
Sepsis	Institute appropriate isolation techniques.
Observe for complications of disease	
Hypocalcemia	Observe for tetany and convulsions.
Hypoglycemia	Check heel blood with Dextrostix.
	Check urine for glycosuria.
Sepsis	Observe for signs of meningitis, especially bulging anterior fontanel.
	Observe for pyarthrosis, usually evidenced by limited movement of affected joint.
	Observe for signs of shock, expecially fall in blood pressure.
Provide emotional support for parents	Allow parents the opportunity to express their feelings.
	Keep parents informed of infant's progress.
	Encourage frequent visiting and participation in care to foster parent-child attachment.

From Whaley LF and Wong DL: Nursing care of infants and children, ed 3, St Louis, 1987, The CV Mosby Co.

Summary of Nursing Actions

NEONATAL HYPOGLYCEMIA

I. Goal
  A. Identification of the newborn at risk
  B. Treatment of the newborn exhibiting hypoglycemia
III. Assessment
  A. Note if newborn comes under the categories of those at risk for hypoglycemia:
    1. Newborns over 8 lb 2 oz (3969 g) or under 5 lb 10 oz (2551 g)
    2. Dysmature infants
    3. Infants of diabetic or prediabetic mothers
    4. Infants of preeclamptic-eclamptic mothers
    5. Polycythemic infants
    6. Cold infants
    7. Infants with severe erythroblastosis fetalis
    8. Infants with congenital heart disease
    9. Infants of mothers who received an infusion of dextrose in a balanced salt solution without insulin during labor, whether the newborn was born vaginally or abdominally.
  B. Do heel-stick test: Dextrostix, Clinistix.
    1. Determine frequency of test by assessing condition of newborn.
      a. For normal term infant, test is done at 45 minutes, 2 hours, and 6 hours of age.
      b. For infant at risk, do test at following intervals: 30 minutes of age, 1½ hours of age, 4 hours of age, 9 hours of age, 12 hours of age, 24 hours of age, and then once daily for 8 days.
  C. Order blood sugar test by laboratory if tests reveal blood glucose concentration levels below 30 mg/dl during the first 72 hours of life or below 45 mg/dl after the first 3 days in the full-term infant (in premature newborns a blood sugar level below 20 mg/dl).
  D. Observe for symptoms of hypoglycemia.
    1. Feeding difficulty, hunger
    2. Apnea
    3. Irregular respiratory effort
    4. Cyanosis
    5. Weak, high-pitched cry
    6. Jitteriness, twitching, eye rolling, convulsions
    7. Lethargy
IV. Potential nursing diagnoses
  A. Potential for injury
  B. Altered nutrition: less than body requirements
  C. Fatigue
  D. Potential for aspiration
  E. Potential activity intolerance
  F. Ineffective breathing pattern
  G. Dysreflexia
  H. Potential altered growth and development
V. Plan/implementation
  A. If suck-swallow reflex is well coordinated, feed the newborn according to hospital protocol. Term infants may be fed at 4 hours of age or earlier, as necessary. Small newborns or those born of diabetic mothers may need to be fed at 1 hour of age. Because newborns' stomach capacity is small, the amount should be small and the feedings frequent.
  B. Some pediatricians prefer early feedings of nonglucose carbohydrates, such as invert sugar or galactose. These preparations are less likely to overstimulate the newborn's pancreas to produce insulin (Whaley and Wong, 1987).
  C. If newborn cannot take fluids by mouth or if blood glucose is below 25 mg/dl, physician will administer 10% glucose in water intravenously.
VI. Evaluation
  A. Newborn suffers no hypoglycemic episodes.
  B. Newborn suffers no brain damage.
  C. Parents understand the condition and are able to establish a positive relationship with the newborn.

Summary of Nursing Actions

NEONATAL HYPOCALCEMIA

I. Goals
  A. To prevent neonatal hypocalcemia
  B. To prevent sequelae attributed to hypocalcemia

II. Priorities
  A. Prompt identification and treatment of neonatal hypocalcemia
  B. Monitor infant to prevent possible return of hypocalcemia

III. Assessment
  A. Identification of infants at risk:
    1. Infants receiving exchange transfusion of blood containing anticoagulant citrate. Citrate combines with calcium, thus depleting ionizable calcium needed for the coagulation process. To anticipate and replace this loss, 10% calcium gluconate is given.
    2. Other conditions that predispose an infant to hypocalcemia include the following:
      a. Perinatal asphyxia (33% of asphyxiated newborns)
      b. Use of bicarbonate to treat acidosis
      c. Diabetic mother (50% of newborns born to insulin-dependent mothers)
      d. Prematurity (33% of neonates born at 37 weeks' gestation or sooner regardless of birth weight)
      e. Preeclamptic-eclamptic mother treated before delivery with magnesium sulfate (a competitive antagonist to calcium)
    3. Tetany of the newborn was formerly a frequent occurrence, when 5- to 10-day-old infants were fed cow's milk.
  B. Within the first 48 hours, hypocalcemia may be exhibited as edema, apnea, intermittent cyanosis, and abdominal distension, but classic symptoms of tetany are absent. Note that these symptoms are similar to those of other neonatal disorders, for example, hypoglycemia and sepsis. Therefore the infant's history must be taken to assist in the correct diagnosis.

IV. Potential nursing diagnoses
  A. Potential for injury
  B. Impaired physical mobility
  C. Potential altered tissue perfusion
  D. Impaired gas exchange
  E. Altered health maintenance
  F. Potential fluid volume deficit on excess
  G. Potential altered nutrition: less or more than body requirements

V. Plan/implementation
  A. Medical therapy: acute care for hypocalcemia consists of calcium gluconate, 10% solution (100 to 150 mg/kg body weight) by intravenous infusion slowly; rapid infusion may cause flushing, vomiting, and circulatory collapse.
    1. Extravasation into surrounding tissue precipitates the calcium, causing necrosis and sloughing. Vitamin D_2 (ergocalciferol) every 24 hours for 2 to 3 weeks may be ordered.
  B. The nurse assists in medical management by monitoring the calcium gluconate infusion and the newborn's heart rate.
    1. If the heart rate is below 100 beats/min, the infusion is discontinued.
    2. A scalp vein is not used; the needle is taped securely at the site, and firm pressure is exerted over the site when the needle is removed to prevent seepage of the calcium gluconate into surrounding tissues.
    3. The needle should be changed every 12 hours for the same reason.
    4. Supportive nursing care includes the following:
      a. Maintenance of normal temperature, hydration, and oxygenation
      b. Reduction of environmental stimuli (e.g., nursing care organized to minimize handling of infant)
      c. Observation for and precautions against seizures
      d. Keeping parents informed of care and progress; providing time for parents to express feelings; encouraging parents to visit frequently and to participate in care of infant

VI. Evaluation
  A. Newborn suffers no episodes of hypocalcemia.
  B. Newborn has no episodes to tetany.
  C. Parents understand the condition and are able to establish a positive relationship with the newborn.

Summary of Nursing Actions

LARGE-FOR-GESTATIONAL-AGE INFANT

I. Goals
  A. For the mother: a satisfying birth
  B. For the newborn: a birth without trauma or injury and a neonatal period without hypoglycemia or hypocalcemia
  C. For the family: a positive birth experience

II. Priorities
  A. Prevention of birth injuries by appropriate choice of delivery method
  B. Prompt identification and treatment of birth injuries
  C. Prompt identification and treatment of hypoglycemia or hypocalcemia
  D. Parental support

III. Assessment
  A. Assess infant for hypoglycemia
    1. Blood glucose level
    2. Symptoms
  B. Assess for gestational age.
  C. After cesarean delivery:
    1. Assess for pallor: usually caused by iatrogenic bleeding
    2. If mother experienced prolonged labor before surgery, assess for anoxia, depressed skull fracture, possible paralyses; later assess for cephalhematoma.
    3. If fetal distress had been noted, observe for meconium aspiration
  D. After vaginal delivery
    1. If fetal distress had been noted, observe for meconium aspiration
    2. Note neurologic problems.
      a. Brachial paralysis: Erb-Duchenne type (symptoms on affected side):
        (1) Arm: abducted and internally rotated
        (2) Wrist: flexed
        (3) Palm: limp, grasp reflex present
        (4) Moro's reflex: asymmetric
      b. Paralysis of phrenic nerve (and usually diaphragmatic paralysis):
        (1) Color: cyanotic
        (2) Breath sounds: diminished
        (3) Respirations: on affected side labored, rapid
        (4) Abdomen: no rise with inspiration
        (5) Cry: weak or hoarse
      c. Facial paralysis (symptoms on affected side):
        (1) Facial contour and movement: asymmetric
        (2) Cheek: flattened
        (3) Eye: open
        (4) Poor suck, drooling of formula on affected side
      d. Brain injury from anoxia, direct trauma, or both:
        (1) Convulsions: clonic, tonic, localized; apneic spells. Symptoms include altered respiratory pattern altered level of consciousness, abnormal eye movements, abnormal chewing movements

        (2) Evidence of increased intracranial pressure: bulging fontanel at rest; wide sutures; especially separation of the coronal and lambdoidal sutures
        (3) Muscle tone; hypotonic; hypertonic
        (4) Reflexes: hyperreflexic, difficult to elicit; absent; asymmetry of response
    3. Orthopedic problems
      a. After vertex delivery: fractured clavicle; symptoms on affected side:
        (1) Arm: decreased or absent movement; pain response on passive movement
        (2) Deformity of clavicle over fracture site is sometimes seen and felt: distal part of clavicle is movable on palpation
      b. After breech delivery: fractured femur; symptoms on affected side:
        (1) Movement: absent; asymmetric Moro's reflex; pain response occurs on passive movement
        (2) Deformity of femur is sometimes seen and felt
    4. Soft tissue trauma
      (a) Abrasions from bony pelvis or forceps
      (b) Echymoses from bony pelvis or forceps
      (c) Petechiae over traumatized area only from bony pelvis or forceps
      (d) After first or second day, cephalhematoma
      (e) Subconjunctival hemorrhage from rupture of scleral capillaries
    5. Miscellaneous
      (a) Long fingernails
      (b) Macerated dry, peeling skin
  E. Assess parental response

IV. Potential nursing diagnoses
  A. Newborn
    1. Potential for injury
    2. Ineffective airway clearance
    3. Impaired gas exchange
    4. Potential for aspiration
    5. Altered nutrition: less or more than body requirements
    6. Altered growth and development
    7. Altered health maintenance
    8. Potential for trauma
    9. Impaired physical mobility
    10. Dysreflexia
    11. Altered tissue perfusion (specify)
  B. Parents
    1. Knowledge deficit
    2. Anxiety
    3. Fear
    4. Ineffective individual coping
    5. Ineffective family coping: compromised
    6. Anticipatory grieving
    7. Spiritual distress

V. Plan/implementation
  A. Treat hypoglcemia.

Summary of Nursing Actions—cont'd

B. Evaluate for and institute appropriate nursing care based on gestational age.

C. After cesarean delivery, record and report observations. Assist physician with treatment.
   1. Possible transfusion.
   2. Preoperative and postoperative care for reduction of depressed skull fracture; reemphasize to parents physician's explanation of cause and management of cephalhematoma, paralyses.
   3. Administer oxygen position infant; medications as necessary.

D. After vaginal delivery:
   1. Facilitate respirations.
   2. Note neurologic problems.
      a. Brachial paralysis: No definitive treatment is given; usually self-limited; position neonate in good body alignment to aid healing; prevent further injury; prevent deformity.
      b. Phrenic nerve paralysis: Position infant with head of mattress up. Place in optimum position to facilitate respiratory effort.
      c. Facial paralysis: If eye stays open, keep moist; close eye and apply patch to protect it from corneal abrasions. Support infant in upright position during feeding. Take extra time to feed. Do not force, since this may cause aspiration.
      d. Brain injury: Order and assist with laboratory tests for differential diagnosis to rule out other causes for convulsions.
         (1) EEG, subdural tap, skull films
         (2) Tests for sepsis; blood culture, urinalysis, lumbar puncture; chest x-ray film
         (3) Tests for metabolic problems
         (4) Tests for structural defects
         (5) O_2 to relieve cyanosis
      e. Position to facilitate respirations. Suction as necessary.
      f. Nutrition: Use nipple with caution; can be fed intravenously.
      g. Intravenous therapy: Administer medications, anticoagulants, antibiotics.
      h. Minimize stimuli: auditory, visual tactile.
   3. Orthopedic problems: Maintain good body alignment to prevent deformity and further injury. Prevent pressure areas on skin.

a. Fractured clavicle: not treated actively.
b. Fractured femur: both legs placed on traction-suspension (Bryant's traction) with or without a spica cast for 3 or 4 weeks until adequate callus is formed.

4. Soft tissue trauma.
   a. Prevent infection through broken skin.
   b. Observe for hyperbilirubinemia as hemorrhagic areas are resolved.

5. Miscellaneous.
   a. Cover hands with mitts to prevent self-inflicted scratches.
   b. Dry, dead skin in bedding will not injure child. Small amounts of lotion may be used; avoid unnecessary bathing.

6. Parental response.
   a. Reinforce, simplify, or clacify physician's explanations of procedures, findings, and medical-surgical management.
   b. Initiate discussion and allow time for mother and father to express feelings about condition of infant, mode of delivery, prognosis, and so on.
   c. Encourage parents to visit, touch, and assist in care of infant when appropriate. Be available to assist parents at crib side. Help parents keep in touch with infant until discharge.

VI. Evaluation
   A. Hypoglycemia is prevented or identified and treated promptly.
   B. Care appropriate to gestational age and needs is instituted.
   C. Injury is identified and treated promptly.
   D. Oxygen needs are met.
   E. Care for neurologic damage is instituted.
   F. Injury from convulsions is prevented.
   G. Sepsis is prevented or identified and treated promptly.
   H. Respirations are facilitated.
   I. Nutritional needs are met.
   J. Orthopedic injuries are identified and treated promptly.
   K. Soft tissue trauma is noted and treated as appropriate.
   L. Self-inflicted scratches are prevented.
   M. Parents' informational and emotional needs are met.

NEONATAL INFECTION

Many maternal infections affect the newborn. The most common are the TORCH infections (see "Maternal Infection" in Unit 6). The nurse must also be knowledgeable about the newborn with acquired immune deficiency syndrome (AIDS). The special care of infants with infection is presented in a summary of nursing actions in this section.

TORCH INFECTIONS AFFECTING NEWBORNS

T   Toxoplasmosis
O   Other: syphilis, varicella, group B β-hemolytic streptococcus, chlamydial infections, hepatitis B, AIDS
R   Rubella
C   CMV infections or cytomegalic inclusion disease (CMID)
H   Herpes simplex

SYMPTOMS AND SYNDROMES ASSOCIATED WITH PEDIATRIC AQUIRED IMMUNE DEFICIENCY SYNDROME (AIDS)

1. Seizure disorders
2. Motor dysfunction
3. Developmental delay
4. Microcephaly
5. Abnormal CT scan
6. Dysmorphic features (in some children)
7. Wasting syndrome
8. Lymphoid interstitial pneumonitis (LIP)
9. Recurrent bacterial infections
10. Encephalopathy
11. Cardiomyopathy
12. Hepatitis
13. Lymphadenopathy syndrome
14. Renal disease
15. Hypergammaglobulinemia
16. Normal ratio of helper to suppressor T cells usually 2:0, although overall number of helper T cells are diminished

This information was current at the time of publication. Because of the dynamic nature of this disease and ongoing research, nurses are encouraged to verify data with current sources.

NURSING CARE OF THE HIV-POSITIVE INFANT*

1. Wear gloves when changing diapers and handling urine specimens.
2. Wear gloves if there is contact with the infant's blood.
3. Wear cover gowns if caring for an infant with copious amounts of secretions.
4. Place diapers, gloves, and articles used to clean the infant in biohazard (usually red) bags for proper disposal.
5. Discard used nipples and bottles.
6. Wash hands with soap and water between sessions of infant contact and after handling infants (even when gloves are worn). This is not an airborne virus, so ordinary soap is effective.
7. Use a 1:10 solution of household bleach to clean any surfaces that come in contact with the infant's blood, feces, urine, or saliva. The solution is effective only for 24 hours; a new solution should be made at that time.
8. Do not cap needles used for intravenous injections or medication administration; dispose of them promptly in puncture-resistant disposable containers.
9. Have disposable resuscitation bags or mouthpieces handy for emergency resuscitation.
10. Basic immunizations may be given to HIV positive infants; however, dead virus vaccine must be used because of the possible immunologic deficits these infants may have.

This information was current at the time of publication. Because of the dynamic nature of this disease and ongoing research, nurses are encouraged to verify data with current sources.

*Institutional procedures may vary; follow the protocol established by your institution.

Summary of Nursing Actions

NEONATAL INFECTION

I. Goals
  A. For the mother: a satisfying birth
  B. For the newborn: a neonatal period in which infection is identified and treated promptly, and if therapy is necessary, no harmful sequelae result
  C. For the family: a satisfying newborn period in which they receive information and support and family-newborn attachment occurs
II. Priorities
  A. Prevent neonatal infection.
  B. Identify and treat neonatal infection promptly.
  C. Facilitate family-newborn attachment.
III. Assessment
  A. Review of prenatal record
  B. Age of onset
  C. Clinical manifestations
    1. Nonspecific: "doesn't look right"; "not doing well"; "poor weight gain"
    2. Organism-specific
      a. *Pseudomonas aeruginosa*: purple necrotic skin lesions
      b. Group B β-hemolytic streptococci:
      c. Herpesvirus type 2: fever, coryza, tachycardia,

hemorrhage, often evidenced by hemoptysis, bloody stools
      d. Gonorrhea: conjunctivitis, unstable temperature, hypotonia, poor feeding behavior
      e. Syphilis; rash, lesions of skin and bone, rhinitis, hepatosplenomegaly
    3. Systemic signs
      a. Respiratory system: apnea; irregular, grunting respirations with retractions
      b. Gastrointestinal system: vomitng; bile-stained diarrhea; abdominal distension; paralytic ileus with no stools; poor suck
      c. Skin: cyanosis, pallor, mottling, jaundice, local lesions
      d. CNS: similar to signs of hypocalcemia, hypoglycemia; that is, lethargy, irritability, tremors, convulsions, coma (increased intracranial pressure if meningitis develops)
      e. Temperature: normal or low or unstable
      f. Hepatomegaly or splenomegaly: notable after well-established sepsis
      g. Hemorrhage

Summary of Nursing Actions—cont'd

D. Laboratory studies
  1. Cultures: blood, umbilical stump, naso-oropharynx, ear canals, skin, CSF, stool, urine
  2. Bilirubin: increased direct (conjugated) bilirubin level, especially if organism is gram negative
  3. Blood studies: for anemia, increased WBC, decreased RBC (an ominous sign)
E. Drug side effects
  1. Penicillin: urticaria, skin rash, pruritus, vomiting, diarrhea, convulsions
  2. Kanamycin (Kantrex): WBCs, RBCs, protein in urine
  3. Polymyxin: proteinuria, irritability
F. Signs of infection with antibiotic-resistant and fungal organisms
G. Sequelae
  1. Meningitis
  2. Pyarthrosis
  3. Septic shock
H. Family responses
VI. Potential nursing diagnoses
  A. Infant
    1. Potential for infection
    2. Altered tissue perfusion (specify type)
    3. Diarrhea
    4. Pain
    5. Potential fluid volume deficit
    6. Altered nutrition: less than body requirements
    7. Altered oral mucous membrane
    8. Impaired gas exchange
    9. Ineffective airway clearance
    10. Ineffective breathing pattern
    11. Impaired skin integrity
    12. Altered patterns of urinary elimination
    13. Ineffective thermoregulation
    14. Potential for injury
  B. Parents
    1. Knowledge deficit
    2. Anxiety
    3. Fear
    4. Ineffective individual coping
    5. Ineffective family coping: compromised
    6. Altered family processes
    7. Powerlessness
    8. Anticipatory grieving
    9. Potential altered parenting
    10. Spiritual distress
V. Plan/implementation
  A. Medical management
    1. Antibiotics
      a. Penicillin, ampicillin, or kanamycin (Kantrex) for treatment of 90% of all organisms; treat for 10 days via intravenous infusion
      b. Gentamicin: especially for gram-negative organisms, such as *Pseudomonas aeruginosa*
    2. Support of physiologic systems
      a. Oxygen
      b. Fluids and electrolytes

c. Warmth
    3. Isolation procedures according to hospital protocol
  B. Nursing management
    1. Recognize signs
    2. Institute preventive measures to block modes of transmission
    3. Calculate dosage of medications accurately
    4. Recognize side effects of medications
    5. Monitor intravenous infusion rate, infusion site; change tubing and dressings at least every day
    6. Monitor optimal thermal environment
    7. Report symptoms of meningitis
  C. Facilitate parents' understanding of newborn's condition, medical and nursing management, expected results of therapies
    1. Clarify misinterpretations or misinformation
    2. Repeat explanations as often as needed
    3. Prepare parents for possible prolonged hospitalization
  D. Care of parents
    1. Encourage parents to express feelings
    2. Encourage parents to visit frequently and participate in newborn's care
    3. Keep parents informed of newborn's progress
  E. Instruct parents about hygiene measures: hand washing, especially after voiding or defecating
  F. Give parents written instruction on the following:
    1. Clinical manifestations
    2. What to report and whom to call
  G. Teach use of and reading of thermometer, if necessary
  H. Support parents
    1. Avoid blaming parents for infant's condition.
    2. Educate parents regarding transmission, treatment, prevention.
    3. Help parents communicate with pediatricians.
    4. Involve parents wiith care if possible. Facilitate early and frequent parent-child contact. Acknowledge positive parent involvement (e.g., interest, cooperation, care of infant).
    5. If nurse feels unprepared or hesitant to provide necessary sexual counseling, as needed for sexually transmitted diseases, parents should be referred to someone else. Avoid critical attitude toward parents.
VI. Evaluation
  A. Sepsis is prevented.
  B. Early signs of sepsis are recognized, and appropriate therapy is instituted.
  C. If therapy is necessary, no harmful sequelae result.
  D. Pathophysiologic sequelae to septicemia are prevented.
  E. Parents are able to form attachment to newborn.
  F. Parents' self-esteem is maintained.
  G. Staff establishes caring relationship with parents to foster their trust and to encourage continuing, active, positive interactions of family with members of health care system.

MATERNAL SUBSTANCE ABUSE

The mother who abuses alcohol or drugs places her fetus and newborn at risk. If prenatal counseling is ineffective or if the woman does not seek prenatal care, the newborn will suffer the consequences. The nurse must be alert to the signs and symptoms of neonatal drug dependence and knowledgeable about interventions for drug withdrawal.

RISKS ASSOCIATED WITH MATERNAL ALCOHOL INGESTION

Amount of Alcohol	Risks
Two or more drinks daily	Intrauterine growth retardation
Includes:	
2 mixed drinks, 1 oz. liquor each	Immature motor activity Increased rate of anomalies
2 glasses of wine, 5 oz. each	Decreased muscle tone Poor sucking pressure
2 beers, 12 oz. each	Increased rate of stillbirths Decreased placental weight
Five or more drinks on occasion	Increased risk of structural brain abnormalities
Six or more drinks daily	Fetal alcohol syndrome

From McCarthy P: Nurs Pract 8:1, 1983. Copyright the Nurse Practitioner: The American Journal of Primary Health Care.

MANIFESTATIONS OF THE PRINCIPAL FEATURES OF FETAL ALCOHOL SYNDROME

Central Nervous System Dysfunction

Intellectual	Mild to moderate mental retardation
Neurologic	Microcephaly (small head size)
	Poor coordination
	Decreased muscle tone
Behavioral	Irritability in infancy
	Hyperactivity in childhood

Growth Deficiency

Prenatal	Less than 3% for length and weight
Postnatal	Less than 3% for length and weight
	Failure to thrive
	Disproportionate-diminished adipose tissue

Facial Characteristics

Eyes	Short palpebral fissures (small eye openings)
	Strabismus, ptosis, myopia
Nose	Short and upturned
	Hypoplastic philtrum (flat or absent groove above upper lip)
Mouth	Thinned upper vermilion (upper lip)
	Retrognathia in infancy (receding jaw)

Abnormalities in Other Systems

Cardiac	Murmurs (atrial septal defects, ventricular septal defects, great-vessel anomalies, tetralogy of Fallot)
Skeletal	Limited joint movements (especially fingers and elbows and hip dislocations)
	Aberrant palmar creases
	Pectus excavatum
Renogenital	Kidney defects
	Labial hypoplasia
Cutaneous	Hemangiomas

From McCarthy P: Nurs Prac 8:1, 1983. Copyright The Nurse Practitioner: The American Journal of Primary Health Care.

Sample Nursing Care Plan

NEONATAL DRUG WITHDRAWAL

ASSESSMENT	NURSING DIAGNOSIS (ND)/ PLAN (P)/GOAL (G)	RATIONALE/ IMPLEMENTATION	EVALUATION
Note maternal drug history: length of drug habit; drug use during pregnancy; time and type of last drug taken. Assess patency of respiratory system: Note cough, swallow, and gag reflex.	ND: Ineffective airway clearance related to mucous or anatomic obstruction. P: Monitor closely and intervene per doctor's orders or established protocols. G: Infant will maintain an	*To maintain an open airway, the nurse will:* Have resuscitative equipment available. Aspirate mouth and nose as indicated. Assess breath sounds frequently. Report tachypnea or signs of	Infant maintains open airway and breathes easily.

Sample Nursing Care Plan—cont'd

ASSESSMENT	NURSING DIAGNOSIS (ND)/ PLAN (P)/GOAL (G)	RATIONALE/ IMPLEMENTATION	EVALUATION
Note sneezing and nasal stuffiness. Note amount and color of mucus. Assess for congenital defects (esophageal atresia). Assess for respiratory distress. Note onset and duration of tachypnea respiratory rate > 60/minutes. Note heart rate frequently during tachypnea episodes. Note presence of respiratory distress (retractions, flaring of nostrils, apnea). Note color—pallor or cyanosis. Note mottling. Note symptoms indicating pathology (heart disease).	ND: Impaired gas exchange related to drug withdrawal effects. P: Monitor closely and intervene per doctor's orders or established protocols. G: Client will be able to maintain adequate ventilation by own respiratory effort.	respiratory distress. Feed slowly in small amounts. Keep head elevated during feeding. *To support and monitor ventilation, the nurse will:* Place infant on cardiopulmonary monitor. Position for respiratory distress (head of bed elevated, prone, or side-lying). Report any increasing distress that alters heart rate or blood pressure. Provide oxygen therapy. Monitor blood gas values or transcutaneous oxygen and carbon dioxide values. Resuscitate and intubate as needed.	Infant able to maintain oxygen intake and respirations by own effort.
Note hyperactive Moro's reflex. Symmetric or asymmetric. Moderately or markedly exaggerated. Has medication affected reflex? Does infant have high-pitched cry? Does crying stop or increase with soothing?	ND: Sensory perceptual alterations related to withdrawal as manifested by increased sensitivity to stimuli. ND: Pain related to withdrawal effects. P: Complete physical examination; intervene per physician's orders or hospital protocols. G: Infant will relax when stimuli is reduced or infant is medicated.	*To reduce CNS excitability, the nurse will:* Group care to allow for uninterrupted rest. Decrease environmental stimuli. Medicate or sedate as ordered. Swaddle infant with blankets, cuddle, and hold close.	Infant relaxes and sleeps. Crying diminishes.

Note tremors:
  Note occurrence with stimuli.
  Note location of tremors.
  Note degree of tremors.
Observe for seizures: onset, origin, body involvement, clonic, tonic, (or both,) eye deviations, skin color.
Note CNS signs: bulging fontanel at rest, increased head circumference, widely spaced sutures, fixation of gaze without blinking.
Note inability to sleep for long intervals.
	ND: Sensory/perceptual alterations related to withdrawal as manifested by seizures.
	ND: Potential for injury related to seizures.
	P: Monitor closely and intervene per physician's orders or hospital procols.
	G: Infant will recover from seizures with minimal or no sequelae.
	
	ND: Sleep pattern disturbance related to with-
		To protect and monitor an infant with seizures, the nurse will:
		Maintain a patent airway.
		Prevent trauma by confining child in a close, soft environment.
		Record and report frequency and duration of seizures.
		Medicate or sedate as ordered.
		Have resuscitative equipment available.
		
		To promote rest, the nurse will:
			Infant recovers from seizures with minimal or no sequelae.
			
			Infant remains asleep for 3- to 4-hour periods.

Continued.

Sample Nursing Care Plan—cont'd

ASSESSMENT	NURSING DIAGNOSIS (ND)/ PLAN (P)/GOAL (G)	RATIONALE/ IMPLEMENTATION	EVALUATION
Assess sleep pattern. Assess effects of medication. Note yawning—onset and frequency.	drawal effect. P: Monitor closely and intervene per physician's orders or hospital protocols. G: Infant will be able to remain asleep for 3 to 4 hours.	Organize care to provide long rest periods. Reduce environmental stimuli. Swaddle infant with blankets, cuddle, or hold close.	
Note suck, swallow, and gag reflex. Note "frantic" suck response. Assess sucking with different types of nipples. Assess for sucking blisters on lip or arms. Assess for causes of poor feeding (esophageal atresia, immaturity, hypoglycemia, sepsis). Note occurrence and frequency of regurgitation. Note intake and output (I&O).	ND: Altered nutrition: less than body requirements, related to inability to ingest or retain food. P: Monitor closely and intervene per physician's orders or hospital protocol. G: Client will ingest and retain sufficient nutrients to promote growth.	*To promote nutritional intake, the nurse will:* Feed small frequent amounts. Position nipple in mouth so that sucking is effective. Keep head elevated during and after feeding. Avoid handling between feeding. Medicate between feedings if possible. Monitor I&O. Correlate intake with condition, growth, and therapy. Protect arms with shirt to prevent sucking blisters. Offer safety pacifier.	Infant ingests and retains sufficient nutrients for growth.
Note signs of dehydration: weight loss, sunken eyes and fontanel, poor skin tugor. Note characteristics of emesis or diarrhea (estimate fluid loss, color).	ND: Fluid volume deficit related to inability to retain fluids. P: Monitor closely and intervene per physician's orders or hospital protocol. G: Client will maintain adequate hydration and not demonstrate signs of dehydration.	*To maintain fluid and electrolyte balance, the nurse will:* Monitor I&O. Weigh every 8 hours or more often if vomiting and diarrhea continue. Give supplementary fluids if indicated for dehydration. Obtain blood for electrolyte levels as ordered.	Infant ingests and retains sufficient fluid or parenteral infusions provide sufficient fluids.
Note reddened areas over bony prominences. Note areas of skin breakdown. Note skin scratches.	ND: Impaired skin integrity related to withdrawal symptoms as manifested by excessive movement causing abrasions of the skin. ND: Potential for injury related to infection. P: Monitor closely and intervene per physician's orders or hospital protocol. G: Client will maintain intact skin free from infection.	*To maintain skin integrity, the nurse will:* Change position frequently. Provide skin care to reddened areas. Pad pressure areas with clothing. Keep fingernails trimmed. If skin is excoriated, treat for possible infection.	Infant's skin will remain intact and free from infection.

HYPERBILIRUBINEMIA

Elevated serum levels, especially of unconjugated (indirect) bilirubin, pose a grave danger to the newborn. Physiologic hyperbilirubinemia may become pathologic and require diagnostic tests and aggressive treatment. This section presents information on the recognition and treatment of hyperbilirubinemia. Commonly performed procedures are included as well as guidelines for client teaching.

Definitions

Rh incompatibility Hemolysis of fetal Rh-positive RBCs; specific antibodies from an Rh negative mother.

ABO incompatibility More common than Rh incompatibility; however, effects are generally less severe. Occurs when type A, B, or AB fetal RBCs cause a type O mother to develop antibodies.

Erythroblastosis fetalis Hemolytic disease of newborn usually caused by isoimmunization resulting from Rh or ABO incompatibility.

Hydrops fetalis Most severe expression of maternal Rh isoimmunization.

Physiologic hyperbilirubinemia Progressive increase in serum levels of unconjugated bilirubin. No bilirubin toxicity develops.

Pathologic hyperbilirubinemia Level of serum bilirubin at which a particular newborn will sustain lesions in the brain tissue (kernicterus), renal tubular cells, intestinal mucosa, and pancreatic cells.

PHASE OF KERNICTERUS

Phase one: the newborn is hypotonic and lethargic and exhibits a poor sucking reflex and depressed or absent Moro's reflex (some infants die during this phase).

Phase two: the newborn develops spasticity and hyperreflexia, often becomes opisthotonic, has a high-pitched cry, and may be hyperthermic. The newborn may convulse.

phase three: at about 7 days of age, the newborn's spasticity lessens and may disappear.

Phase four: after the first month of life, the infant develops sequelae (e.g., spasticity, athetosis, partial or complete deafness, or mental retardation).

Laboratory Analysis

A direct Coombs' test is performed with neonatal cord blood. The neonate's RBCs are "washed" and mixed with Coombs' serum. The test is positive (maternal antibodies are present) if the infant's RBCs agglutinate. The dilution of the specimen of blood at which agglutination occurs (if it does occur) determines the titer of maternal antibodies in fetal serum. The titer determines the degree of maternal sensitization. If the titer is 1:64, an exchange transfusion is indicated.

Procedure 7-6

EXCHANGE TRANSFUSION

DEFINITION

The introduction of whole blood in exchange for 75% to 85% of an infant's circulating blood that is repeatedly withdrawn in small amounts and replaced with equal amounts of donor blood

PURPOSE

1. Reduce serum bilirubin levels
2. Improve oxygen-carrying capacity of the blood:
   a. Remove red cells that are destined for hemolysis by circulating antibodies
   b. Correct the anemia
   c. Remove antibodies (or other causative agents) responsible for hemolysis
3. Correct acidosis

EQUIPMENT

1. Disposable exchange transfusion set
2. Fresh donor's blood (under 3 days old and heparinized), two units on hand in case of error or contamination
3. Monitoring equipment
4. Transfusion record
5. Water bath (38° C [100° F]) to warm the blood
6. Medications: calcium gluconate in 5 ml syringe with no. 24 needle; 50% glucose solution in 10 ml syringe with no. 24 needle; sodium bicarbonate in 10 ml syringe with no. 24 needle
7. Sterile gowns, drapes, gloves, caps, and masks
8. Cleansing solution with sterile cotton pledgets or gauze sponges
9. Adequate lighting
10. Heat source to keep the infant warm

Continued.

Procedure 7-6—cont'd

NURSING ACTIONS	RATIONALE
Identify client and check physician's orders.	To provide the right therapy for the right person.
Wash hands before and after touching client or equipment. Glove, prn.	To prevent nosocomial infection and to implement universal precautions.
Prepare and adjust heat lamps or overhead radiant heat shield; have warmed blankets available for infant.	To prevent cold stress.
Give infant nothing orally for 3 or 4 hours, or stomach contents are aspirated by gastric tube.	To prevent aspiration.
Assemble resuscitative equipment: O_2 source, masks, breathing bag, airways, laryngoscope (extra batteries), endotracheal tube with obturator, suction, medication.	To have readily available if needed for immediate supportive therapy.
Position infant on back and restrain. Take and record vital signs.	To facilitate treatment. Prevents dislodging catheter and tissue trauma. Provides base line to evaluate change.
Assemble electronic monitoring equipment or stethoscope. Attach electrodes, or keep stethoscope over apex of heart. Monitor and record results continuously during procedure.	To identify hazards of procedure that include apnea, bradycardia (100 beats/min or less), cardiac arrhythmia or arrest.
Physician *and* nurse check donor blood: type, Rh, age, and free of sickle cell trait.	To minimize chance of error. Provides donor RBCs that are not affected by maternal antibodies present in the fetal system. Acts as precaution against fatal intravascular sickling.
Run tubing from bottle (bag) through warm water bath to infant.	To avoid cold stress, ventricular fibrillation, vasospasm, or decrease in blood viscosity.
Before starting transfusion, assist physician as necessary	To prevent microbial contamination.
a. Cleanse site of cutdown (jugular or femoral artery) or umbilical stump (umbilical vein).	
b. Drape.	
c. Put on gown and gloves.	
During transfusion:	*During transfusion:*
Physician measures central venous pressure (CVP) before initiating transfusion.	To act as precaution against heart failure from volume overload. Change from 10 to 12 cm pressure is indication to stop and reassess infant's status.
Nurse notes and records time exchange is begun.	To maintain accurate record.
For *each* successive withdrawal of infant's blood *and* injection of donor's blood, nurse records time, amounts in and out, cumulative amounts in and out.	To maintain accurate, continuous record to assist with ongoing procedure and provide index of infant's response.
After 100 ml has been exchanged, physician gives calcium gluconate: nurse monitors heart and respiratory rates and records them.	To minimize possibility of cardiac arrhythmias or arrest.
Nurse records pertinent comments.	To maintain accurate record.
Nurse records medications: time, type, amount, infant response.	To maintain accurate record.
After transfusion (catheter may be removed or left in place with dressing):	To identify complications. Infant is observed to prevent hemorrhage from site and to detect and treat promptly any complications of blood transfusion such as heart failure, hypocalcemia, acute hypercalcemia, hyperkalemia, hypernatremia, hypoglycemia and acidosis,* sepsis, shock, thrombus formation, transfusion mismatch reaction.
Nurse finishes c30ting.	
Nurse continues to observe and record infant's behavior closely for 24 to 48 hours.	
(1) Vital signs: heart rate, respirations, temperatures, pedal pulses	
(2) Lethargy, jitteriness, convulsions	
(3) Dark urine	
(4) Edema	

*Red blood cells continue anaerobic glycolysis with production of acid metabolites after removal from donor. Blood stored for longer than 2 days is likely to contain potentially dangerous levels of potassium and to be more readily subjected to hemolysis.

Procedure 7-7

PHOTOTHERAPY

DEFINITION

The treatment of neonatal hyperbilirubinemia and jaundice by exposing infant's bare skin to intense fluorescent light. The blue range of light accelerates the removal of bilirubin in the skin.

PURPOSE

To reduce levels of unconjugated bilirubin and prevent kernicterus.

EQUIPMENT

Phototherapy unit, eye patches, diaper—a face mask with the wire support removed works effectively (some institutions use disposable diapers).

NURSING ACTIONS	RATIONALE
Wash hands before and after touching infant and equipment. Glove.	To prevent nosocomial infection and to implement universal precautions.
Identify infant.	To ensure that procedure is performed on correct infant.
Undress infant.	To expose as much skin area as possible to light.
Protect infant's eyes with eye patches.	To prevent possible injury to conjunctiva or retina.
Be sure eyes are closed.	To prevent corneal abrasions.
Check eyes for drainage each shift.	To prevent or allow prompt treatment of purulent conjunctivitis, should it occur.
	Research evidence suggests that exposure of the eyes to the phototherapy light units may injure the retina.
Diapering may be accomplished by using a "string bikini," paper face mask with the metal strip removed or a disposable diaper.	To allow optimum skin exposure, yet sufficient to protect genitals and bedding. Metal strip is heated by light and can burn baby's skin.
After placing baby under light, monitor skin temperature. If infant is in incubator, temperature dial on control panel may need to be turned to maintain proper temperature.	To prevent hyperthermia or hypothermia.
	To prevent serious injury, all electric equipment should be grounded, free of defects, and operationally sound to maximize therapeutic effectiveness and to prevent electric shock or burn to the infant or the nurse.
For feeding and especially for parents' visits, discontinue phototherapy and unwrap baby's eyes. Hold for feedings.	To meet need for psychosocial contact and bonding. Parent has opportunity to make eye contact, a necessary activity to develop attachment.
Observe infant's behavior:	To continue surveillance.
Eating and sleeping patterns.	Effect of phototherapy on biologic rhythms uncertain. Data base is needed to differentiate common side effects (loose greenish stools or green urine) from other problems that need treatment. Green color comes from end products of bilirubin.
Loose greenish stools, green urine.	
Replace fluid losses by increasing fluid volume offered to infant by 10 to 20 ml/kg/day.	To prevent dehydration: insensible and intestinal water loss is increased during phototherapy.
Protect skin from excoriation (includes diaper rash).	To prevent infection of broken-down skin areas.
Clean urine and stool off of skin during diaper change.	To prevent harming of skin by chemicals in excreta.
Send serial bilirubins for analysis.	To evaluate level of bilirubin and effectiveness of treatment.
Record time therapy began, note time removed for care, and if therapy was discontinued. Record infant response (e.g., temperature, stools).	To ensure communication with other caregivers.

Guidelines For Client Teaching

HYPERBILIRUBINEMIA

ASSESSMENT

1. Infant, female term newborn, 8 lb 4 oz, 3 days old.
2. Infant bilirubin level is 13.5 mg/dl.
3. Infant breast-feeding.
4. Physician's orders: serial total bilirubin levels; phototherapy.
5. Parents unaware of causes of jaundice and what phototherapy is.

NURSING DIAGNOSIS

Knowledge deficit (parental) related to hyperbilirubinemia and phototherapy.

GOALS

Short-term

To teach parents what hyperbilirubinemia is and why phototherapy is ordered.

Intermediate

To increase parents' ability to evaluate their newborn at home for hyperbilirubinemia.
To reduce parents' anxiety.

Long term

To provide knowledge of hyperbilirubinemia that can be used to prompt treatment for older infants, subsequent infants, and other family members.

REFERENCES AND TEACHING AIDS

Charts, phototherapy equipment, eye mask, paper diaper (or face mask with wire support removed), and printed pamphlets provided by hospital or formula companies for parents to take home and refer to later.

CONTENT/RATIONALE	TEACHING ACTIONS
To review meaning of terms parents will hear: Hyperbilirubinemia: higher levels of bilirubin than normal. Bilirubin: end product of red blood cells when they mature and break down. Jaundice: yellow color of whites of eyes, skin, and mucous membranes caused by circulating bilirubin. Phototherapy: the use of fluorescent light to break down bilirubin in the skin into substances that can be excreted in the feces (stool) or urine.	Seat parents in a quiet place, where they can see charts and talk easily to the nurse. Have chart made with terms spelled out. If possible, have parents hold their wrapped infant for this part of the class.
To review process of excreting bilirubin: When red blood cells (RBCs) break down they release bilirubin. Bilirubin circulates in the blood. In the liver it is combined with another substance. In the combined form it goes by way of the blood to the kidneys and the intestines. It gives the yellow color to urine and the brown color to the stool.	Point to chart depicting process as you explain. Ask for questions. Remind parents this is a process difficult for nurses and physicians to learn, so therefore many questions and repeated explanations are expected.
Before the baby was born, her RBCs were more numerous than ours. They also had a shorter life span, 70 to 90 days instead of 120 days. When the RBCs broke down, the baby's blood carried most of the bilirubin by way of the placenta to the mother's liver to be excreted.	Show picture of baby in utero. Trace route of blood from baby to mother's liver.
After the baby was born, her liver began to take care of all the bilirubin. Even though the baby's liver functions well, it cannot handle the whole load. Bilirubin seeps out of the blood and into the tissues, staining them yellow. The blood level of bilirubin rises quickly up to the fifth day, and then goes down; the jaundice usually clears up by the end of the week.	Point out yellowness of baby's skin. Show chart with approximate amounts of bilirubin and location. Prepare graph illustrating rise and fall of bilirubin over the first week of life.
If the baby is breast-feeding, a certain amount of the jaundice may be caused by the free fatty acids, which interfere with the conjugation of bilirubin. Some babies seem to have extra bilirubin to excrete. The amount in the tissues becomes too great when the blood level reaches 12 mg/dl. There is a danger that the bilirubin at high levels will cause damage to the brain. So your doctor wants the baby to be placed under the Bililight for phototherapy. This will help the baby handle the extra bilirubin and prevent damage to the baby's brain.	Show chart with contents of breast milk and point out the level of free fatty acids. Refer back to chart depicting process of conjugation. Show Bililight equipment. Let parents feel warmth of the light.

Guidelines for Client Teaching—cont'd

CONTENT/RATIONALE	TEACHING ACTIONS
We put eye masks on the baby to keep the light from her eyes.	Demonstrate use of eye mask. Bring infant and place in crib away from Bililight. Apply the eye mask.
We keep the baby undressed so as much light as possible can reach her skin.	Undress baby. Place under Bililight.
We use a paper diaper or the face mask as a small diaper (a "string bikini").	Diaper the infant.
We will take her temperature often so she will not become too hot or too cold.	Take and record temperature. Settle baby comfortably.
We will give her extra water to drink because she will have watery, green stools from the extra bilirubin excreted.	Return to seats and review care. Distribute pamphlets.
We will be taking her out of the Bililight for feedings and cuddling. We will let you know when to come for feedings and to hold her.	
We will be taking blood tests to check the amount of bilirubin and we will let you know the results.	
To reassure parents that they can have questions answered after discharge.	Leave parents with infant. Tell them they can touch her, but not shield her skin from the light.
If you have any questions, ask us any time. We will give you our phone number and you can call at any hour. It is hard not being able to take her home with you.	Demonstrate stroking baby's hand. Return in about 10 minutes to see if there are any questions. Arrange feeding schedule with mother.
	Mother can continue to breast-feed or bring breast milk for feedings she will miss.

EVALUATION Woman (couple) verbalizes understanding of what has been taught and asks appropriate questions.

Summary of Nursing Actions

HYPERBILIRUBINEMIA

I. Goals
  A. For the mother: a satisfying birth
  B. For the newborn: a neonatal period uncomplicated by hyperbilirubinemia
  C. For the family: a positive birth experience

II. Priorities
  A. Prevention of hyperbilirubinemia, or, prompt identification and treatment of hyperbilirubinemia
  B. Education and support of parents of newborn with hyperbilirubinemia

III. Assessment
  A. Review prenatal chart and intranatal record for presence of risk factors.
  B. Assess for hyperbilirubinemia:
    1. If any predisposing factors are present, check to see that cord blood has been sent to laboratory for blood type, Rh, hemoglobin, hematocrit, Coombs test, or other values appropriate for that newborn. Obtain daily hemoglobin and hematocrit values until a stable stage has been reached. Record results.
    2. Note any appearance of jaundice during the first 24 hours; and note degree of jaundice. Test for jaundice, preferably in the daylight, because

there is possible distortion of color from artificial lighting, reflection from nursery walls, etc.
      a. Blanch area over bony area (sternum) with thumb. Skin will look yellow before area is perfused again.
      b. Check conjunctival sacs and buccal mucosa in darker-skinned infants.
    3. Note infant's behavior:
      a. Changes in feeding and sleeping patterns.
      b. Color and consistency of stools; dark, concentrated urine.
      c. Pallor.
      d. Neurologic signs of kernicterus.
    4. Note lab reports on serum bilirubin levels.

IV. Potential nursing diagnoses
  A. Infant
    1. Potential for injury
    2. Impaired gas exchange
    3. Potential activity intolerance
    4. Potential fluid volume deficit
    5. Altered nutrition: less than body requirements
  B. Parents
    1. Knowledge deficit
    2. Anxiety

Continued.

Summary of Nursing Actions—cont'd

    3. Fear
    4. Ineffective family coping: compromised
    5. Ineffective individual coping
    6. Altered family proccesses
    7. Powerlessness
V. Plan/implementation
  A. Record and report jaundice immediately for prompt diagnosis and initiation of treatment.
  B. Maintain phototherapy (see p. 303).
  C. Assist with exchange transfusion.
  D. Support parents.
    1. Keep parents informed (see Guidelines for Client Teaching, "Hyperbilirubinemia," pp. 294-295).
    2. Reinforce explanations of physiologic and pathologic hyperbilirubinemia. Explain need for adequate fluid intake for newborn (e.g., offer water between feedings).
    3. Reinforce physician's explanations regarding disease, its treatment, infant's condition, and possible prognosis.
    4. Teach mother how to identify jaundice and when to call physician, especially if she is discharged with infant soon after delivery.
    5. Involve parents with infant's care when possible.
VI. Evaluation
  A. Perinatal risk factors are prevented.
  B. Infection is prevented.
  C. Early feedings are provided.
  D. Hyperbilirubinemia and its sequela, kernicterus, are absent.
  E. There are minimal or no sequelae from hyperbilirubinemia and its treatment.
  F. Parents understand newborn's condition, therapies, and possible sequelae.

CONGENITAL ANOMALIES

Every year 250,000 infants are born with significant structural and functional disorders. An interdisciplinary team approach is imperative to provide holistic care. Parental disappointment and disillusion and the nurse's own feelings add to the complexity of nursing care.

This section includes information on autosomal aberrations, inborn errors of metabolism, and common sex chromosome abnormalities. Diagnosis and treatment of cardiovascular disorders is presented, along with the danger signs of hydrocephalus, a condition that can be both a symptom and a medical problem in itself.

Table 7-7 *Common Autosomal Aberrations*

Syndrome	Chromosomal Abnormality and Nomenclature	Average Incidence	Major Clinical Manifestations
Cri-du-chat	Deletion of short arm of a B (no. 5) chromosome—46,XY,5p−		Distinctive weak, high-pitched mewlike cry resembling the cry of a cat; small head; hypertelorism; failure to thrive; severe mental retardation—profound with age
Trisomy 13 (Patau's)	Trisomy of a group D (no. 13) chromosome—47,XY,13+	1/15,000	Multiple anomalies, including cleft lip and palate (frequently bilateral); ear malformations; microphthalmia; polydactyly; eye defects; mental retardation; early death
Trisomy 18 (Edwards')	Trisomy of a group E (no. 18) chromosome—47,XY,18+	1/5000	Deformed and low-set ears; micrognathia; rocker-bottom feet; overlapping (index over third) fingers; prominent occiput; hypertelorism; failure to thrive and early death; mental retardation
Trisomy 21 (Down's)	Trisomy of a Group G (no. 21) chromosome—47,XY,21+ (trisomy); 46XY,D−G−, (Dq-Gq)+ (translocation); 46,XY/47,XY,21+ (mosaic)	1/500	Brachycephaly with flat occiput; inner epicanthal folds; small ears, nose, and mouth with protruding tongue; muscular hypotonia; broad, short hands with stubby fingers and simian palmar crease; broad stubby feet with wide space between big and second toes; mental retardation; variable life expectancy

From Whaley LF and Wong DL: Nursing care of infants and children, ed 3, St Louis, 1987, The CV Mosby Co.

Table 7-8 *Some inborn errors of metabolism** *

Disease	Basic Defect	Manifestations	Therapy
Adrenogenital syndrome†	21-hydroxylase deficiency; failure of hydrocortisone synthesis in adrenal cortex	Virilization	Hydrocortisone
Albinism	Deficiency of tyrosinase; failure to convert tyrosine to dopa and, hence, lack of melanin synthesis	Lack of pigment in skin, hair, and eyes; eye defects	None; avoid exposure to sunlight; ophthalmologic care
Crigler-Najjar syndrome	Glycyronyl transferase deficiency; inability to convert indirect bilirubin to direct bilirubin	Jaundice; spasticity; opisthotonos; early death	None
Cystic fibrosis	Unknown; defect in mucus-secreting glands; sweat glands secrete abnormal amounts of sodium chloride	Meconium ileus in newborn; celiac syndrome; pulmonary disease; failure to thrive	Inhalation therapy; antibiotics; pancreatic enzymes
Familial cretinism	Deficiency of iodotyrosine deiodinase	Lethargy; stunted growth; mental retardation	Early administration of thyroid hormone
Galactosemia†	Deficiency of galactose 1-phosphate uridyl transferase; inability to convert galactose to glucose	Failure to thrive; mental retardation; cataracts; jaundice; hepatomegaly; cirrhosis of liver	Eliminate galactose from diet
Glucose 6-phosphate dehydrogenase deficiency (G6PD)	Deficiency of G6PD	Asymptomatic under normal circumstances; hemolytic anemia and jaundice from ingestion of certain drugs (primaquine, acetanilid, sulfanilamide, and naphthalene) and fava beans	Avoid agents that precipitate clinical symptoms
Hypophosphatasia†	Deficiency of alkaline phosphatase	Skeletal abnormalities	None
Maple syrup urine disease†	Defective metabolism of branched chain amino acid	Onset in early infancy; neurologic disorders; odor of urine similar to that of maple syrup	Diet low in branched chain amino acids
McArdle syndrome	Deficiency of muscle phosphorylase	Muscle weakness	Glucagon injections
Phenylketonuria (PKU)	Deficiency of phenylalanine dehydrogenase	Blond hair, blue eyes, fair skin; mental retardation; bizarre behavior	Diet low in phenylalanine
Tay-Sachs disease†	Deficiency of hexosaminidase; defect in synthesis of gangliosides	Progressive neurologic deterioration; blindness: cherry-red spot in macula; early death	None
Tyrosinosis	Deficiency of *p*-hydroxy-phenylpyruvic acid oxidase	Hepatosplenomegaly	None
von Gierke's disease	Deficiency of G6PD; inability to reconvert glycogen to glucose.	Hematomegaly; vomiting; hypoglycemia, convulsions; coma; usually early death	High-protein diet; no definitive therapy
Werdnig-Hoffman syndrome	Unknown; atrophy of anterior horn cells in spinal cord and motor nuclei in brainstem	Usually apparent at birth; "floppy" infant; lies in frog position; fatal in early childhood	Symptomatic

*Autosomal-recessive inheritance pattern.
†Prenatal diagnosis is possible.

Table 7-9 *Common sex chromosome abnormalities*

Syndrome	Chromosomal Nomenclature	Phenotype	X Chromosome	Y Chromosome	Clinical Manifestations
Turner's	45,X	Female	0	0	Short stature; webbed neck; low posterior hairline; shield-shaped chest with widely spaced nipples; sterile, lymphedema of hands and feet in infant
Meta-female	47,XXX (can also be 48,XXXX or 49,XXXXX)	Female	+1 or more	0	Normal female characteristics; usually mentally retarded; mental deficiency in others; fertile
XYY male	47,XYY (can also be 48,XYYY or mosaic)	Male	0	+1 per Y	Usually normal sexual development; tendency to be tall with long head; poor coordination; may demonstrate aberrant behavior
Klinefelter's	47,XXY (48,XXYY, 48,XXXY, 49,XXXXY, etc. mosaics)	Male	+1 or more (1 per X)	+1 per Y	Tall with long legs; hypogenitalism; sterile; may have deficient male secondary sexual characteristics; may demonstrate aberrant behavior

From Whaley LF and Wong DL: Nursing care of infants and children, ed 3, St Louis, 1987, The CV Mosby Co.

Summary of Nursing Actions

NEWBORN WITH CARDIOVASCULAR DISORDER

I. Goals
   A. For the mother: a satisfying birth
   B. For the newborn: a neonatal period in which the cardiovascular disorder is identified and treated promptly
   C. For the family: an experience for which they receive adequate education and support
II. Priorities
   A. Prompt identification and treatment of cardiovascular disorders
   B. Education and support of parents of newborn with cardiovascular disorder
III. Assessment
   A. Mother's previous and present obstetric histories; maternal and paternal medical histories
   B. Cry: weak and muffled, loud and breathless
   C. Color
      1. Cyanotic: usually generalized; increases in supine position; often unrelieved by oxygen; usually deepens with crying; gray, dusky; mild, moderate, severe
      2. Acyanotic: pale, with or without mottling with exertion
   D. Activity level
      1. Restless
      2. Lethargic
      3. Unresponsive except to pain
      4. Lack of movement of arms and legs when crying (severe distress)
      5. Arms flaccid when eating
   E. Posturing
      1. Hypotonic; flaccid even with sleeping
      2. Hyperextension of neck
      3. Opisthotonos

      4. Dyspnea when supine
      5. Knee-chest position favored
   F. Persistent bradycardia (120 beats/min or less) or persistent tachycardia (160 beats/min or more)
   G. Respirations: counted when newborn is sleeping to identify problem early
      1. Tachypnea (60 beats/min or more)
      2. Retractions with nasal flaring or tachypnea
      3. Dyspnea with diaphoresis or grunting
      4. Gasping, followed in 2 or 3 minutes by respiratory arrest if not treated promptly
      5. Grunting with exertion such as crying or feeding by nipple
   H. Feeding behavior
      1. Anorexic
      2. Poor suck: from lack of energy or when unable to close mouth around nipple because of dyspnea
      3. Difficulty coordinating suck, swallow, breathing; pulls away from nipple to take breath
      4. Slow, with pauses to rest
      5. Unable to feed by nipple
IV. Potential nursing diagnoses
   A. Decreased cardiac output
   B. Impaired gas exchange
   C. Altered tissue perfusion (specify type)
   D. Potential for injury
   E. Altered nutrition: less than body requirements
   F. Potential activity intolerance
   G. Ineffective breathing pattern
   H. Altered health maintenance
   I. Sleep pattern disturbance
   J. Altered growth and development
   K. Ineffective breastfeeding

V. Plan/implementation
  A. General care: support respiratory effort and decrease work of heart.
     1. Administer O_2 to relieve cyanosis.
     2. Suction.
     3. Provide warmth.
     4. Position for optimum respiratory effort.
        a. Knee-chest, prone, side-lying
        b. Upright over nurse's shoulder
     5. Omit oral feedings until physician arrives. If oral feedings are ordered, offer small amounts more frequently to avoid overdistention of stomach and compromising respirations and to avoid fatigue.
     6. If oral feedings are discontinued, prepare for gavage feeding or parenteral therapy.
  B. Record and report all findings to provide current data base for continuing therapy.
     1. Degree and extent of cyanosis; palms, earlobes, scrotum (oral mucosa and tongue most reliable)
     2. General body color: pale, grayish, cyanotic
     3. Muscle tone when active and when at rest
     4. Effect of O_2 on cyanosis; how much was needed to relieve symptoms; changes with change in activity level
     5. Heart rate; heart sounds: loudness, location
     6. Respirations
     7. Fatigability

  C. Minimize distress. Painful procedures (e.g., venipuncture) increase distress, especially in cyanotic baby.
     1. Place infant in prone position.
     2. Administer O_2 by mask during procedure.
     3. Keep infant warm.
     4. Request technician to stop before infant begins to gasp.
  D. Prevent stress: infection, hypoglycemia.
  E. Medicate per physician order and observe infant response.
     1. Digitalis preparation: When preparing digitalis dose, second nurse should double-check amount drawn into syringe. Take apical beat; *if heart rate is below 100 beats/min, report to physician before administering drug.*
     2. Give diuretic.
  F. Support parents
VI. Evaluation
  A. Adequate oxygenation of tissues is maintained.
  B. The infant is protected from additional stress, such as infection, inadequate nutrition, and cold.
  C. Corrective or palliative surgery is performed.
  D. Parents have an understanding and beginning acceptance of the problem and its treatment and any necessary continuing care after discharge.
  E. Parents are able to initiate and maintain a positive parent-child relationship.

Table 7-10 *Cardiomyopathy*

Hypertrophic Cardiomyopathy (HCM)	Nonhypertrophic Cardiomyopathy (NHCM)
Diagnostic echocardiogram:	**Diagnostic echocardiogram:**
Myocardium is hypercontractile.	Myocardium is poorly contractile.
Myocardium (right ventricle and interventricular wall) is thickened.	Myocardium is overstretched.
Decrease in size of ventricles.	Increase in size of ventricles.
Outflow tract obstruction (poorly functioning mitral valve).	No outflow obstruction.
Treatment:	**Treatment:**
Medication: β-adrenergic blocker (e.g., propranolol to **decrease** contractility and heart rate)	Medication: cardiotonic (e.g., digoxin to **increase** contractility and **decrease** heart rate)
	Therapy for hypoglycemia/hypocalcemia and polycythemia

DANGER SIGNS

Hydrocephalus

Changes in head size every day
   Width of sutures
   Size and tension of anterior fontanel
   Head circumference
Facial appearance
   Flat, broad bridge of nose
   Bulging forehead
   "Setting-sun" effect as eyes are displaced downward by pressure from accumulating fluid
Neurologic signs
   High-pitched, shrill cry
   Irritability or restlessness
   Poor feeding or changes in feeding pattern from good to poor
   Behavior changes
   Spina bifida

Bibliography

Fanaroff AA and Martin RJ editors: Neonatal-perinatal medicine: diseases of the fetus and infant, ed. 4, St Louis 1987, The CV Mosby Co.

Pernoll ML, Benda GI and Babson SG: Diagnosis and management of the fetus and neonate at risk: a guide for team care, ed 5, St Louis, 1986, The CV Mosby Co.

8

Women's Health and Gynecologic Care

Nursing care of the gynecologic client is preventive, curative, and rehabilitative, and encompasses all age groups. Normal changes, such as menarche and menopause, require supportive nursing care. Abnormal conditions associated with menstruation, sequelae to childbirth, and disorders that may accompany aging challenge the nurse's skill. Comprehensive gynecologic nursing care requires knowledge of fertility management as well as knowledge of the impact of violence on women. Highly technical skills are associated with the nursing care of clients with neoplasia.

Gynecologic problems affect reproductive functions and have an impact on the entire family. The gynecologic nurse assumes the roles of advocate, teacher, and care provider. With education and encouragement, women can become partners in their health care.

GYNECOLGIC AND URINARY CONCERNS

Problems with the female reproductive system may arise at any time during the woman's life. The gynecologic nurse must be knowledgeable about the signs and symptoms of various conditions and the appropriate interventions. This section includes information on general gynecologic care, problems related to menstruation, and the climacterium.

General Gynecologic Concerns

The gynecologic client may seek health care for preventive screening or in response to a problem. Nursing responsibilities include assessment, intervention, and teaching. The following pages provide information on vaginal douching, toxic shock syndrome (TSS), acquired immune deficiency syndrome (AIDS), and urinary incontinence.

Guidelines For Client Teaching

VAGINAL DOUCHING

ASSESSMENT
1. Vaginal douching has been prescribed by the physician.
2. Vaginal douche must be used to deliver medication to the vagina or cervix.
3. Preoperative vaginal douche ordered.

NURSING DIAGNOSIS
Knowledge deficit related to vaginal douching.

GOALS
Short-term
Woman verbalizes understanding of vaginal douching procedure.

Intermediate
Woman implements vaginal douching per physician's order.
Infection is cured or prevented.

Long-term
Woman does not have a recurrence of condition that required vaginal douching.

REFERENCES AND TEACHING AIDS
Printed instructions
Douche equipment

CONTENT/RATIONALE	TEACHING ACTION
To confirm reasons for douching, the nurse reviews: Woman's condition. Physician's order. *To teach safe and effective method of douching* the nurse presents the following: Void and wash hands before douching. Use the following position to place fluid properly:	Provide information and allow time for discussion. Emphasize good hygiene. Use illustration to clarify proper placement of fluids.
1. The optimum position is semirecumbent in a clean tub (after a bath) or in bed. A douche pan may be used in a tub as well. 2. The woman can douche while seated on the toilet; however, the labia should be held together to permit solution to fill the entire vaginal vault. Prepare solution for optimum comfort and effectiveness. The temperature should be 40° to 43°C (105° to 110°F), comfortably warm to the inner aspect of wrist.	Read over the instructions on package of douche medication, answer questions, clarify information.
Allow some solution to flow out of nozzle to lubricate tip, or lubricate with K-Y jelly or other water-soluble lubricant. Hold or place solution container 60 cm (2 ft) above the hips to avoid greater heights, which increase the pressure of the flow. *Do not* use a bulb syringe (or exert excessive force if using a disposable douche with an attached nozzle), fluid or air embolus may result and death may ensue. To bathe the vaginal vault with fluid, insert nozzle upward and backward for 7.6 cm (3 in).	Demonstrate technique to woman and allow her to ask questions. Watch woman give a return demonstration. Discuss how woman will implement method at home; for example, does she have a bathtub, storage space for the equipment? Observe return demonstration of force of fluid flow. Use illustration to reinforce verbal description of anatomic position of vagina and of filling vaginal vault with fluid.
1. Rotate nozzle so that fluid flushes entire mucosa, including that of the posterior fornix. Rotation of the nozzle also reduces the chance of forcing fluid into the cervix. 2. When douching seated on the toilet, hold labia together to fill the vaginal vault, then allow fluid to exit rapidly to flush out debris. Repeat until fluid is used up. 3. Hold labia together for specified period of time if the objective of the douche is to expose the mucosa to medication or moist heat. Sitting up and leaning forward aid in emptying the vagina. For proper care of equipment and to prevent possible spread of infection, wash douche equipment with warm soap and water, and store in a well-ventilated place away from extremes of temperature.	Encourage woman to ask questions. Promote discussion pertaining to the two methods of administration. Make sure woman understands this point. Repeat this instruction if necessary. Use illustration to aid understanding. Stress the importance of keeping the equipment clean and dry.

Continued

Guidelines for Vaginal Douching—cont'd

CONTENT/RATIONALE	TEACHING ACTION
Wash hands to maintain good hygiene.	Discuss simple asepsis with the client (e.g., how bacteria may be transferred from dirty hands to other areas on the body without realizing).

EVALUATION The nurse knows that teaching was effective when woman's return demonstration is accurate, no fluid or air embolus occurs, and there is no spread of infection. Prevention of or resolution of infection may reflect teaching effectiveness.

Toxic Shock Syndrome. Toxic shock syndrome (TSS) is a potentially life-threatening systemic disorder that has three principal clinical manifestations: fever of sudden onset, hypotension, and rash (see box below). The erythematous macular desquamating rash is most prominent on palms and soles. The acute phase to TSS lasts about 4 to 5 days; the convalescent phase, about 1 to 2 weeks.

The CDC (1982) has established diagnostic criteria for TSS that include the above signs plus the following manifestations.

1. Involvement of three or more other organ systems:

System/Area	Manifestations
Gastrointestinal	Nausea; vomiting; diarrhea
Renal	Decreased urinary output; pyuria
Hepatic	Jaundice; abnormal values (increased transaminase)
CNS	Altered sensorium (decreased level of consciousness [LOC]); headache
Respiratory	Adult respiratory distress syndrome (ARDS)
Mucous membranes	Inflammation of vaginal oropharyngeal, and conjunctival membranes
Muscular	Myalgia; weakness
Hematologic	Thrombocytopenia; DIC
Cardiac	Ischemic changes on ECG; decreased left ventricular contractility

2. Serologic laboratory tests for Rocky Mountain spotted fever, leptospirosis, and measles are negative. Cultures positive for *S. aureus* can be obtained from blood, urine, or stool. If primary site of infection is tampon related, positive cultures are obtained from the vagina and cervix.

A toxin (pyrogenic exotoxin C [PEC] or enterotoxin F) secreted by strains of *S. aureus* is the causative factor in TSS. About 9% of women harbor the organism normally in their vaginas; about 1% to 5% of sexually active males have urethral cultures that are positive for *S. aureus* without having the disease. Poor perineal hygiene and lack of handwashing before touching the perineal area may increase risk. Commonly associated conditions that may predispose the person to TSS by providing a portal of entry into systemic circulation include the following:

1. Menstruation
2. Chronic vaginal infection (e.g., herpes)
3. Puerperal endometritis
4. Incisional or soft tissue abscess
5. Skin infection following a bee sting
6. Intravenous (IV) injection of heroin
7. Use of high-absorbency tampons or barrier contraceptives (e.g., sponge, diaphragm) (Berkley et al., 1987); Wolf et al., 1987)
8. Neonatal infection together with maternal infection.

Acquired Immune Deficiency Syndrome (AIDS). Transmission of human immunodeficiency virus (HIV), a retrovirus, occurs primarily through the exchange of body fluids (e.g., blood, semen, perinatal events) (Landesman et al., 1987; Hecht, 1987; Friedland and Klein, 1987). Severe depression of the cellular immune system characterizes acquired immune deficiency syndrome (AIDS). Although the populations at high risk have been well-documented, *all* women should be assessed for the possibility of having been exposed to HIV. AIDS in women is commonly reported at a later stage in the disease. The delay may be in part because women may have symptoms different from those of men (Shaw, 1986). Chronic vaginitis is a common presenting problem.

Delay in diagnosis must be avoided when the woman is pregnant. Exposure to the virus has a significant impact on the woman's pregnancy and newborn feeding method and on the newborn's health status (Klug, 1986). The HIV from infected women is transmitted in three ways (Landesman et al, 1987; Friedland and Klein, 1987):

1. To the fetus as early as the first trimester through maternal circulation
2. To the infant during labor and delivery by inoculation or ingestion of maternal blood and other infected fluids
3. To the infant through breast milk

Urinary Incontinence. Uncontrollable leakage of urine is experienced by many women. Although this condition may be the result of injury sustained during childbirth, other factors may be considered. Five categories of conditions can disturb urinary control (Willson et al., 1987):

1. *Stress urinary incontinence.* The loss of urine occurs with sudden increases in intraabdominal pressure, such as that generated by sneezing, or from sudden jarring movement. The loss is caused by structural injuries to the urethra and bladder neck.

2. *Detrusor dyssynergia.* The incontinence results from involuntary detrusor activity, which is triggered by a variety of stimuli.
3. *Urge incontinence.* Urge incontinence is characterized by the inability to keep from urinating when the urge to void occurs suddenly. Urge incontinence usually is caused by intrinsic disorders of the bladder and urethra, the most common being urethritis and urethral stricture, trigonitis, and cystitis.
4. *Neuropathies.* Neurologic disorders, such as multiple sclerosis, diabetic neuritis, and diseases of or injuries to the spinal cord, disturb the nerve control of bladder function. Such disorders usually cause overflow or uninhibited detrusor incontinence.
5. *Congenital and acquired urinary tract abnormalities.* Urinary tract abnormalities include congenital defects, such as

ectopic ureter, abnormal muscular development of the vesical neck, neurologic disorders, acquired lesions (such as urinary fistulas), and destruction of all or part of the urethra. The incontinence is usually constant and unrelated to voiding, to activity, or to position.

Menstrual Disorders

Disorders associated with menstruation afflict a large percentage of women in the reproductive years. These conditions have a negative effect on the quality of the women's lives and the lives of their families. Three of the most common problems are dysmenorrhea, premenstrual syndrome (PMS), and endometriosis.

Table 8-1   *Dysmenorrhea and Premenstrual Syndrome (PMS): Comparison of Onset and Duration, Range of Response, and Incidence*

	Dysmenorrhea	PMS
Onset and duration	Acute 24-48 hr before or coincident with onset of menses, with pelvic pain that decreases or ends with end of menses	Diffuse 7-10 days before menses; resolves with onset of menses
Range of response	From mild to severe and disabling for 24-48 hr	From awareness of physiologic changes to incapacitation or disruption of life-style
Incidence	Some discomfort: 80% of all women Severe enough to interfere with normal activities for 1-2 days: 35% of older adolescents; 25% of college women; 60%-70% of single women in their 30s and 40s Incapacitation: 10% of all women	5%-95% of all women

Table 8-2   *Classifications of Pelvic Endometriosis*

Classification	Characteristics
Mild	Scattered, fresh lesions (i.e., implants not associated with scarring or retraction of the peritoneum) in the anterior or posterior cul-de-sac or pelvic peritoneum Rare surface implant on ovary, with no endometrioma, without surface scarring and retraction, and without periovarian adhesions No peritubular adhesions
Moderate	Endometriosis involving one or both ovaries, with several surface lesions, with scarring and retraction, or small endometriomas Minimal peritubular adhesions associated with ovarian lesions described Superficial implants in anterior and/or posterior cul-de-sac with scarring and retraction; some adhesions, but no sigmoid invasion
Severe	Endometriosis involving one or both ovaries (usually both) with endometrioma >2 × 2 cm One or both ovaries bound down by adhesions associated with endometriosis, with or without tubal adhesions to ovaries One or both tubes bound down or obstructed by endometriosis; associated adhesions or lesions Obliteration of the cul-de-sac from adhesions or lesions associated with endometriosis Thickening of the uterosacral ligaments and cul-de-sac lesions from invasive endometriosis with obliteration of the cul-de-sac Significant bowel or urinary tract involvement

From Acosta IA et al: Obstet Gynecol 42:19, 1973. Reprinted with permission from The American College of Obstetricians and Gynecologists.

Sample Nursing Care Plan

PREMENSTRUAL SYNDROME (PMS)

ASSESSMENT	NURSING DIAGNOSIS (ND)/ PLAN (P)/GOAL (G)	RATIONALE IMPLEMENTATION	EVALUATION
Single woman exhibiting physiologic and psychologic symptoms of PMS: Temporary water weight gain.	ND: Fluid volume excess related to hormonal influence and fluid retention 10 days before premenstruation. P: Minimize or prevent water weight gain. G: Woman relates a decrease in weight gain caused by water retention.	*To prevent or minimize premenstrual water weight gain the woman will:* Reduce or eliminate salty foods and added salt at the table. Consider pharmaceutical preparations or natural diuretic foods.	Woman will show a reduction in water weight gain and edema premenstrually.
Breast tenderness.	ND: Pain, discomfort in breasts, related to influence of hormones and chemicals in diet. P: Minimize or prevent breast tenderness. G: Woman will relate increased breast comfort.	*To prevent or minimize breast tenderness the woman will:* Decrease caffeine intake in diet. Maintain a balanced diet rich in vitamins and minerals. Wear a comfortable supportive bra.	Woman verbalizes a decrease in breast tenderness.
Depression. Moodiness.	ND: Situational low self-esteem related to hormonal changes before menstrual period. P: Minimize or prevent depression and mood swings. G: Patient will relate less emotional distress.	*To decrease or prevent depression and mood swings the woman will:* Monitor vitamin intake. Avoid alcohol and cigarettes. Get plenty of exercise to decrease stress. Talk about feelings with someone close. Join a support group.	Woman verbalizes an understanding of information presented and experiences less depression. Woman states she feels better about herself since she has become active in a support group.
Craving for sweets.	ND: Altered nutrition: potential for more than body requirements related to hormone-related change in carbohydrate metabolism. P: Use alternative activities and foods to reduce intake of foods high in simple sugars (glucose). G: Woman relates decreased need for and decreased intake of foods high in simple sugars (glucose).	*To minimize wide fluctuation in blood sugar levels, the woman will:* Reduce intake of simple sugars, candy, pastries, table sugar. Eat small, frequent meals and snacks of good nutritious value: i.e., fruit, cheese, etc; maintain a balanced diet. Monitor vitamin intake. Engage in enjoyable activities: social events, jogging or other sports.	Woman reduces intake of simple sugars, replacing sugar and salty snacks with more fruit and protein foods.

Sample Nursing Care Plan

ENDOMETRIOSIS

ASSESSMENT	NURSING DIAGNOSIS (ND)/ PLAN (P)/GOAL (G)	RATIONALE/ IMPLEMENTATION	EVALUATION
Dysmenorrhea with pelvic and abdominal pain which may radiate down thighs or be accompanied by sensation of pelvic fullness. Dysmenorrhea worsens with time.	ND: Pain related to endometriosis. ND: Knowledge deficit related to condition. ND: Body image disturbance, self-esteem disturbance related to symptomatology or diagnosis. P: Assist with diagnosis, meet knowledge needs, and provide opportunity to discuss feelings. G: Pain relieved or minimized; self-esteem is maintained; knowledge needs are met.	*To assist with knowledge needs, self-concept, and pain relief the nurse will:* Assess location, type, and duration of pain; history of discomfort. Provide pain medications as ordered: teach about use and side effects. Teach comfort measures: Heating pad to abdomen. Warm bath. Provide time to discuss feelings. Refer to support group.	Pain is localized and minimized. Woman uses medication correctly. Woman employs comfort measures at home.
Anxiety.	ND: Anxiety, mild to moderate, related to diagnosis. P: Decrease anxiety. G: Woman reports decreased anxiety.	*To decrease anxiety the nurse will:* Discuss feelings and concerns about diagnosis. Provide realistic hope. Be supportive. Provide complete, clear explanation of disease. Provide information about treatment plans. Assist as necessary with decisions about treatment.	Woman's anxiety is decreased through understanding. Woman verbalizes understanding of information presented.
Tiredness or weakness. Anemia.	ND: Activity intolerance related to anemia of hypermenorrhea. P: Relieve anemia and prevent recurrence. G: Blood studies show recovery from anemia; woman performs ADL without becoming overtired.	*To decrease tiredness and weakness secondary to anemia the nurse will:* Teach about and encourage diet high in iron and vitamin C. Provide information on iron supplements, if ordered. Discuss rest periods if possible. Encourage 8 hours of sleep per night.	Woman changes diet to include foods high in iron. Woman takes iron supplements as ordered.
Dyspareunia.	ND: Sexual dysfunction related to endometrial implants in cul-de-sac of Douglas. P: Meet knowledge needs, provide opportunity for discussion, and maintain or improve self-concept. G: Painless sexual intercourse.	*To assist woman to cope with dyspareunia the nurse will:* Assess when pain occurs (during or after intercourse, with deep penetration). Discuss taking pain medication before sexual activity begins. Suggest alternative positions where the woman has greater control over pres-	Woman has painless sexual intercourse.

Continued.

Sample Nursing Care Plan—cont'd

ASSESSMENT	NURSING DIAGNOSIS (ND)/ PLAN (P)/GOAL (G)	RATIONALE/ IMPLEMENTATION	EVALUATION
		sure exerted (woman superior, side lying). Counsel both partners together about need for clear communication before and during sexual intercourse to minimize discomfort and increase pleasure for both.	
Impaired fertility—unknown cause.	ND: Knowledge deficit related to causes of impaired fertility. P: Meet knowledge needs. G: Pregnancy or unimpaired fertility.	*To help woman (couple) cope with impaired fertility the nurse will:* Discuss feelings about having children. Explain realistic potential of pregnancy with various treatments. Be supportive.	Woman (couple) verbalizes understanding of information.
Treatment therapies. Medications.	ND: Knowledge deficit related to treatment of endometriosis. P: Meet knowledge needs. G: Woman understands and takes medications appropriately.	*To explain treatment therapies; the nurse will:* Teach about medication used. Discuss reasons for using this drug. Explain which side effects to observe for and what to do if they occur. Make sure woman has accurate prescription and the right drug. Explain dosage schedule and importance of accuracy in taking.	Women understands about medication and takes the right dose on time.
Surgery.	G: Accurate understanding of treatment regimens.	*To allay fears of surgery, the nurse will:* Teach about laparoscopy. Discuss minor vaginal bleeding afterward. Discuss belching or feeling bloated afterward because intraabdominal carbon monoxide. Teach preoperatively as with other surgery.	Woman comes through surgery with minimal or no problems.

Climacterium

The climacterium is the stage in a woman's life when fertility is decreasing and the menstrual cycle becomes irregular and eventually stops. It also includes the period after ovulation ceases, when symptoms associated with changing hormone levels appear. The physiology of the climacterium is presented in Unit 1.

This normal occurrence is surrounded by myths and is often anticipated with anxiety and fear. Physical and psychologic problems during this period both require skillful and sensitive nursing care. The following sample nursing care plan includes some of the common problems of the climacterium and appropriate nursing interventions.

Sample Nursing Care Plan

NORMAL CLIMACTERIUM

ASSESSMENT	NURSING DIAGNOSIS (ND)/ PLAN (P)/GOAL (G)	RATIONALE/ IMPLEMENTATION	EVALUATION
Vasomotor instability Hot flashes	ND: Pain related to vasomotor disturbances. P: Minimize discomfort, and discuss self-care techniques. G: Woman reports increased comfort. ND: Knowledge deficit related to common symptomatology. P: Discuss symptomatology. G: Woman learns signs and symptoms.	*To help woman understand the climacterium and management of symptoms, the nurse will:* Assess what symptoms woman is experiencing. Discuss physiology of these symptoms. Explain any medications physician orders. Be a good listener. Discuss self-care techniques.	Woman understands these symptoms are normal. Woman uses comfort measures at home.
Night sweats Insomnia	ND: Sleep pattern disturbance related to night sweats and insomnia. P: Minimize or prevent sleep difficulties. G: Woman relates decrease in distress related to sleep pattern disturbance.		
Dizziness Tingling in extremities	ND: Sensory-perceptual alteration related to paresthesia of fingers and toes and dizziness. P: Minimize or prevent problems resulting from paresthesia and dizziness. G: Woman does not experience effects of sensory-perceptual alterations.		
Emotional disturbances Mood swings, irritability Depression Anxiety, nervousness, and agitation	ND: Ineffective individual coping related to the changes of climacterium. P: Assist woman to improve coping mechanisms. G: Woman relates increased ability to accept or cope with changes. ND: Body image disturbance related to changes in body functions. P: Provide opportunity to discuss feelings. G: Woman focuses on positive aspects of this time of her life.	*To facilitate client acceptance of her changing psyche the nurse will:* Discuss stress in the woman's life at the present. Teach relaxation techniques. Teach stress reduction. Validate woman's feelings, reassure her she is not going crazy or losing her mind. Discuss methods to help woman to cope effectively with her changing body and roles in life. Refer woman to support group.	Woman verbalizes problems and discusses possible solutions. Woman uses stress reduction and relaxation techniques.

Continued.

Sample Nursing Care Plan—cont'd

ASSESSMENT	NURSING DIAGNOSIS (ND)/ PLAN (P)/GOAL (G)	RATIONALE/ IMPLEMENTATION	EVALUATION
	ND: Anxiety, mild, related to the stresses of midlife and changing body patterns. P: Relieve anxiety by facilitating verbalization of problems and concerns. G: Woman relates decrease in anxiety.		

Fatigue
  Tiredness
  Weakness
	ND: Increased activity intolerance related to change in body functions and interrupted sleep.
	P: Teach relaxation techniques and stress reduction.
	G: Woman learns and implements self-care techniques.
		To help woman relieve fatigue the nurse will:
		Discuss daily activities.
		Assess use of time.
		Suggest nap in afternoon, if possible.
		Suggest clustering chores, and resting in between.
		Discuss diet.
		Discuss mild exercise.
			Woman understands information presented and uses suggestions at home.

Genital atrophy
  Dyspareunia
  Vaginal discharge
	ND: Sexual dysfunction related to physical and physiologic changes.
	P: Correct or compensate for physical impairments.
	G: Woman expresses satisfaction with sexual activity.
		To help woman in understanding and dealing with these changes the nurse will:
		Discuss sexual patterns.
		Offer suggestions on new positions.
		Discuss use of a lubricating jelly (not Vaseline; water soluble).
			Woman speaks openly with nurse and employs suggestions.

Urinary frequency Stress incontinence	ND: Altered patterns of urinary elimination, related to normal changes or to cystocele. P: Prevent or minimize problems. G: Woman retains normal pattern of urinary elimination.	Teach/encourage Kegel's exercises. Review physiologic and anatomic changes. Review treatment modalities.	Woman retains or regains an acceptable pattern of urinary elimination.
Urinary tract infection	ND: Potential for infection, related to changes in urinary patterns. P: Teach how to prevent infection. G: Woman does not develop infection.	Review prevention of urinary tract infection.	Woman does not develop infection.
Constipation or painful bowel movements	ND: Constipation, related to possible rectocele. P: Teach woman how to minimize or correct problem. G: Woman's bowel elimination pattern resumes within normal limits.	Review self-care techniques of exercise, fluids, diet, routine habits. Discuss physiologic and anatomic basis. Review physician's suggested treatment modalities.	Woman retains or regains her normal pattern of bowel elimination through self-care or surgery.

Sample Nursing Care Plan—cont'd

ASSESSMENT	NURSING DIAGNOSIS (ND)/ PLAN (P)/GOAL (G)	RATIONALE/ IMPLEMENTATION	EVALUATION
Headaches	ND: Pain, related to head-ache. P: Identify cause, mini-mize or prevent pain. G: Woman experiences fewer headaches. Woman uses self-care techniques to cope with headaches.	*To help woman avoid or minimize headaches the nurse will:* Assess type and position of headache. Ascertain when headaches are the worst. Discuss use of medication as ordered by physician.	Headaches are relieved.
Osteoporosis	ND: Knowledge deficit re-lated to causes and pre-vention of osteoporosis. P: Identify those at risk, teach prevention. G: Woman uses self-care techniques and takes medications as ordered.	*To inform woman about causes and prevention, the nurse will:* Explain about estrogen withdrawal. Discuss woman's risk for os-teoporosis. Discuss the part calcium intake plays in pre-venting significant bone loss.	Woman understands infor-mation presented.
Menopause	ND: Knowledge deficit re-lated to cessation of menstruation. P: Teach woman about menopause. G: Woman verbalizes un-derstanding about menopause.	*To teach woman about ces-sation of menstruation, the nurse will:* Discuss importance of birth control at this time. Discuss ovarian function. Discuss cessation of hor-mones and the effects on the body. Point out positive aspects of this time of the woman's life. Dispel old wives tales.	Woman takes on a more positive outlook. Woman does not become pregnant at this time.

IMPAIRED FERTILITY

The inability to conceive and bear a child comes as a surprise to 10% to 15% of otherwise healthy adults. Couples requesting assistance with fertility problems seek acceptance and assistance in coping with and often resolving these problems. Investigation of fertility and identification of the factors responsible for impaired fertility constitute a long and tedious process. The attitude and sensitivity of health care providers lay the foundation for the couple's ability to cope with the diagnostic and therapeutic process.

This section includes information on factors that affect fertility, diagnostic techniques, and therapies. A summary of nursing actions concludes the section.

FACTORS RESPONSIBLE FOR INFERTILITY

Male factor	40% to 50%
Tubal factor	20% to 25%
Ovulatory factor	20% to 25%
Cervical factor	1% to 2%
Uterine factor	1%
Unexplained	10%
Multifactorial	20% to 30%

Table 8-3   *Factors Associated with Fertility and Impaired Fertility*

Factor Required for Fertility	Conditions Associated with Impaired Fertility

Development of reproductive tract is normal.	Congenital or developmental factors
	    Abnormal external genitals (e.g., enlarged clitoris or fused labia) which may suggest masculinization
	    Gynetresia (e.g., absence of vagina or shallow vagina)
	    Vaginal anomalies (e.g., double vagina with single or double cervix and single or double uterus or with one vaginal canal ending blindly, the other vaginal canal ending at entrance to a uterus)
	    Unusual uterus (e.g., congenitally small, or "infantile," uterus)
	    Uterine and tubal defects from exposure to diethylstilbesterol (DES) as embryo/fetus
	    Abnormalities of ovaries (see ovulation)

Ovulation: hypothalamus-pituitary-gonadal axis is normal. An ovum is released from a mature ovarian follicle.	Absence of ovulation
	    Malfunctioning of axis with menstrual irregularities
	    Abnormal ovaries are seen in Turner's syndrome or Stein-Leventhal syndrome
	    Hormonal suppression of hypothalamus-pituitary-gonadal axis with birth control medication
	    Emotional problems (e.g., severe psychoneurosis or psychosis or anorexia nervosa, which may be responsible for anovulatory cycles, commonly associated with amenorrhea or oligomenorrhea)
	    Menstrual irregularities from vigorous exercise (jogging, sports), especially in thin women

Tubal: ovum enters uterine tube promptly after ovulation. Sperm migrate into uterine tube, where fertilization takes place. Fertilized ovum finds its way down tube into endometrial cavity to implant into hormone-prepared endometrium 7 to 10 days after ovulation.	Uterine tube is blocked or its function is altered
	    Blockage of tube by scar tissue formation after infection (pelvic inflammatory disease, ruptured appendix followed by peritonitis) or pelvic surgery
	    Blockage of tube by compression or kinking by abnormal growth such as endometriosis and neoplasms
	    Alteration in tubal motility by birth control medication or from emotional stress

Uterine: endometrium is adequately prepared to receive fertilized ovum.	Uterus is malformed or endometrium is unreceptive to fertilized ovum (malfunction of hypothalamus-pituitary-gonadal axis; presence of endometrial infection; presence of intrauterine device [IUD])
Vaginal-cervical mucus is receptive and supportive to sperm. Cervix is competent.	Absence of mucous characteristics receptive and supportive to sperm Altered vaginal pH from feminine hygiene preparations or douches, infections, antibiotic chemotherapy, disease states (e.g., diabetes mellitus), poor hygiene, or emotional stress Presence of spermicidal foams or other preparations used for contraception Development of antibodies (an immunologic response) against a specific male's sperm (see discussion of sperm, in assessments of the woman and the man)
Sperm are normal, adequate in number, and ejaculated into female reproductive tract.	Sperm "Assessment of the Man," p. 313.
Conceptus develops normally, reaches viability, and is delivered in good condition.	

LAPAROSCOPY

Who: Woman and a driver to take her home

Why: To assess visually the organs in the interior of the abdomen; and to perform minor surgical procedures

How: A small telescope is inserted through a small incision in the anterior abdominal wall using cold fiberoptic light sources that allow for superior visualization of the internal pelvis

When: Laparoscopy is timed depending on the purpose: if tubal patency is to be assessed, it is done 2 to 6 days following cessation of menses; if sites of endometriosis are to be treated, any day of the cycle is appropriate

Where: In a surgical suite with an anesthesiologist present (may be done on an outpatient basis)

Risk:
1. Usually general anesthesia is used
2. A pneumoperitoneum is established by insufflation of carbon dioxide gas via a needle inserted through the abdominal wall
3. Complications are rare (about 1 in 500): infection; electric burns of intraabdominal tissue
4. Postoperative shoulder (referred) pain or subcostal discomfort may occur for a short time

Procedure	Information Sought
• Woman signs informed consent and is prepared verbally for the examination. • Woman is usually admitted a few hours before surgery having taken nothing by mouth (NPO) for 8 hours. • Woman voids just before surgery. • Woman's pubic area is shaved only if examination is likely to be followed by laparotomy. • Anesthesia is given: general anesthesia with intubation; occasionally, local. • Woman is placed in a modified lithotomy position, with the legs at 45 degrees. • The vagina, perineum, and abdomen are prepared and draped, and the area from the umbilicus to the vagina is exposed. • An intrauterine probe is inserted except in cases where intrauterine pregnancy may be present. • A needle is inserted and a pneumoperitoneum with carbon dioxide gas is established to elevate the abdominal wall from the organs creating an empty space that permits visualization and exploration with laparoscope. Rubin's cannula is used for injections of methylene blue dye to assess for tubal patency. The needle may be inserted at lower border of umbilicus. • Examination or procedure is performed. • After surgery, deflation of most of gas is done by direct expression. Trocar (and needle) sites are closed with a single subcuticular absorbable suture or a skin clip, and an adhesive bandage is applied. • Postoperative recovery requires taking of vital signs, assessing level of consciousness, preventing aspiration, monitoring intravenous fluids, and reassuring client regarding shoulder discomfort. Discharge from hospital usually occurs in 4 to 6 hours. • Shoulder or subcostal discomfort (from pneumoperitoneum) usually lasts only 24 hours and is relieved with a mild analgesic. • Caution the woman against heavy lifting or strenuous activity for 4 to 7 days, at which time she is usually asymptomatic.	Findings favorable to fertility: 1. No developmental abnormalities of pelvic structures. 2. No lesions, infections, or adhesions. 3. No complications occur as a result of the examination or procedure. 4. If tubal insufflation is done, the tubes are found to be patent. 5. If there is a reparable problem (e.g., adhesions that are kinking the uterine tubes), the problem is repaired through the laparoscope.

ASSESSMENT OF THE WOMAN

History

1. Duration of impaired fertility: length of contraceptive and noncontraceptive exposure
2. Fertility in other marriages of self or spouse
3. Obstetric
   a. Number of pregnancies and abortions
   b. Length of time required to initiate each pregnancy
   c. Complications of any pregnancy
   d. Duration of lactation
4. Gynecologic: detailed menstrual history and leukorrheal history
5. Previous tests and therapy done for infertility
6. Medical: general medical history including chronic and hereditary disease; drug use
7. Surgical: especially abdominal or pelvic surgery
8. Sexual history in detail: libido, orgasm capacity, techniques, frequency of intercourse, and postcoital practices
9. Psychosomatic evaluation
   a. General
   b. As regards impaired fertility, particularly her reason for seeking advice at this time

Physical Examination

1. General: careful examination of other organs and parts of body; special attention given to habitus, fat and hair distribution, acne
2. Genital tract: state of hymen (full penetration); clitoris; vaginal infection, including trichomoniasis and candidiasis; cervical tears, polyps, infection, patency of os, accessibility to insemination; uterus, including size and position, mobility; adnexae, tumors, evidence of endometriosis

Laboratory Data

1. Routine urine, complete blood count, and serologic test for syphilis; additional laboratory studies as indicated
2. Basic endocrine studies in women with irregular menstrual cycles or in amenorrhea, hirsutism, acne, or excessive weight gain

Irregular Menstrual Cycles	*Amenorrhea*
Protein-bound iodine (PBI) or other thyroid tests	Tomographic x-ray films of skull
17-Ketosteroids	T_4 or other thyroid tests
17-Hydroxycorticoids	17-Ketosteroids
4-Hour glucose tolerance test	17-Hydroxycorticoids
Endometrial biopsy	4-Hour glucose tolerance test
	Endometrial biopsy
	Gonadotropin determination
	Buccal smear and chromosomal studies

   Other laboratory tests added as desired for a more complete diagnosis of endocrine problems
3. RH factor and antibody titer tests—important in abortion and premature delivery problems
4. Sperm antibody agglutination studies. Special laboratory procedure involves obtaining a fresh semen specimen from man and a blood sample from the woman. Sperm are incubated in the blood serum of the woman and checked at intervals for agglutination; the test is negative if no agglutinated sperm are found.

ASSESSMENT OF THE MAN

History

1. Fertility in other marriages of self or spouse
2. Medical: general medical history, including venereal infections, mumps orchitis, chronic diseases, recent fever, drug use
3. Surgical: herniorraphy, injuries to genitals, or other surgery in genital area
4. Occupational: exposure to chemicals, x-ray equipment, or extreme therapy changes; physical nature of occupation; vacations and work habits
5. Previous tests and therapy done for study of impaired fertility
6. Duration of impaired fertility
7. Sex history in detail, with discussion of actual coital techniques; such as frequency and ability to ejaculate
8. Adequacy of erection

Physical Examination

1. General examination: careful examination of other organs and parts of body, with special attention given to habitus, fat and hair distribution
2. Genital tract: penis and urethra; scrotal size; position, size, and consistency of testes; epididymides and vasa deferentia; prostate size and consistency
3. Careful search for varicocele, with man in both supine and upright positions

Laboratory Data

1. Routine urine, complete blood count, and serologic test for syphilis
2. Complete semen analysis—essential
   a. Liquefaction: usually complete within 10 to 30 minutes
   b. Semen volume   2-5 ml (range: 1 to 7 ml)
   c. Semen pH   7.2 to 7.8
   d. Sperm density   20 to 200 million/ml
   e. Normal morphology (%)   ≥60%
   f. Motility (important consideration in sperm evaluation); percentage of forward-moving sperm estimated in relationship to abnormally motile and nonmotile sperm. This requires evaluation by a technician with some degree of experience but as the test provides a more accurate diagnosis; it is well worth the time involved; ≥50% is normal
   g. Cell count: average normal, 60 million or more per milliliter or a total of 150 to 200 or more million per ejaculate; minimum normal standards: 40 million/ml, with a total count of at least 125 million per ejaculate (average of counts on two or preferably three separate specimens)
   NOTE: These values are not absolute, but only relative to the final evaluation of the couple as a single reproductive unit.
3. Additional laboratory studies as indicated
   a. Basic endocrine studies indicated in men with oligospermia or aspermia:
      (1) Tomographic x-ray films of skull
      (2) T_4 or other thyroid tests
      (3) 17-Ketosteroids
      (4) Gonadotropin determination
      (5) 17-Hydroxycorticoids and pregnanediol
      (6) Buccal smear and chromosome studies, for example, Klinefelter's syndrome, XXY sex chromosomes
      (7) Test for sperm antibodies; autoimmunization. Autoimmune antibodies (produced by the man against his own sperm) agglutinate or immobilize sperm is less than 5% of men with impaired fertility
   b. Testicular biopsy, where correct interpretation is available (may give a more accurate diagnosis and prognosis in cases of azoospermia and severe oligospermia), vasography if indicated and available

SUMMARY OF FERTILITY TEST FINDINGS FAVORABLE TO FERTILITY

1. Follicular development, ovulation, and luteal development are supportive to pregnancy:
   a. Basal body temperature, or BBT (presumptive evidence of ovulatory cycles)
      (1) Is biphasic
      (2) Reveals temperature elevation that persists for 12 to 14 days just before menstruation
   b. Cervical mucus characteristics change appropriately during phases of the menstrual cycle
   c. Findings from endometrial biopsies taken at different times during menstrual cycle are consistent with day of cycle
   d. Laparoscopic visualization of pelvic organs verifies follicular and luteal development
2. The luteal phase is supportive to pregnancy:
   a. Levels of plasma progesterone are adequate
   b. Endometrial biopsy findings indicate a secretory endometrium
3. Cervical factors are receptive to sperm during expected time of ovulation:
   a. Cervical os is open
   b. Cervical mucus is clear, watery, abundant, and slippery and demonstrates good spinnbarkheit and arborization (fern pattern)
   c. Cervical examination is negative for lesions and infections
   d. Postcoital test findings are satisfactory (adequate number of live, motile, normal sperm present in cervical mucus)
   e. No immunity to sperm can be demonstrated
4. The uterus and uterine tubes are supportive to pregnancy:
   a. Uterine and tubal patency is documented by
      (1) Passage of carbon dioxide into peritoneal cavity
      (2) Spillage of dye into peritoneal cavity
      (3) Outlines of uterine and tubal cavities of adequate size and shape with no abnormalities
   b. Laparoscopic examination verifies normal development of internal genitals and absence of adhesions, infections, endometriosis, and other lesions
5. Semen is supportive to pregnancy:
   a. Sperm are adequate in number per milliliter of ejaculate
   b. Majority of sperm show normal morphology
   c. Sperm are motile
   d. No autoimmunity exists
   e. Seminal fluid is normal

Table 8-4 *Drug Therapy for Female Infertility*

Drug	Indications	Nursing Actions
Ovulatory Stimulants		
Clomiphene citrate (Clomid; Serophene) (O)—follicular maturing agents	Anovulation caused by hypothalamic suppression (but with an intact hypothalamic-pituitary-ovarian axis)	Counsel regarding oral ingestion of Clomid or Serophene, maintenance of BBT chart for evidence of ovulation, and potential side effects: ovarian cyst formation, vasomotor effects; visual disturbances, partial alopecia, abdominal disturbances, and multiple pregnancies.
Bromocriptine (Parlodel), a synthetic ergot alkaloid	Anovulation caused by elevated levels of prolactin (inhibits release of prolactin)	Counsel regarding oral ingestion of drug with food to reduce its side effects: nausea, vomiting, lightheadedness, dizziness (tolerance develops within a few weeks; menstruation resumes in 75% of women in 6 to 8 weeks). Should not be taken with drugs that elevate prolactin levels, for example, psychotropic agents. Monitor BBT so that drug is discontinued if pregnancy occurs.
Thyroid stimulating hormone (TSH)	Anovulation caused by hypothyroidism	Counsel regarding medical regimen: medication and assessment of blood levels of TSH.
Human menopausal gonadotropin (hMG) (Pergonal; Profasi HP)	Anovulation caused by hypogonadotropic amenorrhea	Administer or test self-injection of hMG.
Gonadotropin-releasing hormone (GnRH), alone or preceded by clomiphene citrate or hMG	Anovulation caused by hypothalamic-pituitary dysfunction, hypothalamic failure, or failure to ovulate with use of Clomid or Serophene	Assist with daily injection or teach woman self-injection. Overall success rate is 15% to 20%.
Hormone Replacement Therapy		
Conjugated estrogens and medroxyprogesterone	Hypoestrogenic condition: high stress level, decreased level of body fat caused by eating disorder (e.g., anorexia nervosa) or excessive exercise	Counsel regarding oral ingestion—estrogens on days 1 to 24 and progesterone on days 15 to 24; possible side effects (e.g., fluid retention); stress reduction and so on.
Hydroxyprogesterone supplementation (vaginal suppositories or IM)	Luteal phase defects	Counsel regarding administration: start 3 to 4 days after estimated ovulation and continue to menses (if no menses, a serum pregnancy test is done).
	Endometriosis	Assist with protocol of care. (see Table 8-2, and Sample Nursing Care Plan, "Endometriosis," pp. 305-306).
Other		
Prednisone (O) (a glucocorticoid)	Congenital adrenal hyperplasia	Counsel regarding oral ingestion regimen and associated side effects.
Danazol	Endometriosis	Assist with counseling woman regarding daily dosages and possible side effects: weight gain, hot flushes, night sweats, decrease in breast size, bloody vaginal discharge, atrophic vaginitis.
Mefenamic acid; Naproxen	Dysmenorrhea with pain, nausea, vomiting, headaches, fainting, diarrhea that are induced by danazol therapy for endometriosis	Counsel regarding need to start therapy 48 hours before onset of dysmenorrhea.
Antimicrobial Therapy	Infection	Implement usual actions when administering antimicrobial medications.

Table 8-5 *Drug Therapy for Male Infertility*

Drug	Indications	Nursing Actions
Testosterone enanthate (Delatestryl) and testosterone cypionate (Depo-Testerone) by injection	Stimulate virilization, especially the adolescent	Teach self-administration, or administer every 2 weeks
hCG (Pregnyl), IM (LH activity)	Virilize a hypogonadotropic male to restore Leydig cell function and spermatogenesis	Administer three times a week, perhaps for 18 months
FSH (human menopausal gonadotropin [hMG], Pergonal or Profasi HP)	Aid hCG for completion of spermatogenesis	Administer three times a week
Bromocriptine (ergot derivative and dopamine agonist, Parlodel)	Treat hypogonadotropic hypogonadism-associated prolactin-producing hypothalamic or pituitary tumors; may reduce the tumor	Counsel regarding oral ingestion with food to decrease side effects: dizziness, fainting, hypotension, headache, nausea, vomiting
Adrenal corticoids specific for the condition	Addison's disease Cushing's disease Congenital adrenal hypoplasia	Practice general medical nursing
Clomiphene citrate (Clomid or Serophene)	Idiopathic subfertility	Counsel regarding oral ingestion every day or every other day in cyclic fashion (25 days followed by 5-day rest period; repeat)
Vitamin C (ascorbic acid, a reducing agent)	Sperm agglutination where there are no autoantibodies	Counsel regarding oral ingestion of 500 mg three times a day indefinitely
Methylprednisolone (Medrol)	Steroid immunosuppression of sperm autoantibodies	Counsel regarding oral ingestion: 96 mg/day for 7 days starting the first regimen on day 21 of the woman's cycle, then every 4 weeks for 3 months
Sputolysin (mucolytic agent)	Increased seminal viscosity; used to wash semen before artificial seminal liquefaction	Counsel regarding use as precoital douching agent by female sexual partner
α-Amylase	Delayed seminal liquefaction	Counsel regarding use as precoital douching agent or cocoa-butter vaginal suppository by female sexual partner

Summary of Nursing Actions

IMPAIRED FERTILITY

I. Goals
  A. To identify factors causing infertility
  B. To treat conditions that are treatable
  C. To maintain client's self-esteem and sense of adequacy as a woman or man
  D. To help client maintain control over his or her destiny through active participation in the decision-making process

II. Priorities
  A. Clients become active partners in the management of their infertility through encouragement, education, and support.
  B. Infertility factors are identified and treated, if possible.

III. Assessment (see Table 8-4)
  A. Interview
    1. Health history
    2. Psychosocial history
    3. Review of systems
  B. Physical examination
  C. Laboratory tests

IV. Potential nursing diagnoses

  A. Body image disturbance
  B. Self esteem disturbance: situational low self esteem
  C. Altered role performance
  D. Personal identity disturbance
  E. Altered family processes
  F. Ineffective individual coping
  G. Ineffective family coping: compromised
  H. Spiritual distress
  I. Powerlessness
  J. Anxiety
  K. Knowledge deficit
  L. Sexual dysfunction
  M. Altered sexuality patterns

V. Plan/implementation
  A. Support person
    1. Greet the woman and her family by name.
    2. Provide privacy as needed while giving instructions for obtaining specimens and changing clothes and while identifying feelings, myths, misinformation, or "magical thinking" about the cause of infertility.
    3. Encourage discussion about the loss of spontane-

Summary of Nursing Actions—cont'd

ity and control over the couple's marital relationship and sometimes over one's progress toward career and goals while undergoing the tests.

4. Explore the couple's support systems, their relationship with the couple, their ages, their availability, and any available cultural or religious support.

5. *If couple conceives,* be prepared for a variety of reactions from anger to joy. Some couples have come to terms with their infertility and have rearranged their lives; pregnancy disrupts the changes.
   a. Assist couple with identification and expression of their feelings.
   b. Offer the same type of care offered to other pregnant couples.
   c. If they choose to continue with the pregnancy, be prepared to offer extra preparation for the realities of pregnancy, labor, and parenthood. *(A history of infertility is considered to be a risk factor for pregnancy.)*
   d. After delivery, offer information about contraception.

6. *If couple does not conceive,* assist physician in assessing their desire to be referred to help with adoption, artificial insemination or in vitro fertilization, or with choosing childlessness.

B. Teacher/counselor/advocate
   1. Assists physician in the identification of the client's gaps in knowledge, clarifies information, and reinforces physician's explanations and instructions.
   2. Acts as the client's advocate by assisting the client to state a concern or question or to request further explanation.
   3. Teaches clients to assess and record BBT and cervical mucus.
   4. Helps physician to assess the client's readiness to learn and her or his level of understanding of infertility, diagnostic tests, and therapy.
   5. Provides written and verbal instructions for specific preparation for tests; provides description of

sensations client may experience during and after procedures.
   6. Helps clients understand and cope with responses/needs commonly associated with infertility.

C. Technician
   1. Utilizes information in boxes to assemble equipment and to assist physician during testing.
   2. Assists with pelvic examination.
   3. Utilizes correct method for obtaining, labeling, and transporting specimens to the laboratory.
   4. Documents and maintains accurate records.

VI. Evaluation
   A. Couple is educated in the anatomy and physiology of the reproductive system.
   B. Couple complies with the investigation of infertility.
   C. Any abnormalities identified through various tests and examinations are treated (e.g., infections, blocked uterine tubes, sperm allergy, varicocele).
   D. Couple receives an estimate of their chances to conceive.
   E. Couple resolves guilt feelings and does not need to focus blame.
   F. If couple conceives, the couple:
      1. Accepts their responses to the pregnancy.
      2. Realigns their goals, aspirations, and identities.
      3. Is comfortable with their decisions regarding this pregnancy (e.g., abortion, continue with pregnancy and keep the child, give the child up for adoption).
   G. If couple does not conceive, the couple:
      1. Decides on an alternative that is acceptable to both of them (e.g., childlessness, adoption, artificial insemination, or in vitro fertilization).
      2. Seeks support as necessary (e.g., RESOLVE, National Organization for NonParents).
   H. Couple finds acceptable methods for handling pressures they may feel from peers and relatives regarding their childless state.
   I. Couple receives list of community agencies that assist with adoptions. (OURS, ARENA) or that provide support (RESOLVE, National Organization for NonParents).

CONTRACEPTION AND FAMILY PLANNING

More than 90% of couples in the United States have used or intend to use some method of birth control. A variety of safe, reliable techniques are available, and the nurse must be knowledgeable about the implications of each method. The client's life-style, religious and cultural beliefs, and commitment all must be considered in the selection of the method. Client teaching is an integral part of nursing care.

This section provides information on "natural" family planning methods, use of the diaphragm, and hormonal contraceptives. Guidelines for client teaching are provided to assist the nurse in ensuring that teaching is comprehensive and effective.

Methods Available Without Prescription

A. Periodic abstinence methods employ a combination of the following:
   1. Rhythm or calendar method.
   2. BBT method
   3. Cervical mucus (Billings, ovulation) method
   4. Sympto-thermal method
   5. Fertility awareness method
   6. Predictor test for ovulation

B. Barrier methods
   1. Condom
   2. Foam
   3. Spermicide
   4. Vaginal sponges

Table 8-6 *Contraceptive Methods and Pregnancies per 100 Women*

Method of Contraception	Contraceptive Failures (number of pregnancies)*
No method	60-80
Calendar only	14-47
Periodic abstinence	1-47
Jellies/creams	4-36
Condom	3-36
Aerosol foams	2-29
Mucous method	1-25
Diaphragm with spermicide	2-20
BBT only	1-20
BBT with intercourse during post-ovulatory time	1-7
IUD	1-6
Combination oral contraceptives	1-3

*The fewer the number of pregnancies, the greater the effectiveness.

Guidelines for Client Teaching

BASAL ("RESTING") BODY TEMPERATURE (BBT)

ASSESSMENT

1. Woman having trouble conceiving for pregnancy.
2. Need for presumptive evidence of ovulation and an adequate luteal (progesterone) phase.
3. Woman interested in learning how to determine her ovulation time.

NURSING DIAGNOSES

Knowledge deficit related to BBT, the procedure to take it and keep a graph.

Potential self-esteem disturbance related to the inability to conceive a child.

Sexual dysfunction related to possible infertility and anovulation.

GOALS

Short-term

Woman learns what BBT is and how to take and record it.

Intermediate

Woman maintains a record of BBT, fever, stress, cervical mucus characteristics.

Long-term

Woman is motivated enough to obtain and maintain BBT graph for several months.

REFERENCES AND TEACHING AIDS

Pamphlets, booklets, diagrams, any printed material depicting the taking and recording of the BBT.
BBT thermometer.

CONTENT/RATIONALE	TEACHING ACTION
To provide content related to BBT: In an ovulating woman, there is a variation in the BBT during the course of her menstrual cycle because of hormones working in her body. The BBT is lower during the first part of the menstrual cycle, the proliferative phase. As ovulation approaches, and the effects of LH and progesterone take over, the BBT rises. If fertilization of the ovum takes place, the BBT remains elevated. However, if fertilization does not take place, the corpus luteum deteriorates and the BBT falls to the lower level again, until the next ovulation occurs.	Discuss BBT with the woman. Show woman a diagram depicting the phases of the menstrual cycle. Discuss the different hormones in the woman's body that are responsible for her menstrual cycle and ovulation. Leave time for questions. Show woman a sample BBT graph and the biphasic line seen in ovulatory cycles.
The BBT thermometer is calibrated in tenths rather than fifths. If woman doesn't want to buy a BBT thermometer, a regular oral thermometer may be used, but it must be left in the mouth under the tongue for 5 minutes.	Show the client the BBT thermometer, and how it is calibrated.
Discuss the procedure woman will follow every day. Before going to bed, shake the thermometer down and leave it on the bedside table. On awakening the following morning, the woman will put the thermometer under her tongue and not move any more. After 3 minutes she	Provide a demonstration. Encourage woman to demonstrate taking and reading the thermometer and how she will graph the temperature while nurse watches. Encourage woman to start a log at the same time that keeps

CONTENT/RATIONALE	TEACHING ACTION
will take the thermometer out of her mouth and replace it on the night stand. On arising, the woman will read the thermometer and record the temperature on the graph. Using a snooze alarm on the woman's clock is a convenient way to time the temperature taking.	track of any other activity that might interfere with her true BBT.

EVALUATION Woman verbalizes understanding of the instructions given, provides a return demonstration, asks appropriate questions, and meets all goals mutually set. When woman returns after 2 or 3 cycles, she brings a completed log and graph and can identify phases of her menstrual cycle by using these data.

Guidelines for Client Teaching

CERVICAL MUCUS CHARACTERISTICS

ASSESSMENT
1. Woman (couple) wants to know how cervical mucus changes with the menstrual cycle.
2. Woman (couple) wants to know how to tell period of maximum fertility by using the changes in cervical mucus.

NURSING DIAGNOSIS
Knowledge deficit related to the changes in cervical mucus during the menstrual cycle and how changes affect fertility.

GOALS
Short-term
Woman learns how to assess for peak mucus sign.

Intermediate
Woman learns to check for mucus several times per day.
Woman learns to record observations daily as to quantity, consistency, color, and sensation from last day of menstrual flow.

Long-term
Woman records findings along with BBT for several menstrual cycles.
Woman (couple) knows when peak mucus sign occurs for maximum fertility.

REFERENCES AND TEACHING AIDS
Pamphlets and booklets distributed by hospitals, clinics, or physicians.
Raw egg white.

CONTENT/RATIONALE	TEACHING ACTION
To provide content related to cervical mucus: Explain to woman (couple) how cervical mucus changes throughout the menstrual cycle. Right before ovulation, the watery, thin, clear mucus becomes more abundant and thick. Feels like a lubricant and can be stretched 5+ cm; this is called spinnbarkheit. This indicates the period of maximum fertility. Sperm deposited in this type of mucus can survive until ovulation occurs.	Show charts of menstrual cycle along with changes in the cervical mucus. Have woman practice with raw egg white. Show findings favorable to fertility.
To teach assessment technique: Explain to woman (couple) that assessment of cervical mucus characteristics is best learned when mucus not mixed with semen, contraceptive jellies or foams, or discharge from infections.	Couple asked to refrain from ejaculation of semen into or near vaginal opening for at least one infection-free cycle.
Woman is to assess cervical mucus several times a day for several cycles. Mucus can be obtained from vaginal introitus, no need to reach into vagina to cervix. Woman records her findings on the same record on which her BBT is entered. Woman records any other events.	**Good hand washing is imperative** to begin and end all self-assessment. From last day of menstrual flow the woman starts her observations. Supply her with a BBT log and graph, if she does not already have one.

EVALUATION Woman (couple) follows your directions, asks appropriate questions, and all goals are met. When woman returns after two or three cycles, she can describe the changes in her cervical mucus during each phase.

USE AND CARE OF THE DIAPHRAGM

Positions for Insertion of Diaphragm

Squatting

This is the most frequently used position and most women find this position satisfactory.

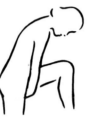

Leg Up Method

A position to suit the convenience of particular women is to raise the left foot (if right hand is used for insertion) on a low stool, and in a bending position the diaphragm is inserted.

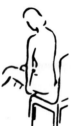

Chair method

A practical method for diaphragm insertion is for the woman to sit far forward on the edge of a chair.

Reclining

In some instances, certain women prefer to insert the diaphragm while in a semi-reclining position in bed.

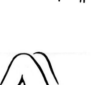

Inspection of Diaphragm

Your diaphragm must be inspected carefully before each use. The best way to do this is:

Hold the diaphragm up to a light source. Carefully stretch the diaphragm at the area of the rim, on all sides, to make sure there are no holes. Remember, it is possible to puncture the diaphragm with sharp fingernails.

Another way to check for pinholes is to fill the diaphragm with water carefully. If there is any problem, it will be seen immediately.

If your diaphragm is "puckered," especially near the rim, this could mean thin spots.

The diaphragm should not be used if you see any of the above; consult your physician.

Preparation of Diaphragm

Your diaphragm must always be used with a spermicidal lubricant in order to be effective. Pregnancy cannot be prevented effectively by the diaphragm alone.

Always empty your bladder before inserting the diaphragm. Place about 2 teaspoonsful of contraceptive gel, contraceptive jelly, or contraceptive cream on the side of the diaphragm that will rest against the cervix (or whichever way you have been instructed). Spread it around to coat the surface and the rim. This aids in insertion and offers a more complete seal. Many women also spread some gel (jelly) or cream on the other side of the diaphragm. See Fig. A.

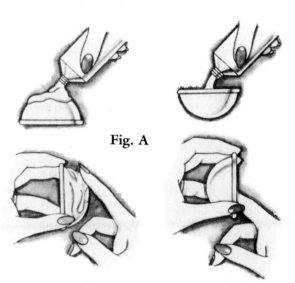

Fig. A

Insertion of Diaphragm

The diaphragm can be inserted as much as 6 hours before intercourse. Hold the diaphragm between your thumb and fingers. The dome can either be up or down, as directed by your physician. Place your index finger on the outer rim of the compressed diaphragm. See Fig. B. Use the fingers of the other hand to spread the labia (lips of the vagina). This will assist in guiding the diaphragm into place.

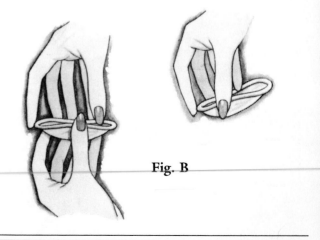

Fig. B

USE AND CARE OF THE DIAPHRAGM—cont'd

Insert the diaphragm into the vagina. Direct it inward and downward as far as it will go to the space behind and below the cervix. See Fig. C.

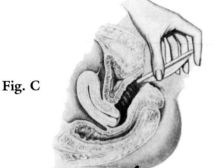

Fig. C

Tuck the front of the rim of the diaphragm behind the pelvic bone so the rubber hugs the front wall of the vagina. See Fig. D.

Fig. D

Directions for Insertion With Diaphragm Introducer

Hold the introducer in either hand. Compress the diaphragm, dome up, with the fingers of your other hand. Place one end of the rim in the grooved end of the introducer. See Fig. E.

Fig. E

Fit the other end of the diaphragm over the notch corresponding to the diaphragm size. See Fig. F. Squeeze approximately 1 tablespoonful of gel, jelly, or cream into the folds of the diaphragm. Spread a small amount around the rim.

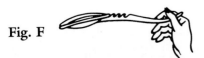

Fig. F

The diaphragm may be inserted while you are lying flat with your legs drawn up. However, any position may be used if more convenient. See positions for insertion of diaphragm.

Insert the diaphragm in a downward direction as far back as it will comfortably go, past the cervix. See Fig. G.

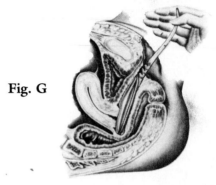

Fig. G

To release the diaphragm, rotate the introducer to the right or left and gently withdraw it. See Fig. H. After the introducer is removed, tuck the front rim of the diaphragm behind the pelvic bone. See Fig. D.

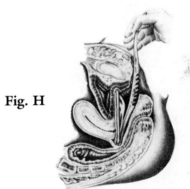

Fig. H

Feel for your cervix through the diaphragm to be certain it is properly placed and securely covered by the rubber dome. See Fig. I.

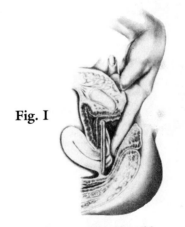

Fig. I

To clean the introducer, wash with mild soap and warm water, rinse and dry thoroughly.

Continued.

USE AND CARE OF THE DIAPHRAGM—cont'd

Final Checking

Whether the diaphragm is inserted manually or with the introducer, the finger test must always be made to see that the outer rim of the diaphragm is tucked firmly behind the pelvic bone (see Fig. D). At the same time, you must check to see that the small round knob of the cervix (mouth of the womb) is securely covered by the rubber dome of the diaphragm. See Fig. I.

Repeated Intercourse

Without removing the diaphragm, an additional applicator-ful of gel (jelly) or cream must be used if intercourse takes place more than 6 hours after the diaphragm has been inserted or for each repeated intercourse. The diaphragm must remain in place for at least 6 hours after the last intercourse.

General Information

Regardless of the time of the month, this method of contraception must be used each and every time intercourse takes place. Your diaphragm must be left in place for at least 6 hours after the last intercourse. If you remove your diaphragm before the 6-hour time period, your chance of becoming pregnant could be greatly increased. You should not leave your diaphragm in place for more than 24 hours, to do so may encourage growth of bacteria that could result in infection or toxic shock syndrome.

Douching is not necessary after the use of the diaphragm. However, if it is desired or recommended by your physician, you must wait the full 6 hours after the last intercourse.

Removal of Diaphragm

The only proper way to remove the diaphragm is to insert your forefinger up and over the top side of the diaphragm, and slightly to the side.

Next, turn the palm of your hand downward and backward hooking the forefinger firmly on top of the inside of the upper rim of the diaphragm, *breaking the suction.*

Pull the diaphragm down and out. This avoids the possibility of tearing the diaphragm with the fingernails. The diaphragm *should not* be removed by trying to catch the rim from *below* the dome. See Fig. J.

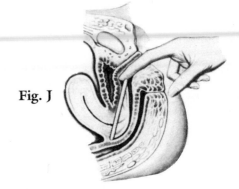

Fig. J

Care of Diaphragm

When using a vaginal diaphragm, avoid using products that may contain petroleum such as certain body lubricants, vaginal lubricants, or vaginitis preparations. These products can weaken rubber.

A little care means longer wear for your diaphragm. After each use the diaphragm should be washed in warm water and Ivory soap. Do not use detergent soaps, cold cream soaps, deodorant soaps, and soaps containing petroleum, since they can weaken the rubber. *Ivory soap should be the only soap used.*

After washing, the diaphragm should be dried thoroughly. All water and moisture should be removed with your towel. The diaphragm should then be dusted with *cornstarch.* Scented talc, body powder, baby powder, and the like, should not be used because they can weaken the rubber. Remember, only *cornstarch* for dusting.

The diaphragm should then be placed back in the plastic case for storage. It should not be stored near a radiator or heat source, or exposed to light for an extended period of time.

Table 8-7   *Risk Factors and Degree of Associated Risk by Age for Users of Oral Contraceptives*

Risk	Age (years)		
	≤29	30-39	≥40
Heavy smokers (≥15 cigarettes)	2	3	4
Light smokers (≤14 cigarettes)	1	2	3
Nonsmokers with no added risk conditions	1	1,2	2
Nonsmokers with added risk conditions	2	2,3	3,4

1 = Use associated with low risk; 2 = use associated with moderate risk; 3 = use associated with high risk; 4 = use associated with very high risk.

Table 8-8 *Hormonal Contraception*

Composition	Route of Administration	Duration of Effect
Combination of an estrogen and a progestin:	Oral	Not more than 24 hours
Biphasic: constant dose of estrogen and an increase in progestin on day 11		
Triphasic: 3 different products on market—in 2, estrogen is constant and progestin varies; in 1, amounts of both vary. Total hormone dose per cycle is lower than in biphasic combinations		
Sequential: estrogen during first half of cycle, progestin during second half; not sold in United States		
Minipill: progestin (norethindrone, 0.35 mg) only	Oral	24 hours
Morning-after pill: estrogen (diethylstilbestrol [DES]) in very high levels—25 mg	Oral	Taken within 72 hours of unprotected coitus during fertile period; because of DES effect on fetus, abortion advised if method fails
Depo-Provera: progestin only (medroxyprogesterone acetate), 150 mg	Intramuscular injection	From 3 to 6 months
Norplant system: progestin (Levonorgestrel) in silastic containers	Implant, subdermal	Up to 5 years

Guidelines for Client Teaching

GENERAL CONTRACEPTIVE METHODS

ASSESSMENT

1. Complete physical assessment and history appropriate for each method.
2. Assessment of woman's (couple's) knowledge of method selected.
3. Assessment of body image.
4. Assessment of motivation needed for method selected.
5. Assessment of life-style and discussion whether method selected fits into daily life.

NURSING DIAGNOSES

Knowledge deficit related to method selected.
Potential for injury related to knowledge deficit or ignorance of method selected.
Potential for infection related to not adhering to proper guidelines of method selected.
Altered nutrition: less than body requirements related to side effects of oral contraceptives.

GOALS
Short-term

Woman (couple) develops a trusting relationship with care provider.
Nurse identifies myths, clarifies information, and dispels misinformation.
Woman (couple) becomes comfortable in the use of the method.
Woman learns relevant information regarding the method being used (i.e., use, action, advantages, disadvantages, side effects, and effectiveness).

Intermediate

Woman (couple) confers with care provider when questions arise regarding use or desire to change to another method.
Women reports side effects or complications or suspected pregnancy immediately.
Woman returns to care provider for periodic checkups or when a change in the method is warranted (e.g., pregnancy is desired, diaphragm needs to be refitted after birth of baby or gain or loss of more than 4.5 kg (10 lb).

Long-term

Woman remains in good health while using chosen method.
Woman achieves desired objective for contraception, that is no children, or desired number of children.
Woman indicates satisfaction with chosen method and care received.

REFERENCES AND TEACHING AIDS

Inserts from packages of chosen method.
Hospital or clinic teaching pamphlets or booklets.
Flip chart showing anatomy of pelvic structures or total body plastic medical model.
Audiovisuals or films for teaching.
Samples of contraceptive device (i.e., BBT charts and thermometer)
Fresh egg white for teaching about cervical mucus.
Mirror.
Handouts of printed material.

Continued.

Guidelines for Client Teaching—cont'd

CONTENT/RATIONALE	TEACHING ACTION
To meet information needs: Provide general discussion about selected method, its mode of action, and reasons for choosing it. Establish basis and direction for cognitive, psychomotor, and affective learning needs. Teach at the client's level without being condescending.	*Encourage general discussion through use of the following:* Provide time, privacy, and assurance regarding confidentiality. Create a receptive, nonjudgmental atmosphere. Consider appropriate cultural/ethnic, intellectual/educational, and developmental factors pertinent to the woman (couple).
Supply information about action, advantages, disadvantages, side effects, and effectiveness.	*Using references and equipment listed above, implement the following:* Discuss information about method selected.
Discuss method, its placement, locus of action.	Indicate on illustration or medical model the placement of the device (IUD, diaphragm, cervical cap or sponge, condom), loci of action (hormonal contraceptive versus diaphragm).
To assist client in developing competence and confidence with chosen method: Learning is reinforced if content is taught in a variety of ways. Time and hands-on experience with chosen method reinforces learning. Confidence and mastery of content and experience before woman leaves the care provider are more likely to result in use of method.	Demonstrate appliance (diaphragm with spermicide), characteristics of "fertile" cervical mucus (egg white), entering temperature on BBT graph, calculating fertile times. Supervise client's return demonstration and practice. Assess client's recall of content taught or its availability on printed material provided.
To reaffirm health care provider's caring and woman's motivation: Review the material presented.	Ascertain that client has appropriate phone numbers for questions and suggest client call back, prn, after implementing method at home.

EVALUATION Woman (couple) demonstrate competence and ask appropriate questions regarding method of choice; goals are met within an appropriate time frame.

STERILIZATION AND ABORTION

Since 1950 voluntary sterilization has grown rapidly in acceptance and is currently the most prevalent method of contraception in the world. Sterilization may be requested by couples who already have the number of children they desire or by those who have decided not to bear children. A summary of sterilization methods follows.

Elective abortion is the purposeful interruption of a previable pregnancy. The control of birth, dealing with human sexuality and the question of life and death, is one of the most highly emotional components of health care. The values, beliefs, and moral convictions of the nurse are involved almost to the same extent as those of the pregnant woman herself. The nurse must be informed and nonjudgmental in educating the woman regarding her options and supporting her in her decision.

Table 8-9 *Summary of Sterilization Methods: Basis for Counseling*

Method and Action	Advantages	Disadvantages and Side Effects	Effectiveness
Woman			
Tubal occlusion: uterine tubes ligated and severed, banded or clipped, or fulgurated, to prevent passage of egg	Abdominal surgery using 2.5 cm (1 in) incision and laparoscopy. Ovaries and endometrium remain intact; menstruation continues	Major surgery with possible complications of anesthesia, infection, hemorrhage, and trauma to other organs. Psychologic trauma in some women. Sperm may enter peritoneal cavity if tubal ligature slips, and ectopic (abdominal) pregnancy may ensue	100% effective if ligatures, bands, or clips do not slip or cut through
Hysterectomy with salpingo-oophorectomy; no egg produced	No further menstruation	Abrupt loss of ovarian hormones, simulating menopause. Possibility of major surgical complications. Pyschologic trauma if there is a perceived loss of femininity and sexuality	100% effective
Man			
Vasectomy: vas deferens ligated and severed or banded to interrupt passage of sperm	Relatively simple surgical procedure. Does not affect endocrine production or function of testosterone. Does not alter volume of ejaculate	Possibility of impotence in some men because of psychologic response to procedure. Reversible in many cases. Even if procedure is reversed, many may remain infertile if he has developed an autoimmune response (antibodies) to his sperm	100% effective after ejaculate is free of sperm that was in vas deferens (about 6 weeks or 10 ejaculations)

Table 8-10 *Interruption of Pregnancy: Basis for Counseling*

Methods*	Advantages	Disadvantages and Side Effects	Effectiveness
First-trimester Procedures			
Menstrual extraction: forced endometrial extraction through undilated cervix	Performed up to 14 days after missed period. No legal prescriptions	Cervical trauma may occur, may lead to incompetence. Hemorrhage	100% if implantation site is not missed
Prostaglandin: Intravenous (IV) administration or injection into cul-de-sac of Douglas or by vaginal suppository or pessary	Stimulates smooth muscle. Causes degeneration of corpus luteum	Requires about 24 hours to take effect. May cause vomiting, diarrhea, chills, local tissue reaction. Retained placenta necessitates D & C	100%
Vacuum (suction) curettage: cannula suction after cervical dilation, under local anesthesia	Effective with relatively few complications: minimum bleeding, minimum discomfort. 5-15 minutes duration. Done on out-of-hospital or same-day surgery basis	Pregnancy 12 weeks or less. Possibility of cervical trauma (decreased if dilation accomplished by insertion of laminaria tent 4-24 hours before procedure); endometrial trauma possible. Hazards: possible uterine perforation, hemorrhage, or infection	100% if implantation site is not missed and if other reproductive tract anomaly (double uterus) does not exist
Dilation and curettage (D & C): cervix dilated, endometrium scraped with spoonlike instrument	Duration of 15 minutes. Usually few complications	Pregnancy 12 weeks or less. Hazards: uterine perforation, infection (25%), effects of general anesthesia, cervical trauma	100% if implantation site is not missed

*Prophylaxis against Rh isoimmunization, $Rh_o(D)$ immune globulin, is given within 72 hours to every Rh-negative, Du-negative, unsensitized (Coombs' negative) woman.

Continued.

Table 8-10, cont'd. *Interruption of Pregnancy: Basis for Counseling*

Methods*	Advantages	Disadvantages and Side Effects	Effectiveness
Second-trimester Procedures			
Intraamniotic infusion: between week 14 and 23 or 24 (uterus in abdominal cavity and sufficient amniotic fluid present)	Does not require laparotomy	Increase in complications proportionately with weeks of gestation	Fetal death within 1 hour of injection; abortion completed within 36-40 hours
Transabdominal extraction: amniotic fluid extracted; replaced with equal amount of saline solution (20%) (or 30% urea in 5% dextrose in water)	Ambulation until labor starts (within 24 hours) and during early labor	Reaction to saline solution (hypernatremia): tinnitus, tachycardia, and headache Water intoxication: edema, oliguria ($\leq$200 mg/8 hours), dyspnea, thirst, and restlessness Induced labor, occasionally explosive with an unripe cervix; fetus passes out of posterior vault of vagina and forms fistula Hazards requiring hospitalization (6% readmitted for complications): Hemorrhage and possible D & C May require postabortal D & C or vacuum extraction as well Fever with sepsis	Two thirds of fetuses aborted within 24 hours
Instillation of 40-45 mg prostaglandins $PGF_2\alpha$, E_2	Labor usually shorter than with saline solution Avoid complications of water intoxication and hypernatremia	May cause vomiting, diarrhea, nausea Fetus may be born alive D & C may be required to remove placental fragments	100%
Dilation and evacuation (D & E)	Hospitalization shortened With skilled operator, complication rate lower than with intraamniotic infusion methods	24 hours before procedure, 2 or 3 laminaria tents used to dilate cervix to required 2 cm Fetus possibly born alive	100%
Second- and Third-trimester Procedures			
Hysterotomy: cesarean incision	Preferred method if woman wishes tubal ligation or hysterectomy to follow	Complications after major surgery—hemorrhage and infection Fetus possibly born alive, opening ethical, moral, religious, and legal problems Mortality risk—combination hysterotomy-hysterectomy 10% greater than with D & C	100%
Hysterectomy: at or before 24 weeks without first emptying uterus	As above	As above	100%

*Prophylaxis against Rh isoimmunization, $Rh_0(D)$ immune globulin, is given within 72 hours to every Rh-negative, Du-negative, unsensitized (Coombs' negative) woman.

Summary of Nursing Actions

INTERRUPTION OF PREGNANCY (ELECTIVE ABORTION)

I. Goals
  A. To use the decision-making process to arrive at a solution acceptable to the woman
  B. To prevent adverse physical or psychologic consequences.
II. Priorities
  A. Providing information and support to assist the woman in decision making
  B. Accurate dating of gestation
  C. Identification of risk factors
  D. Appropriate perioperative management
  E. Follow-up physical and psychologic care
III. Assessment
  A. Interview
    1. Health history: risk factors for continuing the pregnancy (health, fetal abnormality, rape, incest), contraceptive failure, last menstrual period
    2. Psychosocial: social problems, financial hardship, inability to give adequate care to a child, interference with educational/vocational goals, no desire to be a parent at this time.
    3. Review of systems: risk factors for continuing pregnancy (cardiac disease), allergies
  B. Physical examination
    1. Risk factors: concurrent infections, medical disease
    2. Determination of duration of gestation by manual palpation of uterus, measurement of height of fundus
  C. Laboratory tests
    1. Pregnancy test
    2. Blood work: HCT, Hgb, Rh, blood type.
IV. Potential nursing diagnoses
  A. Potential for injury
  B. Potential for infection
  C. Pain
  D. Knowledge deficit
  E. Anxiety
  F. Fear
  G. Powerlessness
  H. Body image disturbance
  I. Personal identity disturbance
  J. Self esteem disturbance: situational low self esteem
  K. Altered family processes
  L. Anticipatory grieving
  M. Altered parenting
  N. Ineffective individual coping
  O. Ineffective family coping: compromised
  P. Spiritual distress
  Q. Altered nutrition: less than body requirements
V. Plan/implementation
  A. Support person
    1. Encourages verbalization of feelings.
    2. Provides information about choices available (having the abortion, carrying the pregnancy to term and then either keeping the child or giving him or her up for adoption; information about the abortion procedure).
    3. Involves family members as appropriate for the woman.
  B. Teacher/counselor/advocate
    1. Instructs client regarding what to expect during procedure, for example, sensations, supportive care.
    2. Ensures that the woman and significant other know and understand the following:
      a. Importance of reporting bleeding that lasts longer than 7 to 10 days
      b. Importance of reporting excessive bright red bleeding with clots
      c. Symptoms of infection to report:
        (1) Nausea or vomiting
        (2) Severe uterine cramping
        (3) Temperature about 100° F (37.8° C)
        (4) Foul odor of vaginal discharge
      d. Careful cleaning of perineal area; wipe front to back after each elimination
      e. That douching, tampons, and coitus should be avoided for 4 to 6 weeks or as indicated by physician
      f. That normal menstrual period should begin in 4 to 6 weeks
      g. Importance of follow-up care
      h. Contraceptive method of choice, since pregnancy is possible within 2 to 3 weeks
  C. Technician
    1. Assists with interview, physical examination, and laboratory tests.
    2. Provides preoperative care: vital signs, blood pressure; abdominal, suprapubic, or perineal cleansing; instruction to empty bladder; sedation per order; intravenous infusion per order.
    3. Provides support to the woman and assists physician during procedure. Monitors vital signs, blood pressure, emotional responses.
    4. Provides postoperative care: vital signs, blood pressure, recovery from medications, bleeding, postdelivery care, RhoGAM injections as ordered, discharge instructions.
VI. Evaluation
  A. Woman arrived at her own decision.
  B. Procedure chosen was appropriate for the duration of gestation.
  C. Perioperative care was given per accepted protocol.
  D. Woman suffers no adverse physical consequences.
  E. Woman suffers no adverse psychologic consequences.
  F. Woman implements postoperative instructions regarding her care.
  G. Woman implements the birth control method suitable for her.
  H. Woman keeps follow-up appointment.

VIOLENCE AGAINST WOMEN

Because of the magnitude of the problem of violence against women, maternity and gynecologic nurses cannot ignore this reality of client care. Prevention, effective nursing actions, and long-term counseling provide the focus for care. The nurse must understand the dynamics of violence against women to provide supportive care to the battered woman or the rape victim.

FIVE CATEGORIES OF RAPE*

Blitz rape: victim and assailant are strangers. A woman pulled into an alley is blitz raped.

Confidence rape: deceit is the major characteristic of confidence rape; for example, the date who uses coersion to obtain sex when the partner is a reluctant, unconsenting acquaintance. This kind of rape is common and seldom reported because the woman is afraid of being considered an accomplice to the rape.

Power rape: the man's victims are usually strangers attacked in a blitz rape. By dominating his victim, the man places the woman in the powerless position he experiences and despises. He fantasizes sexual conquest as a demonstration of his strength and potency. He believes that the woman enjoys the experience.

Anger rape: this is a revenge rape. The assailant uses rape symbolically to punish a significant woman in his life. These are impulse rapes characterized by considerable brutality and trauma.

Sadistic rape: sadism usually characterizes all of the sadistic rapist's relationships. They eroticize their aggression. They abuse and torture the woman until they are completely out of control. In a frenzy, he may commit a "lust murder."

*Modified from Niehaus MA: Rape. In Griffith-Kenney J: Contemporary women's health, Menlo Park, Calif, 1986, Addison-Wesley Publishing Co, Inc.

Table 8-11 *Characteristics of Victim and Abuser*

Victim	Abuser
Childhood Influences	
Many raised to be submissive, passive, and dependent	Raised in family where males rein supreme
Likely to accept traditional female role in marriage	As children may have used violence to problem-solve
Accepts female sex-role stereotypes	Accepts "macho" values
Personality Characteristics	
Attributes beating to some personal inadequacy	Feelings of inadequacy, inferiority, and insecurity
Low self-esteem and feelings of worthlessness	Emotionally immature and/or aggressive (Zdanuk, Harris, and Wisian, 1987)
Learned helplessness reduces problem-solving ability	Extremes in behavior and overreacting
Low tolerance for frustration	Low self-esteem with high degree of self-loathing
Easily upset, critical, aloof, and reserved	Intolerance of having masculinity threatened (White, 1985)
Severe stress reactions and psychophysiologic symptoms	Lacks respect for women
Cannot trust anyone	Poor impulse control
Some attempt suicide	Excessive possessiveness and jealousy (Hillard, 1986)
Feeling that punishment is justified if marriage fails	Some use aggressive sexual attacks to punish and enhance own self-esteem
Lifestyle Factors	
Isolated from family and friends	No particular profession, occupation, or socio-economic group
Totally dependent on husband for financial and emotional support	Often has difficulties at work
	Severely restricts freedom and mobility of wife

Table 8-12 *Myths and Facts About Abuse and Battering*

Myth	Fact
Battering occurs in a small percentage of the population.	Physical assault reportedly occurred in 28% of all American homes in 1976 (Strauss et al., 1980).
Battering occurs only in lower-class families.	Although lower class families have a higher incidence of battering (Gelles, 1979), it also occurs in middle and upper income families. Incidence not really known because of tendency of middle and upper income families to hide their battering.
Battered women like to be beaten and deliberately provoke the attack. They are masochistic.	Women are terrified of their assailants and go to great lengths to avoid a confrontation. In some cases the woman may provoke her husband to release tension that, if left unchecked, might lead to a more severe beating and possible death.
Batterers are uneducated men who are unable to cope with the world.	Many batterers are successful professionals, including politicians, ministers, physicians, and lawyers.
Men who batter their wives also beat their children.	Two thirds of wife-batterers do not beat their children.
Battered women were battered children.	This myth holds true in only a few cases. Most battered women report that their husbands were the first person to beat them.
Alcohol and drug abuse causes battering.	Gelles (1976) and Delgaty (1985) proposed that batterers use alcohol as an excuse to batter and shift the blame from themselves to the alcohol.
Once a battered wife, always a battered wife.	Many women who have battering relationships do not marry again. Those who stay in the relationships do so out of fear and financial dependence. Shelters have long waiting lists.
Batterers and battered women cannot change.	Counseling can effectively help resocialize both batterers and battered women.

Rape Trauma Syndrome

Burgess and Holmstrom (1975) described the progressive manifestations of rape trauma syndrome, presented in the following outline:

A. Acute phase: disorganization
1. Impact reactions, with two styles of response: *expressed,* evidenced in behaviors such as crying or restlessness; and *controlled,* reflected in a calm, composed, or subdued affect
2. Somatic reactions: physical discomfort, skeletal muscle tension, gastrointestinal irritability, and genitourinary disturbance (itching or burning on urination)
3. Emotional reactions: fear, humiliation, degradation, and embarrassment; anger, need for revenge, and self-blame; not uncommonly, mood swings

B. Long-term process: reorganization
1. Increased motor activity: changing residence and/or phone number
2. Nightmares
3. Trauma phobia: fear of indoors or outdoors (depending on site of rape), of being alone, of crowds, or of people walking or standing behind the woman; sexual fears

NEOPLASIA

Neoplasia refers to an abnormal body state characterized by the growth of tumors, benign or malignant. The nurse must know about the various types of tumors, the ways they affect the reproductive organs, and the different interventions available.

The emotional impact of the diagnosis of a tumor, particularly a malignant one, is devastating. Nurses can play a significant role in providing physical and emotional comfort and guidance to women and their families.

Breast Disease

The United States has one of the highest rates of breast carcinoma in the world. The specific risk to an American woman of developing a breast carcinoma in her lifetime is 1 in 10. Therefore, when a woman seeks health care after palpating a lump in her breast, she is justifiably anxious and fearful. The nurse must be supportive regardless of whether the diagnosis is benign or malignant. For the woman with malignant breast disease, the nurse serves as teacher, counselor, and support person.

BENIGN BREAST DISEASE

Mammary dysplasia: fibrocystic breast disease or chronic cystic mastitis—the most common benign breast lesion.

Intraductal papilloma: rare, benign condition that develops within the terminal nipple ducts

Lipoma: common benign tumor that resembles a malignant lesion

Fat necrosis: firm, irregularly shaped mass that causes skin retraction and mimics malignancy

Hypertrophy: often mistaken for mammary dysplasia; usually caused by hormone fluctuation of menstrual cycle

Sample Nursing Care Plan

BREAST CANCER

ASSESSMENT	NURSING DIAGNOSIS (ND)/ PLAN(P)/GOAL(G)	RATIONALE IMPLEMENTATION	EVALUATION
Young woman with advanced breast cancer. Woman states she does not remember hitting her breast so she does not know how she got cancer; she is afraid of surgery, mutilation, and having cancer; and she is afraid of dying.	ND: Knowledge deficit related to diagnosis of breast malignancy. P: Provide time to discuss diagnosis; questions, and concerns. G: Mary speaks of disease in more realistic terms.	*To meet woman's information needs, the nurse will:* Assess readiness to learn. Assess information given to her by the physician. Review information from physician. Provide written materials from American Cancer Society pertaining to her diagnosis.	Woman verbalizes understanding of information presented by both nurse and physician.
Woman is afraid to tell family about diagnosis.	ND: Potential ineffective coping (family and individual) related to condition and its management. P: Facilitate problem-solving and communication between woman and family. G: Woman accepts diagnosis, shares it with family, gains support during illness. ND: Anxiety related to insufficient information of available therapies. P: Provide information. G: Woman makes an informed decision.	*To assist the patient with coping mechanisms, the nurse will:* Bring woman's significant other into clinic to speak to physician. Arrange a meeting among a social worker, the patient and her mate. *To assist the patient in anxiety reduction, the nurse will:* Provide time to discuss feelings and to supply information. Review therapies being considered by physician.	Woman begins to accept her diagnosis. Woman and family support each other and draw strength from one another Woman confirms reduced anxiety and satisfaction with role in decision-making.

Sample Nursing Care Plan—cont'd

ASSESSMENT	NURSING DIAGNOSIS (ND)/ PLAN (P)/GOAL (G)	RATIONALE/ IMPLEMENTATION	EVALUATION
Woman is unaware of available therapies for breast cancer. Mastectomy is therapy of choice. Requests information about postoperative care.	ND: Knowledge deficit related to postoperative care. P: Provide needed teaching and time to discuss feelings, concerns. G: Woman relates accurate understanding of information from preoperative teaching.	*To assist woman to meet learning needs, the nurse will:* Discuss upcoming surgery with physician and woman. Arrange for woman to meet with a woman from Reach to Recovery close to her age. Speak with clergyman. Implement guidelines for client teaching, below.	Woman gains some insight into what the surgery is like, and verbalizes feelings.

Guidelines For Client Teaching

DISCHARGE AFTER MASTECTOMY

ASSESSMENT

1. Woman has had a mastectomy.
2. Woman needs instruction on activities postdischarge.

NURSING DIAGNOSES

Knowledge deficit related to discharge activities after mastectomy.

Potential activity intolerance related to postoperative recovery.

Potential for impaired physical mobility related to mastectomy.

Potential self-care deficit; bathing hygiene, dressing/grooming, related to mastectomy.

Pain, related to postoperative healing.

Body image disturbance related to mastectomy.

Potential for ineffective individual/family coping related to diagnosis of surgery and amputation of breast.

Potential altered sexuality patterns related to impaired self-image and mastectomy.

Potential sensory-perceptual alterations (tactile) of affected arm; hot-cold, numbness, pressure, pain, related to mastectomy.

Body image disturbance related to amputation of breast and diagnosis of cancer.

GOALS

Short-term

Woman takes part in self-care activities.

Woman can verbalize feelings about her surgery and her diagnosis.

Woman begins to use prosthesis in brassiere.

Woman continues exercises at home to strengthen and stretch muscles on affected side.

Intermediate

Woman recognizes symptoms that should be reported to the physician that signal problems.

Woman/couple can verbalize feelings together.

Woman begins to accept altered body image.

Woman assumes complete self-care.

Long-term

Woman has positive body image.

Couple resumes sexual contact.

Woman continues monthly breast self-examination.

Woman keeps follow-up appointments with physician.

REFERENCES AND TEACHING AIDS

Books and pamphlets from the American Cancer Society and Reach to Recovery, Inc. that give instructions on exercises, activities of daily living, tips on dressing, etc.

Continued.

Guidelines For Client Teaching—cont'd

CONTENT/RATIONALE	TEACHING ACTIONS
To counsel woman/couple on care at home: Discuss activities of daily living, hygiene. Daily baths or showers are encouraged. Use of talcum powders and deodorant should be avoided until recovery from surgery and radiation is complete and the physician approves.	Use pamphlets and printed instructions, encourage discussion.
To develop strength and maintain joint mobility: Teach postmastectomy exercises, p. 243.	Demonstrate to the woman/couple the exercises that are most beneficial for her recovery. Usually it will be the ones she has already started while in the hospital. Ask for a return demonstration, guiding her through them and telling her to stop when she experiences pain.
To instruct woman on wound care: Provide information on signs and symptoms that should be reported to the physician immediately.	Following physician's discharge orders, demonstrate wound care; write down the instructions for woman to take home. Provide a list of signs and symptoms that she should report to the physician (i.e., fever, redness, pain, swelling, drainage from wound). Tell woman these are signs of infection.
To assist woman with her bra and the prosthesis: Contact physician or Reach to Recovery representative.	Reinforce teaching done by physician and representative from Reach to Recovery.
To prevent injury: Discuss elevation of the arm on the affected side. Instruct woman to tell others not to use the arm for blood work, injections, etc. Caution woman about possible injury to arm as a result of numbness or decrease in sensation.	Show woman with a picture or diagram how her arm should be elevated on pillows for sleep and periodically during the day. Instruct woman to report swelling of the arm immediately.
To facilitate couple's relationship and maintain self-esteem: Discuss resumption of sexual activity according to physician's orders and how woman is feeling.	Encourage couple to verbalize feelings. Do not push this subject if woman/couple appears uncomfortable with it. Review process of and time frame for grieving.
Discuss follow-up care.	Reaffirm woman's return appointment with physician and emphasize importance of follow-up care.
Provide information on community support systems, nurses, housekeepers, Reach to Recovery, Inc.	Discuss this with the couple.

EVALUATION Woman/couple verbalizes understanding of information presented, asks appropriate questions, and keeps follow-up appointments. All goals are reached within time.

POSTMASTECTOMY ARM EXERCISES*

Exercise: Climbing the Wall

1. Stand facing wall with toes close to wall
2. Bend elbows and place palms of hands against wall at shoulder level
3. Move both hands parallel to each other up the wall as far as possible until incisional pull or pain occur
4. Move both hands down to starting position
5. Goal is complete extension with elbow straight
6. Activities that use the same action: reaching top shelves, hanging out clothes, washing windows, hanging curtains, setting hair

Exercise: Arm Swinging

1. Bend forward from waist, permitting both arms to relax and hang naturally
2. Swing arms together left to right (motion comes from shoulder)
3. Swing arms in circles parallel to floor, clockwise and counterclockwise
4. Stand up slowly

Exercise: Rope Pull

1. Attach a rope over a shower rod or hook
2. Grasp each end of rope, alternately pulling on each end, raising affected arm to a point of incisional pull or pain
3. Shorten rope over time until affected arm is raised almost directly overhead

Exercise: Elbow Spread

1. Clasp hands behind neck
2. Raise elbows to chin level, holding head erect; move slowly and rest when incisional pull or pain occur
3. Gradually spread elbows apart; rest when pull or pain occur

*From American Cancer Society: Reach to Recovery, New York, The Society.

Cancer of the Corpus Uteri and Cervix

About one woman in 100 will develop endometrial cancer in her lifetime. When the cancer is diagnosed in its early stages, surgery is the treatment of choice. The woman who is given the diagnosis and a thorough explanation of the proposed surgical procedure in a caring and sensitive manner is likely to experience an uncomplicated recovery.

Cervical carcinoma is the second most common malignancy of the reproductive tract. A thorough health history identifies the woman at increased risk, and Papanicolaou tests detect about 90% of early cervical neoplasia. Information about the Papanicolaou test and the categories of its results is presented in this section. Treatments for noninvasive and invasive conditions are summarized. The section concludes with a summary of nursing actions for the woman with cancer of the reproductive system.

CANCER OF THE CORPUS UTERI

Endometrial carcinoma is third most frequent cancer, behind breast and colorectal malignancies.

Uterine adenocarcinoma originates from epithelial tissues of the endometrium.

Cancer of the corpus uteri affects mature women; peak incidence is between 50 and 64 years of age.

Factors most important for risk are obesity, nulliparity, and menopause after the age of 52.

Incidence in white women is twice the rate for black women.

Cardinal sign is abnormal uterine bleeding.

Cancer of the corpus uteri is diagnosed by histologic examination.

Treatment is total abdominal hysterectomy (TAH) and bilateral salpingo-oopherectomy (BSO).

Papanicolaou Test. For the woman at average risk, a Papanicolaou test is recommended once every 3 years after two initial negative tests 1 year apart (American Cancer Society, 1984). Papanicolaou test results in the past have been recorded in one of five categories. Since some laboratories still use these categories, they are presented here.

Class I	No abnormal cells present
Class II	Atypical cells are identified; inflammation must be ruled out
Class III	Suspicious abnormal cells present
Class IV	Malignant cells present—carcinoma in situ
Class V	Malignant cells present—invasive cancer

Current practice utilizes a descriptive classification. The descriptive terminology is as follows:

Normal
Metaplasia
Inflammation
Minimal atypia—koilocytosis
Mild dysplasia
Moderate dysplasia
Severe dysplasia—carcinoma in situ
Invasive carcinoma

Reexamination is warranted following treatment for infection. Additional diagnostic procedures (e.g., biopsy) are advised as necessary.

Cervical intraepithelial abnormalities range from simple dysplasia to carcinoma in situ. Three categories of cervical intraepithelial neoplasia (CIN) are recognized (Cashavelly, 1987):

CIN I	Mild dysplasia
CIN II	Moderate dysplasia
CIN III	Severe dysplasia, and carcinoma in situ

TREATMENTS FOR PREINVASIVE CANCER

Cryosurgery is an outpatient or physician's office procedure. It is scheduled within 1 week after cessation of last menstrual period and requires no anesthesia or analgesia. The preferred refrigerant is nitrous oxide. Frozen tissue becomes necrotic and sloughs off in a few days.

Laser surgery: may replace cryosurgery. Carbon dioxide (CO_2) laser is currently used. Epithelial regrowth begins by 3 days. Healing is complete by 6 weeks. For treatment of cervix (relatively insensitive tissue), the woman may need no anesthesia. Some clients complain of a burning or cramping sensation that is tolerable. Two disadvantages are that (1) for tissue other than the cervix, it is too painful to be performed without analgesia or anesthesia; and (2) it takes longer.

Cervical conization is an incision made to include all the abnormal and some normal surrounding tissue. Complications are rare.

TREATMENT FOR INVASIVE CANCER

Radiotherapy may be delivered by radium applications followed by external radiation therapy.

Radical hysterectomy is necessary when radiation is contraindicated or cancer is spread throughout the pelvic organs.

Chemotherapy usually follows surgery. Alkylating, antineoplastic, or nonspecific immunostimulant agents may be used.

Radical vulvectomy and lymphadenectomy are surgical excision of the vulva and dissection of lymph nodes. Preoperative and postoperative teaching and counselling are very important.

Pelvic exenteration is surgical excision of all reproductive organs and adjacent tissues. It includes radical hysterectomy, pelvic node dissection, cystectomy with formation of ileal conduit, vaginectomy, and rectal resection with colostomy. Preoperative and postoperative teaching is of utmost importance. Teaching should include visits by an enterostomal therapist.

Summary of Nursing Actions

CANCER OF FEMALE REPRODUCTIVE ORGANS

I. Goals
  A. For the woman: assistance in accepting the diagnosis, understanding the treatment modalities available, and making informed decisions
  B. For the family: education and counseling so they may provide support to the client
II. Priorities
  A. Identify and treat primary cancer promptly
  B. Identify and treat metastatic lesions
  C. Assess woman's physical and psychologic condition
  D. Help woman and family to become active participants in her care
  E. Prevent secondary problems
  F. Support family coping
III. Assessment
  A. Interview
    1. Family history, predisposing factors, population at risk
    2. Time in childbearing (age, gravidity, parity)
    3. Events preceding symptomatology
    4. Confirmation of diagnosis
    5. Counselling or teaching needed regarding diagnosis
  B. Physical examination
    1. Signs and symptoms of disease
    2. General affect: anxious, upset, uncomfortable, accepting
    3. Vital signs and blood pressure
    4. Existing discomfort: pain, tenderness, bleeding
  C. Laboratory tests
    1. Hemoglobin and hematocrit values

2. Type and Rh factor; cross-match for possible transfusion
3. Urinalysis
4. CBC, WBC, platelets
5. Chest radiograph
6. Any other tests deemed necessary by physician for woman's particular problem, diagnosis, and treatment
IV. Potential nursing diagnosis
  A. Anxiety
  B. Fear
  C. Activity intolerance
  D. Pain
  E. Ineffective family coping: compromised or disabling
  F. Ineffective denial
  G. Defensive coping
  H. Ineffective individual coping
  I. Altered family processes
  J. Fatigue
  K. Potential fluid volume deficit
  L. Anticipatory grieving
  M. Altered health maintenance
  N. Impaired home maintenance management
  O. Hopelessness
  P. Potential for infection
  Q. Potential for injury
  R. Knowledge deficit
  S. Impaired physical mobility
  T. Noncompliance
  U. Altered nutrition: less than body requirements
  V. Parental role conflict

Summary of Nursing Actions—cont'd

W. Potential altered parenting

X. Powerlessness

Y. Altered role performance

Z. Bathing/hygiene self care deficit

AA. Dressing/grooming self care deficit

BB. Feeding self care deficit

CC. Toileting self care deficit

DD. Body image disturbance

EE. Personal identity disturbance

FF. Self esteem disturbance: situational low self esteem

GG. Sexual dysfunction

HH. Altered sexuality patterns

II. Potential impaired skin integrity

JJ. Sleep pattern disturbance

KK. Impaired social interaction

LL. Social isolation

MM. Spiritual distress

NN. Impaired tissue integrity

OO. Altered patterns of urinary elimination

V. Plan/implementation

  A. Technician

    1. Obtain specimen collection, e.g., blood, urine, etc.

    2. Administer medications as ordered.

    3. Start and maintain IV infusions as ordered.

    4. Monitor vital signs, blood pressure, total parenteral nutrition (TPN), level of consciousness (LOC), integument.

    5. Insert retention urinary catheter as ordered.

    6. Provide preoperative and postoperative care as needed.

    7. Hang appropriate blood products when ordered.

    8. Record and report findings promptly.

    9. Monitor chemotherapy as ordered.

    10. If woman to be treated at home, assist with planning.

  B. Support person

    1. Implement care for woman and family.

    2. Give woman and family opportunity to express feelings.

    3. Explain procedures, sensations; answer questions.

    4. Assist woman and family with emotions, anger, acceptance.

    5. Involve family with planning and care.

    6. Provide time for client and family or spouse to be alone.

  C. Teacher/counselor/advocate

    1. Explain all procedures.

    2. Assist client and family in understanding physician's instructions and treatment modalities.

    3. Counsel client regarding disease management.

    4. Refer for social service, support groups, home health care, and homemaker services as appropriate.

    5. Teach woman about signs and symptoms of side effects to drugs, radiation therapy, chemotherapy.

    6. Provide proper environment for rest.

    7. Provide nutritional services for proper diet.

    8. Counsel woman and family about importance of follow-up care.

    9. Reinforce physician's explanations.

    10. Support woman and family in regard to results of tests.

    11. Teach infection prevention.

    12. Provide instruction for use of prosthesis or refer to appropriate service.

VI. Evaluation

  A. Condition is identified promptly, and appropriate therapy is instituted.

  B. Vital signs, blood pressure, nutrition, intake, and output remain within normal limits.

  C. Woman and family come to terms with disease in a positive manner.

  D. Woman and family verbalize understanding of condition, treatment, and prognosis.

    1. Self-concept remains intact.

    2. Spiritual distress is averted.

    3. Sense of power remains intact; she participates in decision-making and in self-care.

  E. Surgical intervention is successful, with no adverse iatrogenic sequelae or nosocomial infections.

  F. Radiotherapy is successful, with minimal adverse reactions.

  G. Chemotherapy is successful, with minimal adverse reactions.

  H. Knowledge needs are met.

  I. Complications are averted.

References

American Cancer Society: Cancer facts and figures, New York, 1984.

Berkley SF et al: The relationship of tampon characteristics to menstrual toxic shock syndrome, JAMA 258(7):908, 1987.

Burgess AW and Holmstrom LL: Crisis and counselling requests of rape victims, Nurs Res 23:196, 1974.

Cashavelly BJ: Cervical dysplasia: an overview of current concepts in epidemiology, diagnosis, and treatments, Cancer Nurs 10(4):199, 1987.

Centers for Disease Control: Toxic shock syndrome, Center for Prevention Services, CDC, Atlanta, 1982.

Delgaty K: Battered women: the issues for nursing, NAACOG Newsletter 12(10):9, 1985.

Friedland, GH and Klein RS: Transmission of the human immunodeficiency virus, 317(18):1125, 1987.

Bibliography

Droegemueller W et al: Comprehensive gynecology, St Louis, 1987, The CV Mosby Co.

Fogel DI and Woods NF: Health care of women: a nursing perspective, St. Louis, 1981, The CV Mosby Co.

Gelles RJ: Abused wives: why do they stay? J Marraige Fam Nov 1976.

Hecht F: Counseling the HIV-positive woman regarding pregnancy, JAMA 257(24)3361, 1987.

Klug RM: AIDS beyond the hospital: children with AIDS, Am J Nurs 86(10):1126, 1986.

Hillard PJ: Physical abuse and pregnancy, Fam Prac Recertification 8(9):89, 1986.

Landesman S et al: Serosurvey of human immunodeficiency virus infection in parturients, JAMA 258(19):2701, 1987.

Shaw NS: Serving your patients in the age of AIDS, Contemp OB/GYN 28(4):141, 1986.

Strauss MA et al: Behind closed doors: Violence in the American family, Garden City, NY, 1980, Anchor Books.

White EC: Chain, chain, change: for black women dealing with emotional abuse, Seattle, 1985, The Seal Press New Leaf Series.

Willson JR et al: Obstetrics and gynecology, ed 8, St. Louis, 1987, The CV Mosby Co.

Wolf PH et al: Toxic shock syndrome, JAMA 258(7):908, 1987.

Zdanyk JM, Harris CC, and Wisian NL: Adolescent pregnancy and incest: the nurse's role as counselor, JOGN Nurs 16(2):99, 1987.

APPENDICES

APPENDIX

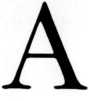

A

Oxytocin Administration Using a Volumetric Infusion Pump

Milliliters per Hour (ml/hr)	Dilution of Oxytocin in IV Fluid (mU min)		
	5 U Oxytocin in 1000 ml Fluid	10 U Oxytocin in 1000 ml Fluid	20 U Oxytocin in 1000 ml Fluid
1.5	0.125	0.25	0.5
3	0.25	0.5	1
6	0.5	1.0	2
9	0.75	1.5	3
12	1.0	2.0	4
15	1.25	2.5	5
18	1.5	3.0	6
21	1.75	3.5	7
24	2.0	4.0	8
27	2.25	4.5	9
30	2.50	5.0	10
33	2.75	5.5	11
36	3.0	6.0	12
39	3.25	6.5	13
42	3.5	7.0	14
45	3.75	7.5	15
48	4.0	8.0	16
51	4.25	8.5	17
54	4.5	9.0	18
57	4.75	9.5	19

Milliliters per Hour (ml/hr)	Dilution of Oxytocin in IV Fluid (mU min)		
	5 U Oxytocin in 1000 ml Fluid	10 U Oxytocin in 1000 ml Fluid	20 U Oxytocin in 1000 ml Fluid
60	5.0	10.0	20
63	5.25	10.5	21
66	5.5	11.0	22
69	5.75	11.5	23
72	6.0	12.0	24
75	6.25	12.5	25
78	6.5	13.0	
81	6.75	13.5	
84	7.0	14.0	
87	7.25	14.5	
90	7.5	15.0	
93	7.75	15.5	
96	8.0	16.0	
99	8.25	16.5	
102	8.5	17.0	
105	8.75	17.5	
108	9.0	18.0	
112	9.25	18.5	
115	9.50	19.0	
118	9.75	19.5	
119	10.0	20.0	

APPENDIX B

Conversion Tables and Equivalents

Conversion of Inches to Centimeters

Inches	Centimeters	Inches	Centimeters
¼	0.635	14½	36.83
½	1.27	15	38.10
1	2.54	15½	39.37
2	5.08	16	40.64
3	7.62	16½	41.91
4	10.16	17	43.18
5	12.70	16½	44.45
6	15.24	18	45.72
7	17.78	18½	46.99
8	20.32	19	48.26
9	22.86	19½	49.53
10	25.40	20	50.80
10½	26.67	20½	52.07
11	27.94	21	53.34
11½	29.21	21½	54.61
12	30.48	22	55.88
12½	31.75	22½	57.15
13	33.02	23	58.42
13½	34.29	23½	56.69
14	35.56	24	60.96

To convert centimeters to inches

Divide the length in centimeters by 2.54.

Example: The average newborn infant measures 50.8 cm;

$$\frac{50.8}{2.54} = 20 \text{ in}$$

To convert inches to centimeters:

Multiply the length in inches by 2.54

Example: The average newborn infant measures 20 in: 20 × 2.54 = 50.8 cm

Approximate Weight Equivalents

Apothecary	Metric
1/600 grain	0.1 mg
1/300 grain *or* 1/320 grain*	0.2 mg
1/200 grain *or* 1/210 grain	0.3 mg
1/160 grain	0.4 mg
1/120 grain	0.5 mg
1/100 grain	0.6 mg *or* 0.65 mg
1/60 grain *or* 1/64 grain	1.0 mg
1/32 grain	2.0 mg
1/20 grain	3.0 mg
1/16 grain	4.0 mg
1/12 grain	5.4 mg
1/10 grain	6.4 *or* 6.0 mg
1/8 grain	8.0 mg
1/6 grain	11.0 mg
1/4 grain	16.0 *or* 15.0 mg
1/3 grain	22.0 *or* 20.0 mg
3/8 grain	24.0 mg
1/2 grain	32.0 *or* 30.0 mg
3/4 grain	50.0 mg
1 grain	64.0 *or* 60.0 mg
1 ½ grains	0.1 g (100 mg)
2 grains	0.128 *or* 0.12 g
2 ½ grains	0.16 *or* 15.0 g
3 grains	0.2 g
4 grains	0.25 g
5 grains	0.32 g
7 ½ grains	0.5 g
10 grains	0.64 *or* 0.6 g
15 grains	1.0 g
1 dram	4.0 g
1 ounce	30.0 g

*Discrepancy occurs because 1 grain = 60 mg, or 1 grain = 64 mg, depending on the source.

Avoirdupois and Imperial Systems

Weight

1 pound (lb) = 16 ounces (oz)

1 oz = 437.5 grains

Height

1 yard (yd) = 3 feet (ft)

1 foot (ft) = 12 inches (in)

Capacity

1 gallon (gal) = 4 quarts (qt) = 8 pints (pt)

1 qt = 2 pt

1 pt = 16 fluid ounces (fl oz)

1 fl oz = 8 drams (or drachm)

1 dram = 60 minims

Fluid Volume

Useful approximate metric and imperial equivalents

1 L = 1.75 pt

1 oz = 30 ml

1 pt = 0.568 L, or 568 ml

1 gal = 4.55 L

Measurements

Domestic	Apothecary	Metric
1 teaspoon	1 dram	4 ml
1 tablespoon	½ fl oz	15 ml
1 teacup	4 oz	120 ml
1 tumbler	8 oz	240 ml

Calculations of Dosages for Infants and Children

Fried's rule:

$$\frac{\text{age in months} \times \text{adult dose}}{150} = \text{Approximate dose for infants}$$

up to 2 years of age

APPENDIX

C

Standard Laboratory Values in the Neonatal Period

1. Hematologic values

		Neonatal
Clotting factors		
Activated clotting time (ACT)		2 min
Bleeding time (Ivy)		2 min
Clot retraction		1-8 min
Clotting time		Complete 1-4 hr
2 tubes		5-8 min
3 tubes		5-15 min
Fibrinogen		150-300 mg/dl*
Fibrinolysin (plasminogen)		Lysis of clot
Partial thromboplastin (PTT)		<90-120 sec
Prothrombin time, one-stage (PT)		12-21 sec
Thromboplastin generation test (TGT)		8-24 sec in 6 min tube

	Term	Preterm
Hemoglobin (g/dl)	17-19	15-17
Hematocrit (%)	57-58	45-55
Sedimentation rate, erythrocytes (ESR) min/hr	0-2	1-5
Reticulocytes (%)	3-7	Up to 10
Fetal hemoglobin (% of total)	40-70	80-90
Nucleated RBC/mm^3 (per 100 RBC)	200(0.05)	(0.2)
Platelet count/mm^3	100,000-300,000	120,000-180,000
WBC/mm^3	15,000	10,000-20,000
Neutrophils (%)	45	47
Eosinophils and basophils (%)	3	
Lymphocytes (%)	30	33
Monocytes (%)	5	4
Immature WBC (%)	10	16

---

1 to *6* from Pierog SH and Ferrara A: Medical care of the sick newborn, ed 2, St. Louis, 1976, The CV Mosby Co. *7* from Bobak IM, Jensen MD, and Zalar MK: Maternity and gynecologic care, ed 4, St. Louis, 1989, The CV Mosby Co.
*dl refers to deciliter (1 dl = 100 ml); this conforms to the SI system: international measurements that have been standardized.

Continued.

2. Biochemical values

		Neonatal
Ammonia		100-150 μg/dl
Amylase		0-1000 IU/hr
Antistreptolysin O titer, group B		
Normal		12-100 Todd units
Recent streptococcal infection		200-2500 Todd units
Bilirubin, direct		0-1 mg/dl
Bilirubin, total	Cord:	<2 mg/dl
	Peripheral blood: 0-1 day	6 mg/dl
	1-2 day	8 mg/dl
	3-5 day	12 mg/dl
Blood gases	Arterial:	pH 7.31-7.45
		P_{CO_2} 33-48 mm Hg
		P_{O_2} 50-70 mm Hg
	Venous:	pH 7.28-7.42
		P_{CO_2} 38-52 mm Hg
		P_{O_2} 20-49 mm Hg
Calcium, ionized		
Calcium, total		
Catecholamines (μg/24 hr)		
Neonatal: norepinephrine, 2-12; epinephrine, 1-2		
Newborn: Norepinephrine, 2-4; epinephrine, 0-1		2.1-2.6 mEq/L
		4-7.0 mEq/L
Ceruplasmin (*p*-phenylenediamine dihydrochloride, 37 C)		
Chloride		
Cholesterol, esters		
Cholesterol, total		
Copper		1-30 mg/dl
Cortisol		95-110 mEq/L
		42% to 71% of total
		45-170 mg/dl
		20-70 μg/dl
AM specimen		15-25 μg/dl
PM specimen		5-10 μg/dl
C-reactive protein (CRP)		0
Creatine		
Creatine phosphokinase (CPK) (creatine phosphate, 30 C)		
Creatinine		0.2-1 mg/dl (higher in females)
Electrophoresis, total protein		10-300 IU/L
		0.3-1 mg/dl
		Preterm: 4.3-7.6 g/dl
		Newborn: 4.6-7.4 g/dl
Preterm: albumin, 3.1-4.2; α₁-globulin, 0.1-0.5; α₂-globulin, 0.3-0.7; β-globulin, 0.3-1.2; γ-globulin, 0.3-1.4		
Newborn: albumin, 3.6-5.4; α₁-globulin, 0.1-0.3; α₂-globulin, 0.2-0.5; β-globulin, 0.2-0.6; γ-globulin, 0.2-1.2		
Fatty acids, free		0.4-1 mg/L
α₁-fetoprotein		0
Fibrinogen		150-300 mg/dl
Glucose, fasting (FBS)		
Hepatitis-associated (Australia) antigen		
Immunoglobulin levels, serum, newborn		
IgG 645-1.244		
IgM 5-30		
IgA 0-11		0
		660-1.439 mg/dl

Iodine, butanol extractable (BEI)
Iodine, T_4-by-column (thyroxine)
Iodine, T_4 (competitive protein-binding thyroxine)
Iodine, total serum organic (PBI)
Iron
Iron-binding capacity (IBC)
17-Ketogenic steroids (17-KGS)
17-Ketosteroids (17-KS)
Lactic dehydrogenase (LDH) (pyruvate, 30 C)
Lipids, total   3-13 µg/dl
Lipoproteins, newborn (mg/dl)   3-12 µg/dl
   Alpha 70-180   3-12 µg/dl
   Beta 50-160   4-14 µg/dl
   Chylo 50-110   100-200 µg/dl
                                                                     60-175 µg/dl
                                                                     2.4 mg/24 hr
                                                                     0.5-2.5 mg/24 hr
                                                                     300-1500 IU/L
                                                                     170-450 mg/dl

Magnesium
Malate dehydrogenase (MDH) (oxaloacetic acid, 37 C)
Phosphatase, acid
Phosphatase, alkaline
Phospholipids
Phosphorus
Potassium   1.4-2.9 mEq/L
Pregnanediol   41-68 IU/L
Protein, total   10.4-16.4 IU/L
Sodium   50-275 IU/L
Transaminases, serum   75-170 mg/dl
                                                                     3.5-8.6 mg/dl
                                                                     4-7 mg/L
                                                                     0 mg/24 hr
                                                                     4.3-7.6 g/dl
                                                                     140-160 mEq/L

   Glutamic-oxaloacetic (SGOT) (aspartate, 30 C)
   Glutamic-pyruvic (SGPT)
Triglycerides   5-70 IU/L
Urea nitrogen (BUN)   5-50 IU/L
Vanillylmandelic acid (VMA)   5-40 mg/dl
                                                                     5-15 mg/dl
                                                                     0-1 mg/24 hr

3. Urinalysis

Volume: 20-40 ml excreted daily in the first few days; by 1 week, 24 hr urine volume close to 200 ml
Protein: may be present in first 2-4 days
Casts and WBCs: may be present in first 2-4 days
Osmolarity (mOsm/L): 100-600
pH: 5-7
Specific gravity: 1.001-1.020

4. Cerebrospinal fluid

Calcium   2-3 mg/L
Cell count   WBCs/mm^3 0-15
                                                                     RBCs/mm^3 0-500

Continued.

Chloride
Color
Glucose
Lactate
dehydrogenase (LDH)
Magnesium
Pándy's test (for excess globulins)
pH (at 37° C)
Pressure
Protein, total
Sodium
Specific gravity
Transaminase, glutamic-oxaloacetic (GOT)
Volume

110-120 mg/L
May be xanthochromic
24-40 mg/dl
5-80 IU/L
3-3.3 mg/dl
Negative
7.33-7.42
50-80 mm Hg
20-120 mg/dl
130-165 mg/L
1.007-1.009
2-10 IU/L
5 ml

5. Cardiorespiratory determinations

Blood pressure at birth
   Term: systolic, 78 mm Hg; diastolic, 42 mm Hg
   Preterm: systolic, 50-60 mm Hg; diastolic 30 mm Hg
Respiratory rate: 30-60 min
Heart rate, fetus
   Baseline: 120-160/min
      Tachycardia: >160 beats/min (with maternal complications)
      Bradycardia: <120 beats/min (with maternal hypotension and hypoxia)
      Acceleration: tachycardia > 160 beats/min with uterine contraction—normal (usually)
   Beat-to-beat variability: disappears with fetal distress
   With uterine contraction
      Early deceleration: bradycardia with onset of contraction—benign
      Variable deceleration: bradycardia due to cord compression—usually benign
      Late deceleration: bradycardia after lag period due to fetal hypoxia—ominous sign
Heart rate, term infant: 140 ± 20 beats/min

6. Urine screening tests for inborn errors of metabolism

Benedict's test: for reducing substances in the urine—glucose, galactose, fructose, lactose; phenylketonuria, alkaptonuria, tyrosyluria, and tryosinosis may give positive Benedict's test.

Ferric chloride test: an immediate, green color for phenylketonuria, histidinemia, and tyrosinuria, a gray to green color for presence of phenothiazines, isoniazid, red to purple color for presence of salicylates or ketone bodies.

Dinitrophenylhydrazine test: for phenylketonuria, maple syrup urine disease, Lowe's syndrome.

Cetyltrimethyl ammonium bromide test: for mucopolysaccharides: immediate positive reaction in gargoylism (Hurler's syndrome); delayed, moderately positive reaction for Marfan's, Morquio-Ullrich, and Murdoch syndromes.

Metachromatic stain (or *urine sediment*): Granules: (free or as inclusion bodies in cells) are seen in metachromatic leukodystrophy; may also be seen rarely in Tay-Sachs and other lipid diseases of the central nervous system.

Amino acid chromatography: Aminoaciduria may be normal in newborns; chromatography may be helpful to detect hypophosphatasia and argininosuccinicaciduria.

Diaper test, Phenistix test, and *Dinitrophenyl-hydrazine (DNPH) test:* simple, inexpensive tests for PKU (phenylketonuria); used for screening; most useful when infant is at least 6 weeks of age.

7. Blood serum phenylalanine tests

Guthrie inhibition assay methods: drops of blood placed on filter paper; laboratory uses bacterial growth inhibition test; phenylalanine level above 8 mg/dl blood: diagnostic of PKU. Effective in newborn period; used also to monitor PKU diet; blood easily obtained by heel or finger puncture; inexpensive; used for wide-scale screening

APPENDIX

D

Relationship of Drugs to Breast Milk and Effect on Infant

Drug	Excreted in Milk	Amount in Milk After Therapeutic Dose	Effect on Infant
Analgesics and antiinflammatory drugs (nonnarcotic)			
Acetaminophen (Datril, Tylenol)	Yes		Detoxified in liver. Avoid in immediate postdelivery period, otherwise no problems with therapeutic dose.
Aspirin	Yes	1-3 mg/dl*	Long history of experience shows complications rare. Can cause interference with platelet aggregation and diminished factor XII (Hageman factor) at birth. When mother requires high, continuing level of medication for arthritis, aspirin is drug of choice. Observe infant for bruisability. Platelet aggregation can be evaluated. Salicylism only seen in maternal overdosing. Mother should increase vitamin C and vitamin K intake.
Donnatal (phenobarbital, hyoscyamine sulfate, atropine sulfate, hyoscine hydrobromide)	Yes		Consider for its component parts. Can be given to children but can accumulate in neonate.
Flufenamic acid (Arlef)	Yes	0.50 μg/ml (mean)†	No apparent effect on infant when maternal dosage was 200 mg, three times a day. Infant able to excrete via urine.
Indomethacin (Indocin)	Yes		Convulsions in breast-fed neonate (case report). Used to close patent ductus arteriosus. Insufficient data as to effect on other vessels. May be nephrotoxic.
Mefenamic acid (Ponstel)	Yes	Trace amounts‡	No apparent effect on infant at therapeutic doses; infant able to excrete via urine.
Naproxen (Naproxyn, synaxyns, naprosine, naxen, proxen)	Yes	1% of maternal plasma; binds to plasma protein	Less toxic in adults than some other organic derivatives.

Modified from Lawrence RA: Breastfeeding: a guide for the medical profession, ed 2, St Louis, 1985, The CV Mosby Co.

*Plasma level was 1-5 mg/dl.

†Shown when mean maternal plasma level was 6.41 μg/ml. Mean level in infant's plasma was 0.12 μg/ml; In infant's urine, 0.08 μg/ml. (Maternal plasma level was 50 times that of infant).

‡0.91 μg/ml mean maternal plasma level showed 0.21 μg/ml mean milk level. Mean infant plasma level was 0.08 μg/ml and mean urine level, 9.8 μg/ml.

Continued.

Drug	Excreted in Milk	Amount in Milk After Therapeutic Dose	Effect on Infant
Oxyphenbutazone (Tandearil)	Yes	In milk of 2 of 55 mothers, 10% to 80% of maternal plasma level	No known effect.
Pentazocine (Talwin)	No		Withdrawal in neonatal period from ingestion during pregnancy.
Phenylbutazone (Butazolidin)	Yes	0.63 mg ml 90 min after 750 mg given IM	Very potent drug; risk to infant not well defined but considerable. Not given directly to children; may accumulate in infant.
Propoxyphene (Darvon)	Yes	0.4% of maternal* dose	Only symptoms detectable would be failure to feed and drowsiness. On daily, around-the-clock dosage, infant could consume 1 mg/day.

Antibiotics

Drug	Excreted in Milk	Amount in Milk After Therapeutic Dose	Effect on Infant
Amantadine (Symmetrel)	Yes	Not defined	Vomiting, urinary retention, rash. Contraindicated.
Ampicillin (Polycillin, Amcill, Omnipen, Penbritin)	Yes	0.07 μg/ml	Sensitivity due to repeated exposure; diarrhea or secondary candidiasis.
Carbenicillin (Pyopen, Geopen)	Yes	0.265 μg/ml 1 hr after 1 g given	Levels not significant. Drug is given to neonate.
Cefazolin (Ancef, Kefzol)	Yes	1.5 μg/ml (0.075% of dose)	Probably not significant.
Cephalexin (Keflex)	No		
Cephalothin (Keflin)	No		
Chloramphenicol (Chloromycetin)	Yes	Half blood level; 2.5 mg/dl	Gray syndrome. Infant does not excrete drug well, and small amounts may accumulate. Contraindicated. May be tolerated in older infant with mature glycuronide system.
Chloroquine (Aralen)	Yes	2.7 mg in 2 days†	Can be used to *treat* child under 6 months of age who is wholly breast fed.
Colistin (Colymycin)	Yes	0.05-0.09 mg/dl	Not absorbed orally.
Demeclocycline (Declomycin)	Yes	0.2-0.3 mg/dl	Not significant in therapeutic doses. Can be given to infants.
Erythromycin (Ilosone, E-Mycin, Erythrocin)	Yes	0.05-0.1 mg/dl; 3.6-6.2 μg/ml	Higher concentrations have been reported in milk than in plasma. Should not be given under 1 month of age because of risk of jaundice. Dose in milk higher when given IV to mother.
Gentamicin	Unknown		Not absorbed from gastrointestinal tract, may change gut flora. Drug is given to newborns directly.
Isoniazid (Nydrazid)	Yes	0.6-1.2 mg/dl‡	Infant as risk for toxicity, but need for breast milk may outweigh risk.
Kanamycin (Kantrex)	Yes	18.4 μg/ml after 1 g given IM	Infant absorbs little from gastrointestinal tract. Infants can be given drug.
Lincomycin (Lincocin)	Yes	0.5-2.4 mg/dl	Not significant in therapeutic doses to affect child.
Mandelic acid	Yes	0.3 g/24 hr after dose of 12 g/day	Not significant in therapeutic doses to affect child.
Methacycline (Rondomycin)	Yes	½ plasma level; 50-260 μg/dl	Same precautions as with tetracycline.
Methenamine (Hexamine)	Yes		Not significant in therapeutic doses to affect child.
Metronidazole (Flagyl)	Yes	Level comparable to serums§	Caution should be exercised because of its high milk concentrations. Contraindicated when infant under 6 months may cause neurologic disorders and blood dyscrasia.
Nalidixic acid (Neggram)	Yes	0.4 mg/dl	Not significant in therapeutic doses beyond neonatal period. Hemolytic anemia in an infant attributed to nalidixic acid in G6PD deficiency or when mother has renal failure.

*Shown by animal experiments. Milk plasma ratio (M/P) = ½.
†Peaks in 6 hr.
‡Same concentration in milk as in maternal serum.
§Gives serum levels in infants of 0.05 to 0.4 μg/ml.

Drug	Excreted in Milk	Amount in Milk After Therapeutic Dose	Effect on Infant
Nitrofurantoin (Furadantin)	Yes	Trace to 0.5 µg/ml	Not significant in therapeutic doses to affect child except in G6PD deficiency.
Novobiocin (Albamycin, cathomycin)	Yes	0.36-0.54 mg/dl	Infant can be given drug directly.
Nystatin (Mycostatin)	No	Not absorbed orally	Can be given to infant directly
Oxacillin (Prostaphlin)	No		
Para-aminosalicylic acid	No		
Penethamate (Leocillin)	No	27-74 µg/dl	Animal study suggests it be avoided
Penicillin G, benzathine (Bicillin)	Yes	10-12 units/dl	Clinical need should supersede possible allergic responses.
Penicillin G, potassium	Yes	Up to 6 units/dl; 1.2-3.6 µg/dl	Infant can be given penicillin directly. Parents should be told to inform physician that infant has been exposed to penicillin because of potential sensitivity.
Pyrimethamine (Daraprim)	Yes	0.3 mg/dl (3% of dose)	Significant in therapeutic doses when infant under 6 months and entirely breast-fed.
Quinine sulfate	Yes	0-0.1 mg/dl after maternal dose of 300-600 mg	In therapeutic doses, no effect on child except rare thrombocytopenia.
Sodium fusidate	Yes	0.2 µg/ml	Not significant in therapeutic doses to affect child.
Streptomycin	Yes	Present for long periods in slight amounts when given as dihydrostreptomycin	Not to be given more than 2 weeks. Ototoxic and nephrotoxic with long use. Is given to infants directly.
Sulfanilamide	Yes	9 mg/dl after dose of 2-4 g/24 hr	Not significant in therapeutic doses; may cause a rash or hemolytic anemia. Should be avoided for first month after delivery.
Sulfapyridine	Yes	3-13 mg/dl after dose of 3 g/24 hr	To be avoided; has caused skin rash.
Sulfathiazole	Yes	0.5 mg/dl after dose of 3 g/24 hr	Not significant in therapeutic doses to affect child after 1 month of age.
Sulfisoxazole (Gantrisin)	Yes	Concentration similar to plasma level	To be avoided during first month after delivery; may cause kernicterus.
Tetracycline HC1 (Achromycin, Panmycin, Sumycin)	Yes	0.5-2.6 µg/ml after dose of 500 mg four times a day	Not enough to treat an infection in an infant. May cause discoloration of the teeth in the infant; the antibiotic, however, may be largely bound to the milk calcium. Do not give longer than 10 days or repeatedly.
Anticoagulants			
Coumarin derivatives Dicumarol (bishydroxycoumarin) Warfarin (Panwarfin)	Yes	Probably little but may be cumulative*	Monitor prothrombin time. Give vitamin K to infant. Discontinue if surgery or trauma occurs. Drug of choice if mother to continue nursing.
Ethyl biscoumacetate (Tromexan)	Yes	0-0.17 mg/dl†	Hemorrhage around umbilical stump and cephalhematoma reported Prothrombin normal in infants with hemorrhage. Vitamin K has no effect. Contraindicated while nursing.
Heparin	No		Heparin ineffective orally.
Phenindione (Hedulin)(Dindevan)	Yes		Breast milk a major route of excretion. Reports of serious hemorrhage in infant. Prothrombin times prolonged in infant. Contraindicated while nursing.
Anticonvulsants and sedatives‡			
Barbital (Veronal)	Yes	8-10 mg/L after 500 mg dose	May produce sedation in infant, in general, barbiturates pass into milk but do not sedate infant. Watch for symptoms.
Carbamazepine (Tegretol)	Yes	60% of plasma levels‖	Animal studies show lack of weight gain, unkempt appearance.

*Reports conflict.
†No correlation with disage, continues in milk after plasma clear.
‡All barbitals appear in breast milk.
‖When plasma 13.0 µmole/L, 7.5 µmole/L in milk.

Continued.

Drug	Excreted in Milk	Amount in Milk After Therapeutic Dose	Effect on Infant
Chloral hydrate (Noctec, Somnos)	Yes	Up to 1.5 mg/dl	No significant symptoms, can be given to infants directly.
Phenytoin (Dilantin)	Yes	1.5 to 2.6 μg/ml after 300 mg/24 hr dose	One case of hemolytic reaction reported. Other infants appear to tolerate the small doses. Therapeutic plasma level 10-20 μg/ml.
Mephenytoin (Mesantoin)(hydantoin homologue of mephobarbital)	Unknown		Detoxified in liver. No information.
Pentobarbital (Nembutal)	Yes		Depends on liver for detoxification so may accumulate in first week of life until infant is able to detoxify. No problem for older infant in usual doses.
Phenobarbital (Luminal)	Yes	0.1-0.5 mg when plasma level 0.6-1.8 mg	Sleepiness and decreased sucking possible. On usual analeptic doses infants alert and feed well. On hypnotic doses infants depressed and difficult to rouse.
Phensuximide (Milontin)			No specific data.
Primidone (Mysoline)	Yes		Causes drowsiness and decreased feeds. May cause bleeding due to hypoprothrombinemia. Infant needs vitamin K. Avoid drug during lactation.
Sodium bromide (Bromo-Seltzer and across-the-counter sleeping aids)	Yes	Up to 6.6 mg/dl	Drowsy, decreased crying, rash, decreased feeding.
Trimethadione (Tridione)			No specific data.
Antihistaminics Brompheniramine (Dimetane) Diphenhydramine (Benadryl) Methdialzine (Tacaryl) Tripelennamine (Pyribenzamine)	Yes	No specific data available; all pass into milk	Drug is used in neonates. May cause sedation, decreased feeding, or may produce stimulation and tachycardia. Should avoid long-acting preparations, which may accumulate in infant. When combined with decongestants, may cause decrease in milk.
Autonomic drugs Atropine sulfate*	Yes	0.1 mg/dl	Hyperthermia, atropine toxicity, infants especially sensitive; also inhibits lactation. Infant dose 0.01 mg/kg.
Carisoprodol (Soma, Rela)	Yes	2-4 times maternal plasma level	Blocks interneuronal activity in descending reticular formation and spinal cord; drowsiness, hypotonia, poor feed.
Ergot (Cafergot)	Yes	Unknown	90% of infants had symptoms of ergotism: vomiting and diarrhea to weak pulse and unstable blood pressure. Short-term therapy for migraine should not exceed 6 mg. Cafergot also contains 100 mg caffeine.
Mepenzolate bromide (Cantil)	No		Postganglionic parasympathetic inhibitor used to diminish gastric acidity and decrease spasm of colon. Oral absorption low.
Methocarbamol (Robaxin)	Yes	Minimum	Too little in milk to produce effect.
Neostigmine	No		No known harm to infant.
Propantheline bromide (Pro-Banthine)	No	Uncontrolled data indicate no measurable levels	Drug rapidly metabolized in maternal system to inactive metabolite. Mother should avoid long-acting preparations, however.
Scopolamine (Hyoscine)	Yes		Usually given as single dose and of no problem to neonate. No data on repeated doses.
Cardiovascular drugs Diazoxide (Hyperstat)			Arteriolar dilators and antihypertensive, only given IV, not active orally.
Dibenzyline†			No data available
Digoxin	Yes	0.96-0.61 ng/m‡	Dixogin 20% bound to protein; infant receives <1/100 of dose. If mother at toxic level of 5 ng/ml, milk would have a 4.4 ng/ml and infant would receive only ½₀ daily dose.

*Ingredient in many prescription and nonprescription drugs.
†α-blocking agent.
‡Peak level occurs 4-6 h after dose given. Maternal plasma level was higher, M/P = 0.9 and 0.8; infant's plasma level was 0.

Drug	Excreted in Milk	Amount in Milk After Therapeutic Dose	Effect on Infant
Guanethidine (Ismelin)*	Yes		Not significant in therapeutic doses to affect child.
Hydralazine (Apresoline)	Yes		Jaundice, thrombocytopenia, electrolyte disturbances possible.
Methyldopa (Aldomet)*	Yes		Galactorrhea. No specific data except as affects mother's milk production.
Propranolol (Inderal)†	Yes	40 ng/ml of maternal plasma‡	Insignificant amount. Infants reported had no symptoms noted. Should watch for hypoglycemia and/or "β-blocking" effects.
Quinidine	Yes		Arrhythmia may occur.
Reserpine (Serpasil)||	Yes		May produce galactorrhea, lethargy, diarrhea, or nasal stuffiness.
Cathartics			
Aloin	Yes	Low	Occasionally caused colic and diarrhea in infant.
Anthraquinone laxatives such as dihydroxyanthraquinone (Dorbane and Dorbantyl)	Yes	High	Caused colic and diarrhea in infant.
Calomel	No	None	None.
Cascara	Yes	Low	Caused colic and diarrhea in infant.
Milk of magnesia	No	None	No effect.
Mineral oil	No	None	No effect
Phenolphthalein	Unknown	Unknown||	Reported to cause symptoms in some.
Rhubarb	Unknown	None	None in syrup form. Fresh rhubarb may give symptoms of colic and diarrhea.
Saline cathartics	No	None	No effect.
Senna	No	None	None.
Stool softeners and bulk-forming laxatives	No	None	No effect.
Suppositories (for constipation)	No	None	Not absorbed
Diagnostic materials and procedures			
Barium		No	Not absorbed
Iopanoic acid (Telepaque)	Yes		Not sufficient to produce problem in infant on single dose. Does contain iodine radical.
Radioactive compounds			
Radioactive sodium	Yes	0.5% to 1.3% of dose/L¶	Diminished after 24 hr; discontinue nursing 24 hr.
[^{67}Ga] citrate	Yes		Discontinue nursing until ^{67}Ga has cleared, usually 24 hr.
^{125}I, ^{131}I	Yes	M/P = 0.13 μCi/0.002 μCi**	^{131}I content in milk proportional to amount of milk. Most excreted in 24 hr. Discontinue nursing for 48 hr or check milk before resuming feeding if under 48 hr.
^{90}Sr	Yes	M/P = 1/10	Less than in cow's milk. Bottle infant doubles stores in 1 month.
^{99m}Tc	Yes		Reported to clear in 6-22 hr. Discontinue breast-feeding 24 hr. ^{99m}Tc preferentially picked up by breast tissue.
Tuberculin test	No		Tuberculin-sensitive mothers can adoptively immunize their infants through breast milk, and that immunity may last several years.
X-ray films	No		No effect.

Continued.

*Adrenergic blocking agent.
†β-blocking agent.
‡Total daily dose to infant via milk is 15-20 μg.
§Adrenergic blocking agent.
\|\|Reports differ.
¶Peak in 2 hr; detectable for 96 hr.
**27% of dose in 48 hr.

Drug	Excreted in Milk	Amount in Milk After Therapeutic Dose	Effect on Infant
Diuretics			
Acetazolamide (Diamox)	Probable	No specific data available but probably similar to sulfonamide	Acts as enzyme inhibitor on carbonic anhydrase non-bacteriostatic sulfonamide. Observe only for dehydration and electrolyte loss by monitoring urine and turgor.
Furosemide (sulfamoylanthranilic acid) (Lasix)	No		Drug is given to children under medical management.
Mercurial diuretics (Dicurin, Thiomerin)	Yes		In addition to diuretic effect, there is risk of mercury deposition. However, drug not absorbed orally.
Spironolactone (Aldactone)	Yes	Canrenone, a metabolite, appears	Acts as antagonist of aldosterone; causes sodium excretion and potassium retention. The metabolite apparently has some activity.
Thiazides (Diuril, Enduron, Esidrix, Hydrodiuril, Oretic, Thiuretic tables)	Yes	>0.1 mg/dl*	Risk of dehydration and electrolyte imbalance, especially sodium loss, which would require monitoring. Watching weight and wet diapers and taking an occasional specific gravity reading of the urine and serum sodium would indicate status of infant. Risk, however, is extremely low, May suppress lactation due to dehydration in mother.
Environmental agents			
Aldrin	Yes	Varies by location	Not a reason to wean from breast. No need to test milk unless inordinate exposure.
Benzene hexachloride (BHC)	Yes	Varies by location	Not a reason to wean from breast. No need to test milk unless inordinate exposure.
Dichlorodiphenyltrichloroethane (DDT or DDE)	Yes	Varies by location	Not a reason to wean from breast. No need to test milk unless inordinate exposure.
Dieldrin	Yes	Varies by location	Also found in permanently mothproofed garments. Avoid these. Not a reason to wean.
Hexachlorobenzene (HCB)	Yes	Varies by location	Not a reason to wean from breast. No need to test milk unless inordinate exposure.
Heptachlorepoxide	Yes	Varies by location	Not a reason to wean from breast. No need to test milk unless inordinate exposure.
Methyl mercury	Yes	500-1000 ng/ml†	Infant blood level 600 ng/ml in heavy exposure. Only in excessive exposure is testing and/or weaning necessary.
Polybrominated biphenyl (PBB)	Yes	Varies by location	If mother at high risk from the environment or the diet, milk sample should be measured. If level in milk is high, then breast-feeding should be discontinued. Those at risk are (1) workers who handle PBB/PCB and (2) individuals who eat game fish from contaminated waters. Crash diets mobilize fats and should be avoided especially if PBB or PCB present.
Polychlorinated biphenyl (PCB)	Yes	Varies by location	
$^{90}Sr, ^{89}Sr$ (strontium)	Yes	1/10 of that in maternal diet	Cow's milk has six times as much as human milk. Cow's milk-fed infant doubles amount in body in 1 month.
Heavy metals			
Arsenic	Yes	Can be measured for given woman	Can accumulate. Check infant's blood level if there is reason to suspect exposure.
Copper	Yes		
Fluorine	Yes		Monitor for excessive dose.
Gold thiomalate (Myocrisin)	Yes	0.022 µg/ml when mother given 50 mg/week	No proteinuria or aminoaciduria observed
Halothane	Yes	2 ppm	Nursing mothers who work in environment with halothane should be checked.
Iron	Yes		

*Linear relationship between plasma and milk. In 1 L of milk at 0.1 mg/dl there would be 1 mg/24 hr. Infant dose is 20 mg/kg/24 hr.
†M/P = 8.6% in heavy exposure.

Drug	Excreted in Milk	Amount in Milk After Therapeutic Dose	Effect on Infant
Lead	Unknown		Nursing contraindicated if maternal serum 40 μg; conflicting reports, breast milk not always cause of lead poisoning in breast-fed infant.
Magnesium	Yes		Not sufficient to be toxic.
Mercury	Yes		Hazardous to infant.
Hormones and contraceptives			
Carbimazole (Neo-Mercazole)	Yes		Antithyroid effect may cause goiter.
Chlorotrianisene (Tace)	Yes		Has estrogenic effect although does not change consistency of milk. May have feminizing effect on infant.
Contraceptives (oral) Ethinyl estradiol Mestranol 19-Nortestosterone Norethindrone (Norlutin) Norethynodrel (Enovid)	Yes		May diminish milk supply. May decrease vitamins, protein, and fat in milk. One author showed no difference when mothers took norethindrone. Most significant concern is long-range impact of hormone on young infant, which is not certain. Reports of feminization of infant.
Corticotropin	Yes		Destroyed in gastrointestinal tract of infant. No effect.
Cortisone	Yes		Animal studies show 50% lower weight than controls and retarded sexual development and exophthalmos.
Dihydrotachysterol (Hytakerol)			May cause hypercalcemia; need monitoring of infant serum and urine calcium.
Epinephrine (Adrenalin)	Yes		Destroyed in GI tract of infant.
Estrogen	Yes	0.17 μg/dl after 1 g	Risks as with oral contraceptives.
Fluoxymesterone (Halotestine, Ora-Testryl, Ultrandren)	Yes		Suppress lactation; masculinizing
Insulin	Unknown		Destroyed in gastrointestinal tract.
Liothyronine (Cytomel)	No		Synthetic form of natural thyroid.
Medroxyprogesterone acetate (Provera)	No		
Phenformin HCl	Yes	Minimum	Not sufficient to cause symptoms in infant. Does not cause hypoglycemia in normal infants. No case reports available.
Prednisone	Yes	0.07–0.23% dose/L after 5 mg dose*	Minimum amount not likely to cause effect on infant in short course.
Pregnanediol	Yes		Unknown risk as with other female hormones over a long period of time.
Tolbutamide (Orinase)	Yes		Not recommended in the childbearing years.
Narcotics			
Codeine		0 to trace after 32 mg every 4 hr (6 doses)	No effect in therapeutic level and transient usage. Can accumulate. Individual variation. Watch for neonatal depression.
Heroin	Yes		13 of 22 infants had withdrawal. Historically breast-feeding had been used to wean addict's infant. This is no longer recommended.
Marijuana (*Cannabis*)	Yes		Shown in laboratory animals to produce structural changes in nursing child's brain cells; impairs DNA and RNA formation. Infant at risk of inhaling smoke during feeding or when held by person who is smoking.
Meperidine (Demerol)	Yes	>0.1 mg/dl†	Trace amounts may accumulate if drug taken around the clock when infant is neonate. Watch for drowsiness and poor feeding
Methadone	Yes	0.03 μg/ml or 0.023–0.028 mg/24 hr‡	When dosage not excessive, infant can be breast-fed if monitored for evidence of depression and failure to thrive.

*0.16 μg/ml after 10 mg dose; 2.67 μg/ml after 2 hr.
†Plasma 0.07–0.1 mg/dl.
‡Mother received 50 mg/24 hr; M/P = 0.83. Peak level 4 hr after oral dose. Results obscured if addict also taking the herbal root golden seal.

Continued.

Drug	Excreted in Milk	Amount in Milk After Therapeutic Dose	Effect on Infant
Morphine	Yes	Trace	Single doses have minimum effect. Potential for accumulation. May be addicting to neonate. Breast feeding no longer considered appropriate means of weaning infant of an addict.
Percodan (oxycodone [derived from opiate thebaine] aspirin, phenacetin, caffeine)	Yes		Consider for its component parts. In neonatal period sleepiness and failure to feed, which increase maternal engorgement and neonatal weight loss, have been observed, probably caused by oxycodone.

Psychotropic and mood-changing drugs

Drug	Excreted in Milk	Amount in Milk After Therapeutic Dose	Effect on Infant
Alcohol	Yes	Similar to plasma level	Ordinarily no problem and can be therapeutic in moderation, infants are more susceptible to effects. Chronic drinking reported to cause obesity in infant. Ethanol in doses of 1-2 g/kg to mother causes depression of milk-ejection reflex (dose dependent). No acetaldehyde found in infants.
Amphetamine	Yes		Has caused stimulation in infants with jitteriness, irritability, sleeplessness. Long-acting preparations cumulative.
Benzodiazepines* Chlordiazepoxide HCl (Librium)	Yes		Not sufficient to affect infant first week when glucuronyl system needed for detoxification. May accumulate. Older infant, no apparent problem.
Diazepam (Valium)	Yes	90 μg/L†	Detoxified in glucuronyl system. In first weeks of life may contribute to jaundice. Metabolite active. Effect on infant: hypoventilation, drowsiness, lethargy, and weight loss. Single doses over 10 mg contraindicated during nursing. Accumulation in infant possible.
Pineazepam	Yes	Metabolite, 5-11.2 ng/ml; pineazepam, >1.0 ng/ml‡	No data, probably similar to diazepam.
Haloperidol (Haldol)	Yes	Unknown	A butyrophenone antidepressant; animal studies in nurslings show behavior abnormalities.
Lithium carbonate (Eskalith, Lithane, Lithonate)	Yes	⅓-½ maternal plasma level§	Measurable lithium in infant's serum. Infant kidney can clear lithium; however, lithium inhibits adenosine 3':5:-cyclic monophosphate, significant for brain growth. Also affects amine metabolism. Real effects not measurable immediately. Report of cyanosis and poor muscle tone and ECG changes in nursing infant.
Monoamine oxidase (MAO) inhibitors (Eutonyl, Nardil)			Inhibits lactation.
Meprobamate (Miltown, Equanil)	Yes	2-4 times maternal plasma level	If therapy continued, infant should be followed closely.
Penfluridol‖	Yes	Unknown	Animal studies show learning abnormalities in sucklings. This is a potent long-acting oral neuroleptic drug.
Phenothiazines Chlorpromazine (Thorazine)	Yes	⅓ plasma level¶	Can be safely nursed; minimum in milk. Increase maternal prolactin. No symptoms in infants reported; 5-year follow-up showed infants normal.
Mesoridazine (Serentil)	Yes	Minimum	
Piperacetazine (Quide)	Yes	Minimum	Probably no effect.
Thioridazine (Mellaril)	Yes	No information	Thioridazine is less potent in general than other phenothiazines. Probably quite safe.
Trifluoperazine (Stelazine)	Yes	Minimum	

*Alcohol enhances effect of this group.

†10 mg or less yields 45 mg of diazepam/ml and 85 ng of metabolite/ml. P/M ratio is variable. Mean P/M ratio of diazepam is 6.14; of metabolite is 3.64. Effect lasts about 4 days.

‡Both drug and active metabolite appear for about 4 days after dose.

§0.030 mmol/L in infant's serum, 0.57 mmole/L in infant's urine. Milk level was half of maternal serum level in one case report.

‖Neuroleptic drug.

¶If dose <200 mg, milk contains bare trace. Dose of 1200 mg showed trace.

Drug	Excreted in Milk	Amount in Milk After Therapeutic Dose	Effect on Infant
Tricyclic antidepressants	Yes		Apparently no accumulation. No infants that have been observed showed symptoms. Watch for depression or failure to feed. Increase maternal prolactin secretion.
Amitriptyline HC1 (Elavil)	Yes	Minimum amounts	
Desipramine HC1 (Norpramin, Pertofrane)	Yes	Minimum amounts	
Imipramine HC1 (Tofranil)	Yes	0.1 mg/dl*	
Stimulants			
Caffeine	Yes	1% of dose	Accumulates when intake moderate and continual. Causes jitteriness, wakefulness, and irritability. Caffeine present in may hot and cold drinks. Consider if infant very wakeful.
Theobromine	Yes	3.7-8.2 mg/L after 240 mg dose†	No adverse symptoms observed in the infants. Chocolate most common cause of exposure.
Theophylline	Yes	10% of maternal dose‡	Irritability, fretfulness.
Thyroid and antithyroid medications			
Carbimazole (Neo-Mercazole)	Yes		May cause goiter.
Methimazole (Tapazole)	Yes	M/P >1	Inhibits synthesis of thyroid hormone but does not inactivate existing thyroid. Can inhibit infant thyroid. ⅛ grain/day of thyroid can be given to infant simultaneously.
Potassium iodide	Yes	3 mg/dl§	May alter thyroid function of infant; may cause goiter in infant.
Propylthiouracil	Yes	0.077% of dose	Risk of goiter and agranulocytosis. With present microtechniques for T_3, T_4 and TSH, close monitoring of infant is possible, as with methimazole.
Radioactive iodine^{125}I, ^{131}I (as a treatment)	Yes	M/P >1	*Treatment* doses are excreted via the breast for 1-3 weeks. Milk can be checked by Geiger counter if there is a question. Breast feeding should be discontinued until milk is clear.
Thiouracil	Yes	9-12 mg/d‖	Same as for propylthiouracil
Thyroid and thyroxine	Yes		Does not produce adverse symptoms on long-range follow-up. Noted to improve milk supply of hypothyroid mothers. No contraindication.
Miscellaneous			
Cyclophosphamide	Yes	Present¶	Antineoplastic agent. Any amounts contraindicated.
DPT	Yes	Minimum	Does not interfere with immunization schedule.
Methotrexate	Yes	Minor route of excretion: M/P = 0.08/1.0	Antimetabolite. Infant would receive 0.26 μg/dl, which researchers consider nontoxic for infant.
Nicotine	Yes	Mean 91 ppb (20-512 ppb)**	Decreases milk production. No apparent effect on infant—perhaps a tolerance is developed in utero. Smoking may interfere with let-down reflex if smoking started before onset of a feeding.
Poliovirus vaccine	No		Live vaccine taken orally. Not necessary to withhold nursing 30 min before and after dose. Provide booster after infant no longer nursing.
Rh antibodies	Yes		Destroyed in gastrointestinal tract; not effective orally.
Rubella virus vaccine	Yes	Minimum	Will not confer passive immunity. Mother should not be given vaccine when at risk for pregnancy.
Smallpox vaccine	No		Exposure is by direct contact. Live virus. No longer given.

*Plasma level 0.2-1.3 mg/dl.
†113 g chocolate bar.
‡M/P = 0.7.
§Dose was 325-650 mg three times a day.
‖Maternal plasma level was 3.4 mg/dl after a 1 g dose; M'P = 3.
¶Single 500 mg IV dose in milk at 1,3,5, and 6 h after injection.
**At ½-1½ packs/day. Large variation from single donor.

Index

A